Recent Titles in This Series

(*Continued in the back of this publication*)

Applied Problems of Radon Transform

American Mathematical Society
TRANSLATIONS
Series 2 • Volume 162

Applied Problems of Radon Transform

Simon Gindikin
Editor

American Mathematical Society
Providence, Rhode Island

С. Г. Гиндикин (редактор)

Приложения преобразования Радона

Translated from an original Russian manuscript by D. DEART
Translation edited by SIMEON IVANOV

ABSTRACT. The aim of this collection is to acquaint the reader with recent work in this area that was done in what was formerly the Soviet Union. The papers in this collection are devoted to mathematical problems that are related to applications. In some cases these problems are problems of practical tomography; in other cases they are theoretical problems that originated in tomography. However, in all these papers the main emphasis is on the mathematical aspects of the problem.

1991 *Mathematics Subject Classification*. Primary 44–02, 44A12, 65R10, 92C55

Library of Congress Cataloging-in-Publication Data

Prilozhenii͡a preobrazovanii͡a Radona. English.
Applied problems of Radon transform/S. G. Gindikin, editor.
p. cm. — (American Mathematical Society translations, ISSN 0065-9290; ser. 2, v. 162)
Includes bibliographical references.
ISBN 0-8218-7508-6 (acid-free paper)
1. Tomography—Mathematics. 2. Radon transforms. I. Gindikin, S. G. (Semen Grigor′evich)
II. Title. III. Series.
QA3.A572 ser. 2 vol. 162
[RC78.7.T6]
510 s—dc20
[616.07′57′0151] 94-27251
CIP

∞ The paper used in this book is acid-free and falls within the guidelines
established to ensure permanence and durability.
♻ Printed on recycled paper.

This volume was typeset using $\mathcal{A}_{\mathcal{M}}\mathcal{S}$-TEX,
the American Mathematical Society's TEX macro system.

10 9 8 7 6 5 4 3 2 1 98 97 96 95 94

Contents

Amer. Math. Soc. Transl.
(2) Vol. **162**, 1994

Time Series Analysis and Grassmannians

V. M. Buchstaber

Introduction

We consider the well-known problem of constructing a model (approximation) for a time series $f = (f_1, \dots, f_N)$ in the class of functions of the form

$$g(t) = \sum_{k=1}^{K} a_k(t) e^{\lambda_k t} \sin(\omega_k t + \varphi_k), \tag{1}$$

where the $a_k(t)$ are polynomials. Attempts to solve this problem using the least square method meet substantial difficulties [**1**]. The only methods that really work in practical application are those that extensively use additional information about the form and the number of terms in the sum in (1) (methods of polynomial approximation, spectral analysis, etc.). One of the first important examples of a realization of such an approach is the solution of the problem about the modeling of the gas expansion laws using sums of damping exponents. This solution was found by Gaspard Riche de Prony back in 1795. His method essentially uses the fact that exponents are eigenfunctions of the shift operator $t \to t + \Delta t$.

In the present paper we develop a method of multidimensional unfolding that enables us to use statistical analysis of the original time series in order to estimate the contribution of various terms in (1), and, most important, their number, prior to applying complicated approximation algorithms.

A multidimensional (n-dimensional) unfolding of the time series $f = (f_1, \dots, f_N)$ is a piecewise-linear curve X_f in the n-dimensional Euclidean space $\mathbb{R}^n$ that consecutively joins the vectors $X_q \in \mathbb{R}^n$, $q = 1, \dots, p = N - n + 1$, determined by length n segments $X_q' = (f_q, \dots, f_{q+n-1})$ of the original series. By going from the time series f to its n-dimensional unfolding we can use the geometry of unfolding for the analysis of f.

For example, the analysis of one- and two-dimensional projections of the curve X_f using the projection pursuit method [**2**] enables us to get an idea about the character of distinctions between projections of the unfolding of the original series and projections of unfoldings of various components of the discrete model expression (1).

We say that the n-rank of the time series f does not exceed r if there exists an r-dimensional plane $L \subset \mathbb{R}^n$ such that $X_f \subset L$. Below we prove the following results.

- Let $N_1 \geq N + n$. The series $f = (f_1, \dots, f_N)$ can be completed to a series $\widetilde{f} = (f_1, \dots, f_N, \widetilde{f}_{N+1}, \dots, \widetilde{f}_{N_1})$ whose n-rank does not exceed $r < n$ if and only if

$$f_m = \sum_{s=1}^{l} c_{l-s+1} f_{m-s}, \qquad l \leq r,$$

for all $m = l + 1, \dots, N$.
- Let g be the series $g = (g_1, \dots, g_N)$, where $g_q = g((q-1)\Delta t)$ for a function $g(t)$ of the form (1). Then the n-rank of g does not exceed r for all $n > r$, N, and Δt if and only if $g(t)$ is a solution of an ordinary differential equation

$$\sum_{q=0}^{r} b_q \frac{d^q}{dt^q} g(t) = c \tag{2}$$

with constant coefficients $b_0, \dots, b_r, c$.

Let L be an r-dimensional plane in $\mathbb{R}^n$. For a given time series f denote by $X_f(L)$ the orthogonal projection of the unfolding X_f to L. It is clear that $X_f(L)$ is a piecewise linear curve in $\mathbb{R}^n$ with nodes $(X_1(L), \dots, X_p(L))$. Denote

$$\rho_n(f, L) = \|X_f - X_f(L)\|^2 = \frac{1}{p} \sum_{q=1}^{p} \|X_q - X_q(L)\|^2,$$

where $\|\cdot\|$ is the standard Euclidean metric in $\mathbb{R}^n$. Let us consider the Grassmann manifold $G'(r, n)$ of all r-dimensional planes in $\mathbb{R}^n$. Using the n-dimensional unfolding X_f, we obtain the function

$$\rho_n(f)\colon G'(r, n) \to \mathbb{R}^1, \quad \rho_n(f)(L) = \rho_n(f, L).$$

Denote

$$r_n(f) = \inf_{L \in G'(r,n)} \rho_n(f, L).$$

Below we use the principal component method **[2]** to compute $r_n(f)$ and to describe the set $\mathscr{L}_n(f, r)$ of all r-dimensional planes where the function $\rho_n(f)$ takes the value exactly $r_n(f)$. We suggest an algorithm for the construction of a time series $f(L, r)$ for each piecewise linear curve $X_f(L)$ and prove that for a time series $f_*(r) = f(L_*, r)$, $L_* \in \mathscr{L}_n(f, r)$, the following theorem holds.

If $g(t)$ is a solution of the equation (2), *then*

$$\|f - g\|_\mu^2 \geq \|f - f_*(r)\|_\mu^2,$$

where μ is a natural Euclidean metric (*to be defined below*) *in the space T of all time series T with N samples* (*or marks*).

Therefore, $\|f - f_*(r)\|_\mu^2 = \delta_r$ gives a *lower* bound to the quality of the approximation of the series f in the class of functions of the form (1) satisfying equations of the form (2) without applying algorithms for estimation of the parameters λ_k, ω_k, φ_k, and the coefficients of the polynomials $a_k(t)$. In particular, we obtain a lower bound to the order of the equation (2) if we need an a priori approximation error of order less than a given threshold δ.

Additional possibilities occur in the visual analysis of deviations of values of the series f from the values of the series $f(r)$, thus allowing us to select terms in the model (1). This is especially important, since in general parameters in this model are dependent.

The theory described in this paper is realized as a software package that is used to solve the following problems of ecological monitoring:

(1) Modeling of time series (construction of a model of a time series using sampling data).
(2) Description of the dynamics of sampling anomalies (deviation from model times series).
(3) Detection of structural changes of a time series (dynamics of parameters of model times series)

Practical results are described in [**3–5**]. Some of these results are presented in Figures 1–4 to illustrate the main ideas of the paper.

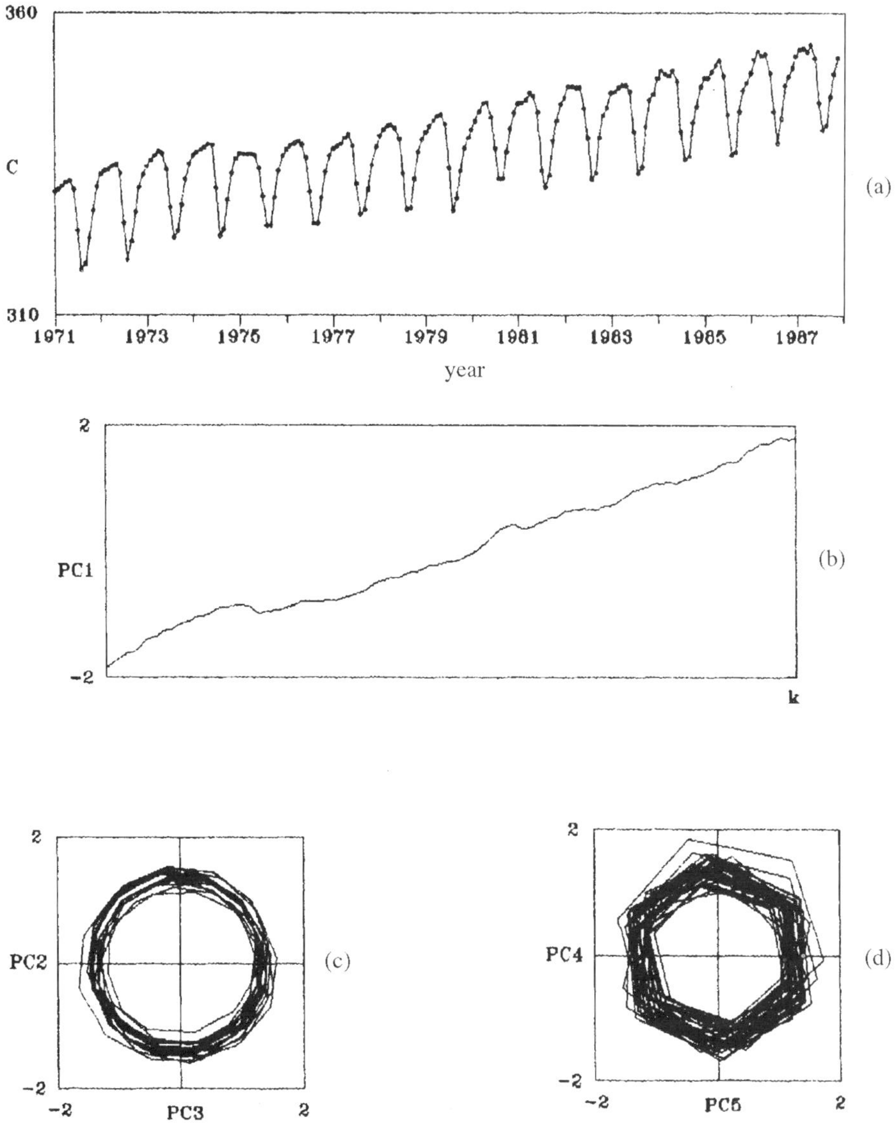

FIGURE 1

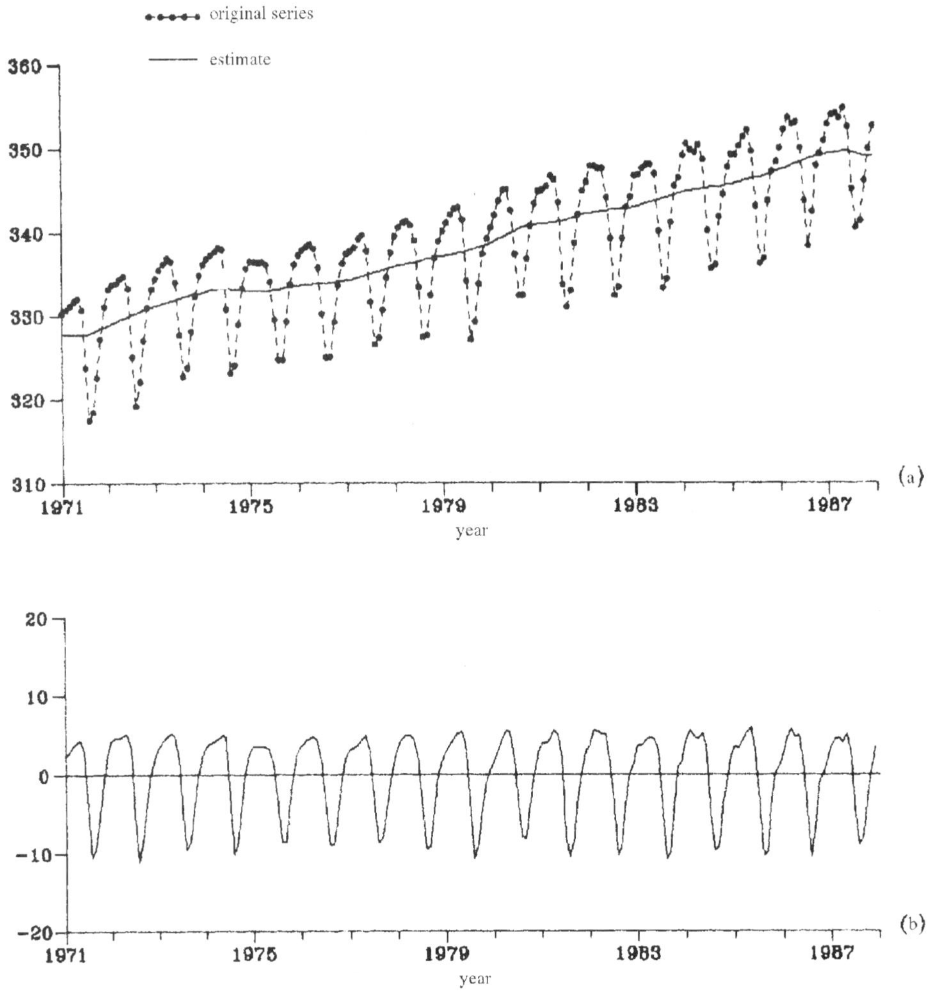

FIGURE 2

§1. Main definitions and general results

Let $f(t)$ be the time series under investigation, $f(t) = (f_1, \dots, f_N)$, where $f_q = f((q-1)\Delta t)$, $q = 1, \dots, N$.

DEFINITION 1. A piecewise linear curve $X_f \subset \mathbb{R}^n$ with nodes $X_1, \dots X_p$, where $X'_q = (f_q, \dots, f_{q+n-1})$, is called the *n-dimensional unfolding* of the time series $f(t)$.

Here and later by a vector $X \in \mathbb{R}^n$ we mean a column vector, and by X' we denote the corresponding row vector.

First, let us consider n-dimensional unfoldings of model time series. Without loss of generality below we assume that $\Delta t = 1$. 1. $g(t) = a^t$, *where* $a > 0$. We have $a^{t+\tau} = a^t a^\tau$, so that

$$X'_1 = (1, \dots, a^{n-1}), \dots, X'_q = (a^{q-1}, \dots, a^{q+n-2}) = a^{q-1} X'_1.$$

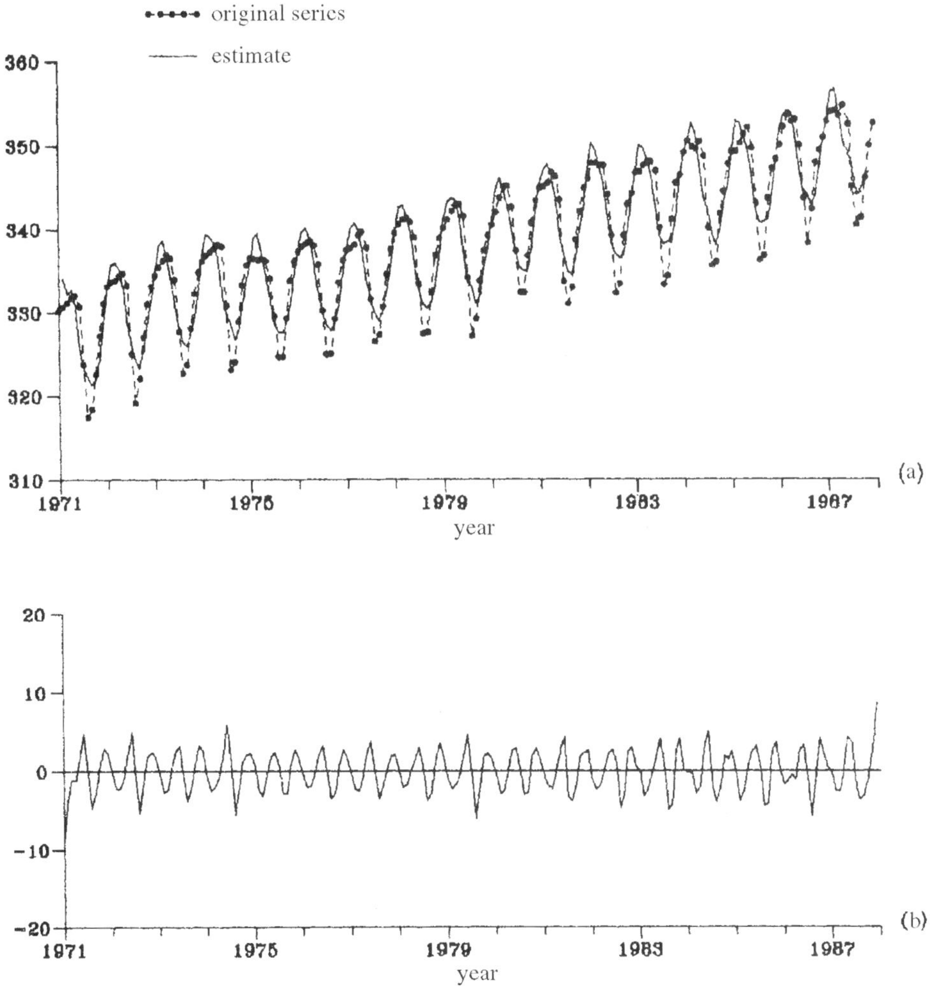

FIGURE 3

Therefore for all n and N we have $X_{g(t)} \subset L \subset \mathbb{R}^n$, where L is the line in $\mathbb{R}^n$ with the director vector $X_1/\|X_1\|$.

2. $g(t) = \sin(\omega t + \varphi)$, *where* ω *and* φ *are parameters.* We have

$$g(t+\tau) = g(t)\cos(\omega\tau) + g(t + \pi/(2\omega))\sin(\omega\tau).$$

Denoting

$$Y_1' = (1, \cos\omega, \dots, \cos\omega(n-1)), \qquad Y_2' = (0, \sin\omega, \dots, \sin\omega(n-1))$$

we have

$$X_q = \sin(\omega(q-1)+\varphi)Y_1 + \cos(\omega(q-1)+\varphi)Y_2, \qquad q = 1, \dots, p.$$

Therefore $X_{g(t)} \subset L \subset \mathbb{R}^n$, where L is the two-dimensional plane spanned by the vectors Y_1 and Y_2.

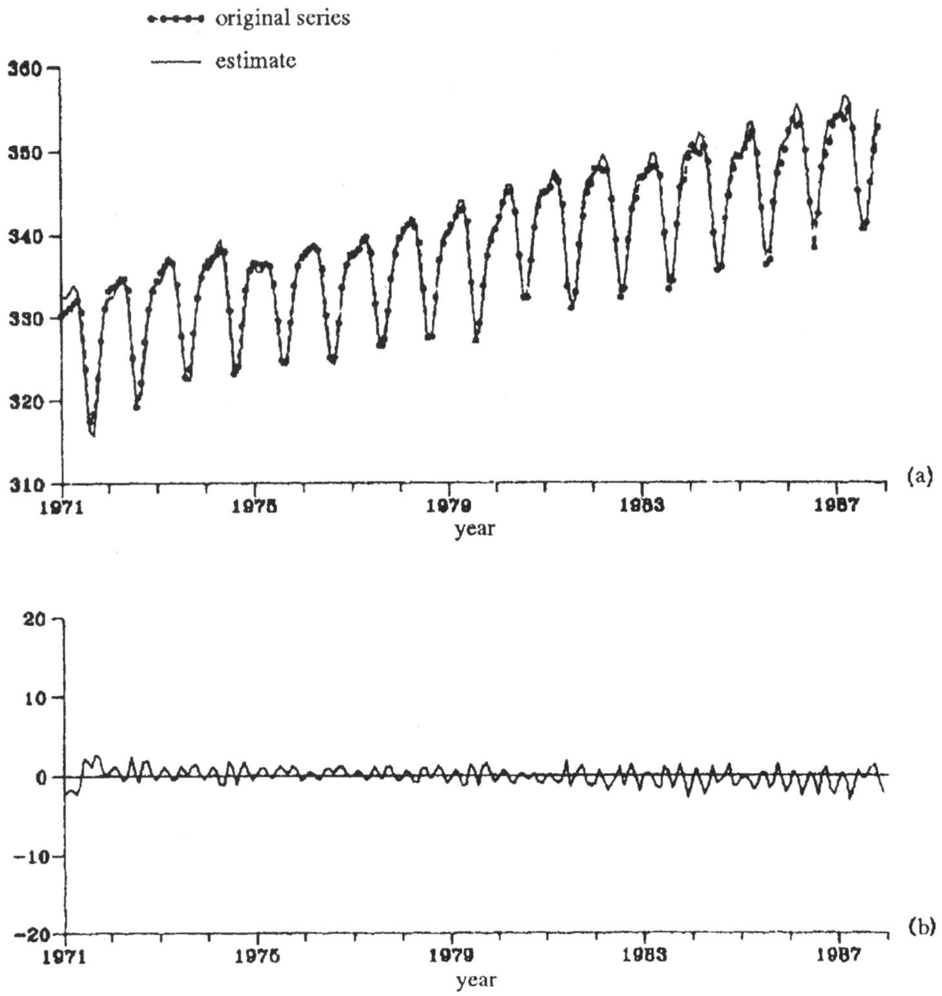

FIGURE 4

Let us note that

$$\langle Y_1, Y_2\rangle = \sum_{m=0}^{n-1} \cos(m\omega)\sin(m\omega)$$

$$= \frac{1}{2}\sum_{m=0}^{n-1} \sin(2m\omega) = \tfrac{1}{2}\csc(\omega)\sin(n\omega)\sin((n-1)\omega).$$

In particular, in the case $\omega = 2\pi/n$ the vectors Y_1 and Y_2 are orthogonal and for $N \geq 2n+1$ the unfolding X_g is the right n-gon in the plane L.

In Figure 1 projections of the 12-dimensional unfolding of the actual time series are presented. Figure 1c indicates the existence of a cycle with $\omega = 2\pi/12$, and

Figure 1d indicates the existence of a cycle with $\omega = 2\pi/6$. Deviation of the projection of the curve from the right 12-gon and the right 6-gon allows us to judge anomalies of sampling data.

3. $g(t) = \sum_{k=0}^{m} b_k t^k$. We have

$$g(t+\tau) = \sum_{k=0}^{m} g^{(k)}(t) \frac{\tau^k}{k!},$$

where

$$g^{(k)}(t) = \frac{d}{dt} g^{(k-1)}(t), \qquad k \geq 1.$$

Denote

$$Y_1' = (1, 1, \dots, 1),$$
$$Y_k' = (0, 1/(k-1)!, \dots, (n-1)^{k-1}/(k-1)!), \qquad k = 2, \dots, m+1.$$

Since $g^{(m)}(t) = m! b_m = \text{const}$, we get

$$X_q = \sum_{k=0}^{m-1} g^{(k)}(q-1) Y_{k+1} + m! b_m Y_{m+1},$$

so that for $n \geq m$ we have $X_{g(t)} \subset L \subset \mathbb{R}^n$, where L is an m-dimensional subspace containing the vectors $Y_1, \dots, Y_{m+1}$.

A common feature of all these model time series is that the corresponding n-dimensional unfoldings lie in some subspaces L whose dimension does not depend on n and N. These model time series belong to the class of functions that possess an addition formula of the form

$$g(t+\tau) = \sum_{k=0}^{m} \varphi_k(t) \psi_k(\tau) \tag{3}$$

for some m and some functions $\varphi_k(t)$, $\psi_k(t)$. Denote

$$Y_k' = (\psi_k(0), \dots, \psi_k(n-1)).$$

Then the addition formula for $g(t)$ shows that the nodes of the n-dimensional unfolding $X_{g(t)}$ can be written in the form

$$X_q = \sum_{k=0}^{m} \varphi_k(q-1) Y_k,$$

so that if one of the functions $\varphi_k(t)$ is a constant, say $\varphi_0(t) \equiv 1$, then $X_{g(t)} \subset L \subset \mathbb{R}^n$, where L is a subspace in $\mathbb{R}^n$ of dimension not exceeding m.

Let us consider now the case when a function $g(t)$ with the addition formula (3) has m derivatives and the functions $\psi_k(t)$, $k = 1, \dots, m$, also have m derivatives.

Differentiating (3) l times with respect to τ and substituting $\tau = 0$, we get

$$g^{(l)}(t) = \sum_{k=0}^{m} \varphi_k(t) \psi_k^{(l)}(0).$$

Therefore, under the condition $\varphi_0(t) \equiv 1$ formula (3) shows that the $m+1$ functions $g(t) - \psi_0(0)$, $g'(t) - \psi_0'(0), \dots, g^{(m)}(t) - \psi_0^{(m)}(0)$ belong to the m-dimensional linear space generated by the functions $\varphi_k(t)$, $k = 1, \dots, m$, i.e., are linearly dependent. Therefore, there exist constants $b_0, \dots, b_m$ such that

$$\sum_{q=0}^{m} b_q (g^{(q)}(t) - \psi_0^{(q)}(0)) \equiv 0$$

Denoting

$$\mathfrak{D} = \sum_{q=0}^{m} b_q \frac{d^q}{dt^q},$$

we get $\mathfrak{D}g(t) = c$, where $c = \sum_{q=0}^{m} b_q \psi_0^{(q)}(0)$. The theory of ordinary differential equations shows that $g(t)$ must be of the form (1).

Therefore the class of functions of the form (1) coincides with the class of functions that have sufficiently many derivatives and possess the addition formula (3).

An arbitrary piecewise linear curve Y in $\mathbb{R}^n$ with nodes $Y_1, \dots, Y_p$ is described by a table

$$Y = \begin{pmatrix} y_{11} & \cdots & y_{1p} \\ y_{21} & \cdots & y_{2p} \\ \cdots & \cdots & \cdots \\ y_{n1} & \cdots & y_{np} \end{pmatrix}$$

where $Y_q' = (y_{1q}, \dots, y_{pq}) \in \mathbb{R}^n$.

Definition 2. We say that *the rank of a curve Y does not exceed r* if there exists an r-dimensional plane $L \subset \mathbb{R}^n$ such that $Y_q \in L$ for all $q = 1, \dots, p$.

We note that the definition of the rank of a curve does not depend on the choice of a basis in $\mathbb{R}^n$.

Let us consider the scattering matrix $T(Y)$ of the curve Y:

$$T(Y) = \sum_{q=1}^{p} (Y_q - \overline{Y})(Y_q - \overline{Y})',$$

where

$$\overline{Y} = \frac{1}{p} \sum_{q=1}^{p} Y_q.$$

The principal components theory **[2]** immediately implies the following result.

Lemma 1. *The rank of the curve Y does not exceed r* ($\operatorname{rk} Y \leq r$) *if and only if $\lambda_s = 0$ for all $s > r$, where $\lambda_1 \geq \lambda_2 \geq \cdots \geq \lambda_n \geq 0$ are the eigenvalues of the scattering matrix $T(Y)$.*

Definition 3. We say that *the n-rank of the time series $f(t)$ does not exceed r* if $\operatorname{rk} X_f \leq r$, where X_f is the n-dimensional unfolding of $f(t)$.

To the unfolding X_f of a time series f there corresponds the table $X_d = (x_{ij})$, $1 \leq i \leq n$, $1 \leq j \leq p$, with $x_{ij} = f_{i+j-1}$, so that X_f is a Hankel matrix **[6]**. Evidently, this special form of the table X_f is not preserved under coordinate changes. We describe an approach to the analysis of properties of the unfolding $X_f \subset \mathbb{R}^n$, hence also of the series f, that essentially uses a fixed ordering of coordinates in the Euclidean space $\mathbb{R}^n$.

We need the notion of the Schubert symbol, which plays the central role in the construction of a cell decomposition of Grassmann manifolds. We will follow the book [7]. Consider in $\mathbb{R}^n$ the chain of subspaces $\mathbb{R}^0 \subset \mathbb{R}^1 \subset \cdots \subset \mathbb{R}^k \subset \cdots \subset \mathbb{R}^n$, where $\mathbb{R}^k$ consists of all vectors of the form $(y_1, \ldots, y_k, 0, \ldots, 0)$. Each l-dimensional plane $W \subset \mathbb{R}^n$ passing through the origin define a sequence of numbers

$$0 \leq \dim(W \cap \mathbb{R}^1) \leq \dim(W \cap \mathbb{R}^2) \leq \cdots \leq \dim(W \cap \mathbb{R}^n) = l.$$

Evidently, two consecutive numbers in this sequence differ by at most 1. Therefore, the nondecreasing function

$$\varphi(k) = \dim(W \cap \mathbb{R}^k), \qquad k = 0, \ldots, n,$$

has exactly l discontinuity points. Therefore, for a given plane W we get a sequence of numbers $1 \leq \sigma_1 < \sigma_2 < \cdots < \sigma_l \leq n$, where σ_i is uniquely determined from the conditions

$$\varphi(\sigma_i) = i, \quad \varphi(\sigma_i - 1) = i - 1.$$

This sequence is called the *Schubert symbol* of the plane $W \subset \mathbb{R}^n$. The following general result holds.

An l-dimensional plane $W \subset \mathbb{R}^n$ has a Schubert symbol $\sigma_1 < \sigma_2 < \cdots < \sigma_l$ if and only if it possesses an orthogonal basis $W_1, \ldots, W_l$ such that $W_k \in \mathbb{R}^{\sigma_k}$ and the σ_kth coordinate of the vector W_k equals -1 for all $k = 1, \ldots, l$.

The indicated basis in the plane W is determined uniquely, and we will call vectors W_k of this basis the *Schubert vectors* of the plane W.

Now let us consider a time series f whose n-rank does not exceed $r \leq n-1$. Then there exists a r-dimensional plane L such that $X_q \in L$ for all $q = 1, \ldots, p = N - n + 1$. Any vector $X \in L$ can be uniquely represented in the form $X = \widetilde{X} + \xi$, where $\widetilde{X}$ is the orthogonal projection of X to the r-dimensional plane $\widetilde{L}$ which is parallel to L and passes through the origin $0 \in \mathbb{R}^n$, and ξ is a vector that is orthogonal to L and does not depend on X. Denote by $L^{\perp}$ the $(n-r)$-dimensional subspace that is orthogonal to $\widetilde{L}$. Associate to $L^{\perp}$ its Schubert symbol $\sigma_1 < \sigma_2 < \cdots < \sigma_{n-r}$ and the corresponding orthogonal basis $W_1, \ldots, W_{n-r}$ of Schubert vectors. By construction, for any Schubert vector $W_k = (w_{k1}, \ldots, w_{k,\sigma_k - 1}, -1, 0, \ldots, 0)$ we have

$$\langle X_q, W_k \rangle = \sum_{j=1}^{\sigma_k - 1} w_{kj} f_{q+j-1} - f_{q+\sigma_k-1} + w_{k0} = 0,$$

where $w_{k0} = -\langle \xi, W_k \rangle$. Denote $q + \sigma_k - 1 = m$, $q + j - 1 = m - s$. We obtain

$$(7) \qquad f_m = \sum_{s=1}^{\sigma_k - 1} w_{k,\sigma_k - s} f_{m-s} + w_{k0}, \qquad m = \sigma_k, \ldots, p_k, \quad k = 1, \ldots, n-r,$$

where $p_k = N - n + \sigma_k$. For the Schubert symbol we have

$$n - r - 1 \leq \sum_{k=1}^{n-r-1} (\sigma_{k+1} - \sigma_k) = \sigma_{n-r} - \sigma_1 \leq n - \sigma_1,$$

so that $\sigma_1 \leq r + 1$. Therefore, we have proved that if the n-rank of a time series f

does not exceed $r \leq n-1$, then there exist constants $c_0, c_1, \dots, c_l$, $l \leq r$, such that

$$(8) \qquad f_m = \sum_{s=1}^{l} c_{l-s+1} f_{m-s} + c_0, \qquad m = l+1, \dots, N-n+l+1.$$

Indeed, it suffices to take $(c_1, \dots, c_l, -1, 0, \dots, 0) = W_1$ and $l = \sigma_1 - 1$ for any r-dimensional plane L that contains the unfolding X_f.

Formula (8) allows us to compute the numbers $\widehat{f}_m$ for $m = N-n+l+2, \dots, N$. In general, this values should not coincide with the corresponding terms of the series f_m. The following simple example allows a better understanding of the situation.

Consider the series $(0,1,2,3,4,2)$. Its three-dimensional unfolding has the nodes

$$X_1 = (0,1,2), \quad X_2 = (1,2,3), \quad X_3 = (2,3,4), \quad X_4 = (3,4,2).$$

Simple computations show that the 3-rank of this series equals 2, the Schubert symbol of the line in R^3 which is orthogonal to the two-dimensional support L of the unfolding is $\sigma_1 = 2$, and the corresponding Schubert vector is $(1,-1,0)$. According to (8), we have

$$f_m = f_{m-1} + 1 \quad \text{for } m = 2,3,4,5, \qquad f_6 \neq \widehat{f}_6 = f_5 + 1.$$

The time series $\widetilde{f} = (\widetilde{f}_m)$ of length $\widetilde{N} > N$ is called *the extension of the series* $f = (f_m)$ *of length* N if $\widetilde{f}_m = f_m$ for all $m \leq N$.

In the assumptions and notation of (8) one can easily see that if

$$f_m \neq \sum_{s=1}^{l} c_{l-s+1} f_{m-s} + c_0$$

for $m = N-n+l+2 \leq N$, then the n-rank of *any* extension $\widetilde{f}$ of the series f is greater than r. The possibility of extending a time series without increasing the n-rank is described in the following lemma.

LEMMA 2. *Let $r \leq n-1$ and $N_1 > N+n$. A given series $f = (f_1, \dots, f_N)$ admits an extension $\widetilde{f} = (\widetilde{f}_1, \dots, \widetilde{f}_{N_1})$ with the n-rank not exceeding r if and only if there exist constants $c_0, c_1, \dots c_l$, $l \leq r$, such that*

$$f_m = \sum_{s=1}^{l} c_{l-s+1} f_{m-s} + c_0$$

for all $m = l+1, \dots, N$.

PROOF. Let $\widetilde{f}$ be an extension of the series f with the n-rank of $\widetilde{f}$ not exceeding r. Then there exist constants $c_0, \dots, c_l$ that provide the representation (8) for the series $\widetilde{f}$. As was shown earlier, this formula holds for all m such that $l+1 \leq m \leq N_1 - n + l + 1$. In particular, it holds for $l+1 \leq m \leq N$, since, by the conditions of the lemma, $N < N_1 - n + l + 1$. Conversely, let the required formula hold for all $m = l+1, \dots, N$. Using this formula, we construct an extension $\widehat{f}$ of length $\widehat{N}$ and prove that for each $\widehat{N} > N$ the n-rank of this extension does not exceed r.

Consider the n-dimensional unfolding $X_{\widetilde{f}} = (X_1, \dots, X_p, \dots)$. Formula (8) implies the formula

$$X_q = \sum_{s=1}^{l} c_{l-s+1} X_{q-s} + c_0, \qquad q \geq l+1. \tag{9}$$

We have

$$X_{q+1} - X_q = c_l X_q + \sum_{s=1}^{l-1} (c_{l-s} - c_{l-s+1}) X_{q-s} - c_1 X_{q-l}.$$

Therefore,

$$X_{q+1} = \sum_{k=0}^{l} \lambda_k X_{q-k},$$

where $\lambda_0 = 1 + c_l$, $\lambda_k = (c_{l-k} - c_{l-k+1})$ for $1 \leq k \leq l-1$, and $\lambda_l = -c_1$. Since $\sum_{k=0}^{l} \lambda_k = 1$, for any $q \geq l+1$ the node X_{q+1} of the unfolding $X_{\widetilde{f}}$ lies in the l-dimensional subspace spanned by the first $l+1$ nodes $X_1, \dots, X_{l+1}$. Since $l \leq r$, the n-rank of $\widetilde{f}$ does not exceed r. The lemma is proved. □

For the above examples of model time series

$$a^t, \quad \sin(\omega t + \varphi), \quad P_s(t) = \sum_{l=0}^{s} b_l t^l$$

we have for arbitrary Δt, n, and N

$$\begin{aligned} &\operatorname{rk}_n a^t \leq 1 && \text{for any } a > 0, \\ &\operatorname{rk}_n \sin(\omega t + \varphi) \leq 2 && \text{for any } \omega \text{ and } \varphi, \\ &\operatorname{rk}_n P_s(t) \leq s && \text{for any } b_0, \dots, b_s. \end{aligned}$$

DEFINITION 4. We say that the *absolute rank* of a continuous time signal f does not exceed r if for any Δt, n, and N the rank of the corresponding time series does not exceed r.

As we have shown earlier, the absolute rank of the continuous time signal $f(t)$ does not exceed r if and only if $f(t)$ is a solution of an ordinary differential equation

$$\sum_{k=0}^{r} b_k \frac{d^k f(t)}{dt^k} = C,$$

where C and b_k, $k = 1, \dots, r$, are some constants.

Using the notion of the absolute rank of a time series $f(t)$ we can introduce, for fixed Δt, n, N, a filtration in the set $\mathfrak{MD}$ of real solutions of ordinary differential equations with constant coefficients as follows:

$$\mathfrak{MD}_1 \subset \mathfrak{MD}_2 \subset \cdots \subset \mathfrak{MD}_n = \mathfrak{MD},$$

where $\mathfrak{MD}_r$ is the set of time signals with absolute rank not exceeding r.

§2. Nonparametric modeling of time series from projections of their unfoldings

Consider the set $\mathfrak{M}(p,n) = \mathfrak{M}$ of all piecewise linear curves with p nodes in the space $\mathbb{R}^n$. Introduce in $\mathfrak{M}$ the structure of the Euclidean space $\mathbb{R}^{pn}$ in such a way that if $Y_1 = (Y_{11}, \dots, Y_{1p})$, and $Y_2 = (Y_{21}, \dots, Y_{2p})$ are two curves, then

$$\|Y_1 - Y_2\|^2 = \frac{1}{p}\sum_{q=1}^{p} \|Y_{1q} - Y_{2q}\|^2,$$

where $\|\cdot\|^2$ is the standard Euclidean distance in $\mathbb{R}^n$.

In the space $\mathfrak{M} \sim \mathbb{R}^{pn}$ we have the filtration $\mathfrak{M}_1 \subset \mathfrak{M}_2 \subset \dots \subset \mathfrak{M}_n = \mathfrak{M}$, where $\mathfrak{M}_r$ is the set of curves with rank not exceeding r.

DEFINITION 5. The curve $X(r) \in \mathfrak{M}_r$ is called a *projection* of a given curve $X \in \mathfrak{M}$ to $\mathfrak{M}_r$ if

$$\|X - X(r)\|^2 = \min_{Y \in \mathfrak{M}_r} \|X - Y\|^2.$$

The theory of principal components **[2]** gives the following theorem.

THEOREM 1. *For any curve $X \in \mathfrak{M}$ we have*

$$X(r) = \overline{X} + V(r)V'(r)X,$$

where $\overline{X}$ is a constant curve $(\overline{X}, \dots, \overline{X})$ and $V(r)$ is the matrix composed of column vectors $V_1, \dots, V_r$, where $V_s \in \mathbb{R}^n$ are the eigenvectors of the scattering matrix $T(X)$ with eigenvalues λ_s ordered in such a way that $\lambda_1 \geq \lambda_2 \geq \dots \geq \lambda_r \geq \dots \geq \lambda_n \geq 0$.

PROOF. Denote

$$\rho(X, \mathfrak{M}_r) = \min_{Y \in \mathfrak{M}_r} \|X - Y\|^2.$$

Consider the following function $\rho(X, L)$ on the Grassmannian $G'(r,n)$ of all r-dimensional planes in $\mathbb{R}^n$:

$$\rho(X, L) = \|X - X(L)\|^2 = \frac{1}{p}\sum_{q=1}^{p} \|X_q - X_q(L)\|^2,$$

where $X_q(L)$ is the orthogonal projection of the node X_q of the curve X to the plane L and $X(L)$ is the curve with nodes $(X_1(L), \dots, X_p(L))$. It is clear that

$$\rho(X, \mathfrak{M}_r) = \min_{L \in G'(r,n)} \rho(X, L).$$

Let $G(r,n)$ be the Grassmannian of all r-dimensional planes in $\mathbb{R}^n$ passing through the origin 0. Recall that $G(r,n)$ is a compact smooth manifold of dimension $r(n-r)$. There exists a canonical map $G'(r,n) \to G(r,n)$, which sends the plane L to the unique plane $\widetilde{L}$ that is parallel to L and passes through the origin. Using this map we can identify $G'(r,n)$ with the manifold of pairs $(\widetilde{L}, \xi) \in G(r,n) \times \mathbb{R}^n$, where $\xi \in \mathbb{R}^n$ is a vector that is orthogonal to $\widetilde{L}$. For $L = (\widetilde{L}, \xi)$ denote by $L^{\perp}$ the plane which is orthogonal to $\widetilde{L}$. We have

$$X_q(L) = X_q(\widetilde{L}) + \xi, \qquad \overline{X} = \frac{1}{p}\sum_{q=1}^{p} X_q = \overline{X}(\widetilde{L}) + \overline{X}(L^{\perp}).$$

Therefore

$$(X_q - X_q(L)) = [(X_q - \overline{X}) - (X_q - \overline{X})(\widetilde{L})] + (\overline{X}(L^{\perp}) - \xi). \tag{10}$$

Substituting (10) into the formula for $\rho(X, L)$, we obtain

$$\rho(X, L) = \rho(X - \overline{X}, \widetilde{L}) + \|\overline{X}(L^{\perp}) - \xi\|^2.$$

Let us remark that by $\overline{X}$ we denote both the average vector of the curve X and the constant curve $(\overline{X}, \dots, \overline{X})$. Therefore,

$$\rho(X, (\widetilde{L}, \overline{X}(L^{\perp})) = \rho(X - \overline{X}, \widetilde{L}) \le \rho(X, (\widetilde{L}, \xi))$$

for all curves X, all r-dimensional planes $\widetilde{L}$, and all vectors $\xi \in \widetilde{L}$. Therefore,

$$\rho(X, \mathfrak{M}_r) = \min_{\widetilde{L} \in G(r,n)} \rho(X - \overline{X}, \widetilde{L}).$$

Choose an orthonormal basis in the subspace $L^{\perp} \subset \mathbb{R}^n$ and form the matrix $P(\widetilde{L})$ whose columns are vectors of this basis. By construction,

$$\|(X_q - \overline{X}) - (X_q - \overline{X})(\widetilde{L})\|^2 = \|P(\widetilde{L})'(X_q - \overline{X})\|^2.$$

Using the identity

$$\|P(\widetilde{L})'(X_q - \overline{X})\|^2 = \operatorname{tr}(P(\widetilde{L})'(X_q - \overline{X})(X_q - \overline{X})'P(\widetilde{L})),$$

where $\operatorname{tr}(\cdot)$ is the trace of the matrix, we see that

$$\rho(X - \overline{X}, \widetilde{L}) = \operatorname{tr} P(\widetilde{L})'T(X)P(\widetilde{L}). \tag{12}$$

The scattering matrix $T(X)$ is symmetric and nonnegative definite. In $\mathbb{R}^n$ we consider an orthonormal basis formed by eigenvectors $V_1, \dots, V_n$ of the matrix $T(X)$ ordered by the decreasing of the corresponding eigenvalues.

Let $\widetilde{L}_*$ be the r-dimensional plane with the basis formed by vectors $V_1, \dots, V_r$. Then the vectors $V_{r+1}, \dots, V_n$ form a basis in $L_*^{\perp}$. Denote by $V(r)$ the matrix formed by the column vectors $V_1, \dots, V_r$, and by $V(n-r)$ the matrix $P(\widetilde{L}_*)$ formed by the columns $V_{r+1}, \dots, V_n$. By construction,

$$T(X)P(\widetilde{L}_*) = P(\widetilde{L}_*)\Lambda(n-r),$$

where $\Lambda(n-r)$ is the diagonal matrix with entries $\lambda_{r+1}, \dots, \lambda_n$. Therefore,

$$\rho(X - \overline{X}, \widetilde{L}_*) = \sum_{k=1}^{n-r} \lambda_{r+k}.$$

Now standard methods of linear algebra using formula (12) written in the basis $V_1, \dots, V_n$ easily show that

$$\min_{\widetilde{L} \in G(r,n)} \rho(X - \overline{X}, \widetilde{L}) = \rho(X - \overline{X}, \widetilde{L}_*).$$

The theorem is proved. □

Denote $\sum_{k=1}^{n-r} \lambda_{k+r} = r_n(X)$, and consider the set of planes

$$\mathscr{L}_n(X;r) = \{\widetilde{L} \in G(r,n) : \rho(X - \overline{X}, \widetilde{L}) = r_n(X)\}.$$

If $\lambda_r > \lambda_{r+1}$, then $\mathscr{L}_n(X;r)$ consists of a single plane $\widetilde{L}_*$. If $\lambda_r = \lambda_{r+1}$, we can find $k_1 \geq 0$ and $k_2 \leq n$ such that $k_1 < r < k_2$ and

$$\lambda_{k_1} \neq \lambda_r, \quad \lambda_{k_1+1} = \lambda_r, \quad \lambda_{k_2} = \lambda_r, \quad \lambda_{k_2+1} \neq \lambda_r.$$

Let $W_1 \subset \mathbb{R}^n$ be the k_1-dimensional subspace with the basis $V_1, \dots, V_{k_1}$, and $W_2 \subset \mathbb{R}^n$ the k_2-dimensional subspace with the basis $V_1, \dots, V_{k_2}$. Then

The set $\mathscr{L}_n(X;r)$ consists of all r-dimensional subspaces in $\mathbb{R}^n$ that contain the subspace $W_1 \subset W_2$ and are contained in W_2.

Therefore, the projection of a curve X to $\mathfrak{M}_r$ is determined uniquely if and only if $\lambda_r > \lambda_{r+1}$. If $\lambda_r = \lambda_{r+1}$, the role of the projection can be played by any curve of the form $\overline{X} + X(\widetilde{L})$ with $\widetilde{L} \in \mathscr{L}_n(X;r)$.

Let us note that for $X = X_f$ we gave the description of the set $\mathscr{L}_n(f;r)$ mentioned in the Introduction.

We identify the space of all time series with N samples with a linear space of dimension N given with a fixed basis.

DEFINITION 6. A time series $g_Y = (g_1, \dots, g_N)$ is called a *projection* of a given curve $Y \in \mathfrak{M}$ to the space of time series T if

$$\| Y - X_{g_Y} \|^2 = \min_{f \in T} \| Y - X_f \|^2,$$

where X_{g_Y} and X_f are the n-dimensional unfoldings of time series g_Y and f.

THEOREM 2. (a) *For a curve $Y \in \mathfrak{M}$, its projection g_Y to the space of time series T is of the form $g_Y = (g_1, \dots, g_N)$, where*

$$g_s = \begin{cases} \dfrac{1}{s} \sum\limits_{l=1}^{s} y_{l,s-l+1}, & 1 \leq s \leq n, \\ \dfrac{1}{n} \sum\limits_{l=1}^{n} y_{l,s-l+1}, & n \leq s \leq p, \\ \dfrac{1}{N-s+1} \sum\limits_{l=1}^{N-s+1} y_{l+s-p,p-l+1}, & p \leq s \leq N. \end{cases}$$

Recall that $p = N - n + 1$.

(b) *Let X_f be the n-dimensional unfolding of a time series f. Then for any curve $Y \in \mathfrak{M}$ we have*

$$\|X_f - Y\|^2 = \|X_f - X_{g_Y}\|^2 + \|X_{g_Y} - Y\|^2.$$

Now we consider the following distance in the space of time series T. Let $f = (f_1, \dots, f_N)$ and $g = (g_1, \dots, g_N)$ be two time series. For a fixed n set

$$\|f - g\|_\mu^2 = \frac{1}{N} \sum_{s=1}^{N} \mu_s (f_s - g_s)^2,$$

where

$$\mu_s = \begin{cases} s/n, & 1 \leq s \leq n, \\ 1, & n \leq s \leq p, \\ (N-s+1)/n, & p \leq s \leq N \end{cases}$$

Let us comment on the choice of the distance in the space of time series T. Passing from a series f to its n-dimensional unfolding X_f, we get a linear map $i: T \to \mathfrak{M}$, $i(f) = X_f$. Choosing the standard Euclidean metric $\|Y_1 - Y_2\|$ in $\mathfrak{M} \sim \mathbb{R}^{pn}$, we define a metric in T in such a way that the imbedding i preserves the distance up to a factor. In this case the form of the weight function is uniquely determined by the condition

$$\|f - g\|_\mu^2 = (p/nN)\|X_f - X_g\|^2.$$

To conclude this comment, we present a construction of a class of metrics in the space T of time series that satisfy all principal results of this paper. We choose systems of positive weights $\alpha = (\alpha_1, \dots, \alpha_n)$, $\beta = (\beta_1, \dots, \beta_p)$, and define the following Euclidean metrics in $\mathbb{R}^n$ and in $\mathfrak{M}$:

$$\|Y_1 - Y_2\|_\alpha^2 = \sum_{k=1}^{n} \alpha_k (y_{k1} - y_{k2})^2, \qquad Y_1, Y_2 \in \mathbb{R}^n,$$

$$\|X - Y\|_{\alpha,\beta}^2 = \sum_{q=1}^{p} \beta_q \|X_q - Y_q\|_\alpha^2,$$

where $X = (X_q)$, $Y = (Y_q) \in \mathfrak{M}$. Consider the characteristic polynomials of weight systems α and β

$$\alpha(z) = \sum_{k=1}^{n} \alpha_k z^{k-1}, \qquad \beta(z) = \sum_{q=1}^{p} \beta_q z^{q-1}$$

and define the weight system $\gamma = (\gamma_1, \dots, \gamma_N)$ corresponding to the polynomial $\gamma(z) = c\alpha(z)\beta(z)$, where $c = \text{const}$. We recall that $p = N - n + 1$, so that $(n-1) + (p-1) = N - 1$. Introducing in the space T of length N time series the metric

$$\|f - g\|_\gamma^2 = \sum_{m=1}^{N} \gamma_m (f_m - g_m)^2,$$

we see by a straightforward computation that

$$\|f - g\|_\gamma^2 = c\|X_f - X_g\|_{\alpha,\beta}^2.$$

Definition 6′. A time series $g_Y = (g_1, \dots, g_N)$ is called an *(α, β)-projection* of a curve $Y \in \mathfrak{M}$ to the time series space T if

$$\|Y - X_{g_Y}\|_{\alpha,\beta}^2 = \min_{f \in T} \|Y - X_f\|_{\alpha,\beta}^2.$$

Theorem 2′. (a) *Let $g_Y = (g_1, \dots, g_N)$ be an (α, β)-projection of a curve $Y \in \mathfrak{M}$. Then*

$$g_m = \frac{1}{\gamma_m} \sum \alpha_k \beta_q y_{kq}, \qquad m = 1, \dots, N,$$

where the summation is over all k, q such that $k + q = m + 1$, $1 \le k \le n$, $1 \le q \le N - n + 1$.

(b) *Let $f = (f_1, \dots, f_N)$ be the n-dimensional unfolding of a time series. Then for any curve $Y \in \mathfrak{M}$ we have*

$$\|X_f - Y\|_{\alpha,\beta}^2 = \|X_f - X_{g_Y}\|_{\alpha,\beta}^2 + \|X_{g_Y} - Y\|_{\alpha,\beta}^2.$$

Here g_Y is the (α, β)-projection of the curve Y described in (a).

The proof of Theorem 2′ is based on the following identity, which admits a direct verification. Let $\{x_j\}$ and $\{\lambda_j\}$, $j = 1, \ldots, J$, be two number sequences with $\sum_{j=1}^{J} \lambda_j = s_\lambda \neq 0$. Then for any number y we have

$$\sum_{j=1}^{J} \lambda_j (x_j - y)^2 = \sum_{j=1}^{J} \lambda_j (x_j - x_\lambda)^2 + s_\lambda (x_\lambda - y)^2,$$

where

$$x_\lambda = \frac{1}{s_\lambda} \sum_{j=1}^{J} \lambda_j x_j.$$

Let us note that, together with our main metric μ with the characteristic polynomial of the system of weights equal to $(1/N)\mu(z) = c\alpha(z)\beta(z)$, where

$$c = \frac{p}{nN}, \qquad \alpha(z) = \frac{1 - z^n}{1 - z}, \qquad \beta(z) = \frac{1}{p}\frac{1 - z^p}{1 - z},$$

a practically important metric is the metric γ with the characteristic polynomial $\gamma(z) = \alpha(z)\beta(z)$, where

$$\alpha(z) = \left(\frac{1+z}{2}\right)^{n-1}, \qquad \beta(z) = \left(\frac{1+z}{2}\right)^{p-1}.$$

Now we continue the exposition for the case of the metric μ.

For a fixed r and our time series f, denote by X_* the projection of the n-dimensional unfolding X_f to $\mathfrak{M}_r$ and by f_* the projection of X_* to $\mathcal{T}$ (see Definitions 1, 5, 6). Theorems 1 and 2 imply that the time series f_*, as a nonparametric model of the series f, has the following extermal properties.

COROLLARY 1. *For any curve $Y \in \mathfrak{M}_r$,*

$$\|f - f_*\|_\mu^2 + (p/nN)\|X_{f_*} - X_*\|^2 \leq \|f - g_Y\|_\mu^2 + (p/nN)\|X_{g_Y} - Y\|^2$$

COROLLARY 2. *If g is a time series of rank not exceeding r, then*

$$\|f - g\|_\mu^2 \geq \|f - f_*\|_\mu^2 + (p/nN)\|X_{f_*} - X_*\|^2.$$

The proof follows from the fact that if $Y = X_g$, then $g_Y = g$.

§3. Main results

THEOREM 3. *If the rank of a time series g does not exceed r, then for our time series f we have*

$$\|f - g\|_\mu^2 \geq \|f - f_*\|_\mu^2.$$

Therefore we have an algorithm for the construction of nonparametric approximations $f_*(r)$, $r = 1, \ldots, n-1$, of a time series f (see Theorems 1 and 2), and can compute the errors

$$\delta_r = \|f - f_*(r)\|_\mu^2.$$

Theorem 3 implies that if $\delta_r > \delta$, where δ is some threshold, then for the approximation of the time series f by functions of the form

$$g(t) = \sum a_k(t) e^{\lambda_k t} \sin(\omega_k t + \varphi_k)$$

with $\operatorname{rk} g(t) \leq r$ we get

$$\|f - g\|_\mu^2 > \delta.$$

Hence, we have a lower bound for the approximation error even before applying algorithms for the estimation of the parameters λ_k, ω_k, φ_k and the coefficients of the polynomials $a_k(t)$, which in general is a hard nonlinear problem that can have a nonunique solution (see [**1**, Chapter 11]).

Let us note in conclusion that the bounds δ_r can be improved using iterations of the algorithm. Denote $f = f_{(0)}$, $f_{(1)} = f_*, \dots, f_{(m)} = f_{(m-1)*}, \dots$, Then we have the following improved estimate.

THEOREM 4. *If the rank of a time series g does not exceed r, then for the series f and for an arbitrary $m \geq 1$ we have*

$$\|f - g\|_\mu^2 \geq \|f - f_{(1)}\|_\mu^2 + \|f_{(1)} - f_{(2)}\|_\mu^2 + \dots + \|f_{(m-1)} - f_{(m)}\|_\mu^2.$$

COROLLARY 3. $\|f_{(m-1)} - f_{(m)}\|_\mu \to 0$ *as* $m \to \infty$.

The proof follows from the fact that the sequence $f_{(m)}$, $m = 0, 1, \dots,$ does not depend on g, so that the number sequence

$$\sum_{k=1}^{m} \|f_{(k-1)} - f_{(k)}\|_\mu^2,$$

is bounded from above (by Theorem 4) and monotone increasing.

References

1. S. L. Marple, Jr., *Digital spectral analysis with applications*, Prentice Hall, Englwood Cliffs, NJ, 1987.
2. S. A. Aĭvazyan, V. M. Buchstaber, I. S. Yenyukov, and L. D. Meshalkin, *Applied statistics, classification, and reduction of dimensionality*, "Finansy i Statistika", Moscow, 1989. (Russian)
3. M. Ya. Antonovskiĭ, V. M. Buchstaber, and L. S. Veksler, *Application of multivariant statictical analysis for the detection of structural changes in the series of monitoring data*, Working paper WP-91-31, IIASA, Laxenburg, 1991.
4. ______, *Application of multivariant statictical analysis for the detection of structural changes in the time series of ecological monitoring data*, Problems of Ecological Monitoring and Modelling of Ecological Systems, vol. 15, Gidrometeoizdat, St-Petersburg, 1993. (Russian)
5. ______, *Detection of changes in the properties of monitoring time series by the methods of multivariant statictical analysis*, Problems of Measurements of Parameters of Hydroacoustical and Geophysical Fields and Information Processing, NPO "VNIIFTRI", Moscow, 1992. (Russian)
6. F. R. Gantmakher, *Theory of matrices*, 2nd ed., "Nauka", Moscow, 1966; English transl. of 1st ed., Chealsea, New York, 1959.
7. J. W. Milnor and J. D. Stasheff, *Characteristic classes*, Princeton Univ. Press, Princeton, NJ, 1974.

Amer. Math. Soc. Transl.
(2) Vol. **162**, 1994

Inversion of the Generalized Radon Transform

A. S. Denisyuk

Introduction

We consider the following problem of integral geometry. Let X be a region in the Euclidean space $\mathbb{R}^n$ and let there be given a family Y of k-dimensional submanifolds $(1 \le k \le n)$ in it. On each submanifold $y \in Y$ let a density σ_y be defined. To a function $f(x)$ in the region X we associate its *k-dimensional generalized Radon transform*

$$R_k f(y) = \int_y f(x)\sigma_y. \tag{0.1}$$

The problem is to reconstruct the original function f from $R_k f$ (see **[3]**). The classical case corresponds to the situation when Y is the manifold of hyperplanes in $\mathbb{R}^n$ and σ_y is the Lebesgue measure on the hyperplane y. In this case explicit inversion formulas are known **[3, 11, 8]** that go back to Radon's paper **[20]**.

The one-dimensional Radon transform is called the *ray transform*. There are similar inversion formulas for a family of lines in $\mathbb{R}^n$ **[11]**. However, in this case for $n = 3$ the function $R_1 f$ depends on a larger number of parameters than the original function f. Therefore we can formulate the problem of reconstructing the function f from the values of its ray transform on an n-dimensional family of lines.

The corresponding problem in complex spaces was studied by I. M. Gel′fand and M. I. Graev in **[12]**. Those n-dimensional families of lines in $\mathbb{C}^n$ that allow a local inversion formula for the ray transform were called *admissible complexes*. In $\mathbb{R}^n$, a local inversion formula for the ray transform just cannot exist, but the geometry of a family plays an important role in the inversion formula.

For example, ray transform inversion formulas are known for the family of lines in $\mathbb{R}^3$ that intersect a given curve $\gamma \subset \mathbb{R}^3$ (see **[5, 21, 14, 1, 15, 8]**. The manifold K of lines intersecting a given curve is *characteristic*, i.e., at each point $y \in K$ it is tangent to a conical subbundle $\Sigma \subset TY$, where Y is the manifold of all lines in $\mathbb{R}^3$. The fiber of Σ at a point $y \in Y$ is defined by the formula $\Sigma_y = \bigcup_{x \in y} T_y Y_x$, where $Y_x \subset Y$ is the set of all lines passing through x. V. P. Palamodov has conjectured that explicit ray transform inversion formulas can be found for an arbitrary n-dimensional characteristic complex of lines in $\mathbb{R}^n$.

Characteristic complexes were studied in the paper **[5]**. In particular, it was proved that in a neighborhood of a generic line an n-dimensional characteristic complex of lines in $\mathbb{R}^n$ consists of lines intersecting a given curve $\gamma \subset \mathbb{R}^n$ if $n > 3$, whereas for $n = 3$ it consists either of lines intersecting a given curve $\gamma \subset \mathbb{R}^3$ or of lines tangent to a given surface $W \subset \mathbb{R}^3$. It turns out that for an arbitrary characteristic

0065-9290/94/$1.00 + $.25 per page

complex of lines in $\mathbb{R}^n$ one can, starting from integrals over lines, obtain integrals over hyperplanes. Thus, the inversion problem for the ray transform is reduced to the inversion of the Radon transform.

This construction can be extended to families of curves and, more generally, to families of k-dimensional ($1 \leq k \leq n-2$) surfaces. In this case the problem is reduced to the inversion of the generalized Radon transform for hypersurfaces that form a more general family than those considered in **[7, 13, 17]**.

The present paper consists of three sections. In §1 we consider a general family of hypersurfaces. If a condition that we call the completeness condition for a family of hypersurfaces is satisfied, we obtain a formula that gives the inverse of R_{n-1} up to a smoothing pseudodifferential operator. We also give the asymptotic expansion of the symbol of such an operator. The completeness condition is the condition that for each point $x \in X$ one can find an $(n-1)$-dimensional subfamily of hypersurfaces passing through x such that for any conormal vector $\omega \in T_x^* X$ there exists a unique hypersurface $H_{x,\omega}$ from this family such that ω is orthogonal to $H_{x,\omega}$, and, in addition, x is the only point that belongs to all these hypersurfaces. Our approach to the problem is close to the approach in the paper of Beylkin **[13]**.

In §2 we describe the additional integration method for the reduction of the k-dimensional ($1 \leq k \leq n-2$) generalized Radon transform to the inversion of the generalized Radon transform for hypersurfaces. The completeness condition for a family of k-dimensional manifolds is sufficient for the applicability of this method.

We devote §§3 and 4 to applications of the methods from §2 in various situations; §3 contains explicit inversion formulas for the ray transform for n-dimensional characteristic complexes of lines in $\mathbb{R}^n$.

In §4 this method is applied to the complex consisting of geodesics of a Riemannian metric that intersect a given curve. We present an explicit formula that defines an operator inverting the ray transform up to a smoothing operator. Another approach to a similar problem was considered by Greenleaf and Uhlmann in **[16]**.

The author is grateful to his thesis advisor V. P. Palamodov for formulation of the problems and constant help and attention.

§1. Inversion of the generalized Radon transform for a family of hypersurfaces

Let X be a region in the Euclidean space $\mathbb{R}^n$. Denote by $S^*X \cong X \times S^{n-1}$ the bundle of unit conormal vectors; let S^{n-1} be the $(n-1)$-dimensional unit sphere and U a smooth manifold of dimension $n-1$.

DEFINITION 1.1. A family of hypersurfaces in a region $X \subset \mathbb{R}^n$ is said to be *complete* if it can be defined by a mapping $\varphi\colon S^*X \times U \to X$ such that for any point $(x, \omega) \in S^*X$ the following conditions are satisfied:

(1) the mapping $\varphi(x, \omega, \cdot)\colon U \to X$ is an immersion and the surface $H_{x,\omega} = \operatorname{Im}(\varphi(x, \omega, \cdot))$ passes through the point x orthogonally to ω for a value of the parameter $u = u(x, \omega)$ that depends smoothly on (x, ω);

(2) $\operatorname{rank}(d_{x,\omega}\varphi) = n$ for $u \neq u(x, \omega)$.

We define the generalized Radon transform $R_{n-1}\colon C^\infty(X) \to C^\infty(S^*X)$ by the formula

$$R_{n-1}f(x, \omega) = \int_U f(\varphi(x, \omega, u)) a(x, \omega, u) \rho_{x,\omega},$$

where $\rho_{x,\omega}$ is the volume element on $H_{x,\omega}$ that is naturally induced by the Euclidean metric on X and $a \in C^\infty(S^*X \times U)$ satisfies the condition that for any $(x,\omega) \in S^*X$ the function $a(x,\omega,\cdot)$ has a compact support.

Define the back projection operator

$$R^*_{n-1}g(x) = \frac{1}{2(2\pi)^{n-1}} \int_{S^{n-1}} g(x,\omega)b(x,\omega)\Omega,$$

depending on a weight $b \in C^\infty(S^*X)$, Ω being the standard volume element on the unit sphere S^{n-1}.

THEOREM 1.2. *Let there be given a complete family of hypersurfaces in a region $X \subset \mathbb{R}^n$, and let $a(x,\omega,u(x,\omega)) \neq 0$ and $b(x,\omega) = 1/a(x,\omega,u(x,\omega))$. Then for any function $f \in C^\infty(X)$ we have*

$$(-\Delta)^{(n-1)/2} R^*_{n-1} R_{n-1} f = f + Kf,$$

where Δ is the Laplace operator, R_{n-1} is the generalized Radon transform, R^*_{n-1} is the back projection with weight b, and K is a classical pseudodifferential operator of order -1.

PROOF. We define a family of functionals $\delta_{x,\omega} \in \mathscr{E}'(\mathbb{R}^n)$ by the formula

$$\langle \delta_{x,\omega}, \psi \rangle = R_{n-1}\psi(x,\omega), \qquad \psi \in \mathscr{E}(\mathbb{R}^n).$$

Then

$$R_{n-1}f(x,\omega) = \frac{1}{(2\pi)^n} \int \widetilde{f}(\xi)\widetilde{\delta}_{x,\omega}(-\xi)\, d\widetilde{\xi},$$

where $\widetilde{f}(\xi) = \int f(x)\exp(-i\langle \xi, x\rangle)\,dx$ is the Fourier transform of the function $f(x)$ and $\widetilde{\delta}_{x,\omega}(\xi)$ is the Fourier transform of $\delta_{x,\omega}$.

Therefore,

$$\begin{aligned} R^*_{n-1}R_{n-1}f(x,\omega) &= \frac{1}{2(2\pi)^{2n-1}} \int_{\mathbb{R}^n} \widetilde{f}(\xi) \left(\int_{S^{n-1}} \widetilde{\delta}_{x,\omega}(-\xi) b(x,\omega)\Omega \right) d\xi \\ &= \frac{1}{(2\pi)^n} \int \widetilde{f}(\xi) A(x,\xi)\, d\xi, \end{aligned}$$

where

$$A(x,\xi) = \frac{1}{2(2\pi)^{n-1}} \int_{S^{n-1}\times U} e^{i\lambda\langle \theta, \varphi(x,\omega)\rangle} a(x,\omega,u) b(x,\omega)\Omega \otimes \rho_{x,\omega}, \tag{1.2}$$
$$\lambda = |\xi|, \qquad \theta = \xi/|\xi|.$$

Let us use the stationary phase method (see **[12**, §7.7]). Up to a function that decreases faster that any power of λ, the integral (1.2) is equal to the sum of integrals over neighborhoods of critical points of the phase $g(x,\theta,\omega,u) = \langle \theta, \varphi(x,\omega,u)\rangle$. A point $(\omega,u) \in S^{n-1} \times U$ is a stationary point for g if and only if

$$\frac{\partial g}{\partial \omega} \equiv \left\langle \theta, \frac{\partial \varphi}{\partial \omega}(x,\omega,u) \right\rangle = 0 \quad \text{and} \quad \frac{\partial g}{\partial u} \equiv \left\langle \theta, \frac{\partial \varphi}{\partial \omega}(x,\omega,u) \right\rangle = 0.$$

Property (2) of Definition 1.1 shows that $u = u(x,\omega)$, whereas property (1) of Definition 1.1 shows that either $\omega = \theta$ or $\omega = -\theta$. Therefore, the phase of the integral (1.2) has exactly two stationary points $P_\pm = (\pm\theta, u(x,\pm\theta))$, which depend smoothly on the parameters x and θ. It turns out that both these points are nondegenerate, $g(x,\theta,\pm\theta,u(x,\pm\theta)) = \langle\theta,x\rangle$. Applying Theorem 7.7.6 from **[12]**, we obtain

$$A(x,\xi) \simeq e^{i\langle x,\xi\rangle} \sum_{j=1}^{\infty} \frac{a_j(x,\theta)}{|\xi|^{j+n-1}} \quad \text{as } |\xi| \to \infty, \tag{1.3}$$

where $a_j(x,\theta) = a_j^+(x,\theta) + a_j^-(x,\theta)$; $a^\pm$ corresponds to the critical point $P_\pm$.

Therefore, $R_{n-1}^* R_{n-1}$ is a classical pseudodifferential operator (with a polyhomogeneous symbol) of order $1-n$ (see **[12, §18.1]**).

Let us now prove the nondegeneracy of the critical points and compute a_0. Fix (x_0,ξ_0). Consider the point $P_+ = (\theta, u(x,\theta))$. For the second points the arguments are similar.

Introduce Cartesian coordinates $x = (x_1,\dots,x_n)$ on X in such a way that $x_0 = (0,\dots,0)$, $\theta_0 = \xi_0/|\xi_0| = (0,\dots,0,1)$. It is clear that the value of $a_0(x_0,\theta_0)$ is independent of the coordinates on $S^{n-1}\times U$.

Introduce coordinates $v = (v^1,\dots,v^n)$ and $u = (u^1,\dots,u^n)$ on $S^{n-1}\times U$ in such a way that $u(x_0,\theta_0) = 0$ and hypersurfaces close to H_{x_0,ω_0} have the conormal vector $v = (v^1,\dots,v^{n-1},\sqrt{1-v^2})$, $v = \sum (v^i)^2$, and are parametrized as follows:

$$\varphi(x,\omega,\cdot)\colon u \mapsto \begin{pmatrix} u^1 + F_1(v,u) \\ \dots \\ u^{n-1} + F_{n-1}(v,u) \\ -\left(\sqrt{1-v^2}\right)^{-1} \sum_{i=1}^{n-1} u^i v^i + F_n(u,v) \end{pmatrix}$$

with $F_j(v,0) \equiv 0$ and $(\partial F_j/\partial u^i)(v,0) \equiv 0$; $j = 1,\dots,n$; $i = 1,\dots,n-1$.

Therefore, we are computing the first term of the asymptotic expansion, as $\lambda \to \infty$, of the integral

$$I(\lambda) = \frac{1}{(2\pi)^{n-1}} \int e^{i\lambda g(v,u)} B(v,u)\, dv\, du;$$

here

$$g(v,u) = F_n(u,v) - \left(\sqrt{1-v^2}\right)^{-1} \sum_{i=1}^{n-1} u^i v^i,$$

$$B(v,u) = \frac{a(x,\omega(v),u)}{2a(x,\omega(v),0)} \sqrt{\frac{l(u,v)}{1-v^2}},$$

and $l(u,v)$ is the determinant of the metric tensor on $H_{x,\omega}$ induced in a standard way by the Euclidean metric on X expressed in local coordinates $u = (u^1,\dots,u^{n-1})$. The integration is over a neighborhood $W \subset S^{n-1}\times U$ of the point P_+ with coordinates $(0,0)$ that is a critical point of the phase g. By Theorem 7.7.6 from **[12]** we have

$$a_0^+(x,\theta) = \frac{1}{\sqrt{|\det Q^+|}} e^{(i\pi/4)\operatorname{sgn} Q^+} B(v,u)\,|_{v=0,u=0},$$

where Q^+ is the Hessian of the phase function g at the point P_+.

The matrix Q^+ can be interpreted as the second quadratic form of the embedding $\varphi_x\colon S^{n-1}\times U \supset W \to S^*X$, $\varphi_x(\omega,u) = (\varphi(x,\omega,u), n(x,\omega,u))$, where $n(x,\omega,u)$ is the unit conormal vector to $H_{x,\omega}$ at the point $\varphi(x,\omega,u)$; $n(x,\theta,u(x,\theta))=\theta$. Therefore, the ratio

$$\sqrt{\frac{l(u,v)}{(1-v^2)|\det Q^+|}}\Bigg|_{v=0,u=0}$$

in the formula for a_0 does not depend on the choice of the local coordinates v and u.

In our coordinates, the matrix Q^+ has the form

$$Q^+ = \begin{pmatrix} \mathbb{O} & -\mathbb{E} \\ -\mathbb{E} & \mathbb{F} \end{pmatrix} \tag{1.4}$$

where

$$\mathbb{F} = \left(\frac{\partial^2 F}{\partial u^k \partial u^l} \Big|_{v=0,u=0} \right), \qquad k,l = 1,\dots,n-1,$$

$\mathbb{E}$ is the unit $(n-1)\times(n-1)$ matrix and $\mathbb{O}$ is the zero $(n-1)\times(n-1)$ matrix. Since $|\det Q^+| = 1$, the critical point P_+ is nondegenerate.

Let us consider a continuous family of matrices

$$Q_t^+ = \begin{pmatrix} \mathbb{O} & -\mathbb{E} \\ -\mathbb{E} & t\mathbb{F} \end{pmatrix}, \qquad t\in[0,1].$$

Since $|\det Q_t^+| = 1$, $\operatorname{sgn} Q^+ = \operatorname{sgn} Q_1^+ = \operatorname{sgn} Q_0^+ = 0$. Therefore, $a_0^+(x,\theta) = 1/2$. Similarly, $a_0^-(x,\theta) = 1/2$. Adding up these two equalities, we get $a_0(x,\theta) = 1$, so that

$$R_{n-1}^* R_{n-1} f = (-\Delta)^{(1-n)/2} f + K_1 f,$$

where K_1 is a classical pseudodifferential operator of order $-n$. Applying the operator $(-\Delta)^{(n-1)/2}$ to both parts of the last equality, we complete the proof of the theorem. □

Now we compute the symbol of the operator K. By the Morse lemma (see **[12,** Lemma C.6]), for any point $(x,\theta)\in S^*X$ one can introduce coordinates $z = (z^1,\dots,z^{2n-1})$ (depending smoothly on the parameters (x,θ)) in some neighborhood $W\subset S^{n-1}\times U$ of the point P_+ such that P_+ has zero coordinates and

$$g(v(z),u(z)) = \frac{1}{2}\langle Q^+ z, z\rangle, \qquad \det \left\| \frac{\partial z}{\partial(v,u)} \Big|_{v=0,u=0} \right\| = 1,$$

where $g(v,u) = \langle \theta, \varphi(x,\omega(v),u)\rangle$ and the matrix Q^+ is defined in (1.4).

In a neighborhood $W\subset S^{n-1}\times U$ of the point P_+ we define a symmetric quadratic form $\widetilde{Q}^+ \in S^2T^*W$ (depending smoothly on the parameters (x,θ)), $\widetilde{q}_{ij}^+(z) = q_{ij}^+$, where $\widetilde{q}_{ij}^+$ and q_{ij}^+ are entries of the matrices $\widetilde{Q}^+$ and Q^+, respectively, and z are coordinates defined in the Morse lemma. To the form $\widetilde{Q}^+$ we associate a second order differential operator $L_{x,\omega}^+$ acting in some local coordinates $y=(y^1,\dots,y^{2n-2})$ near the point P_+ by the formula

$$L_{x,\omega}^+ f = \frac{1}{\sqrt{|\det \widetilde{Q}^+|}} \sum_{i,j=1}^{2n-2} \frac{\partial}{\partial y^i}\left(\widetilde{q}_+^{ij} \sqrt{|\det \widetilde{Q}^+|}\, \frac{\partial}{\partial y^j} f \right)$$

and the density $\kappa_+ = \sqrt{|\det \widetilde{Q}^+|}\cdot |dy^1\cdots dy^{2n-1}|$, where $f\in C^\infty(W)$, and $\widetilde{q}_+^{ij}$ are the entries of the matrix inverse to $\widetilde{Q}^+$. Similarly, in a neighborhood of the point P_- we define a differential operator $L^-_{x,\omega}$ and a density κ_-.

THEOREM 1.3. *Under the conditions of Theorem* 1.2 *the symbol of the operator* K *has the asymptotic expansion*

(1.5)

$$\sigma_K(x,\xi) \simeq \sum_{j=1}^{\infty} \frac{1}{2j!}\left(\frac{i}{2|\xi|}\right)^j \left[(L^+_{x,\theta})^j \left(\frac{a(x,\omega,u)}{a(x,\omega,u(x,\theta))} \cdot \frac{\Omega \otimes \rho_{x,\omega}}{\kappa_+}\right)_{\substack{\omega=\theta \\ u=u(x,\theta)}} + (L^-_{x,\theta})^j \left(\frac{a(x,\omega,u)}{a(x,\omega,u(x,-\theta))} \cdot \frac{\Omega \otimes \rho_{x,\omega}}{\kappa_-}\right)_{\substack{\omega=-\theta \\ u=u(x,-\theta)}}\right]$$

PROOF. Since neither side of (1.5) depends on local coordinates, it is convenient to rewrite the integral (1.2) in the coordinates $z = (z^1, \dots, z^{2n-2})$ from the Morse lemma and to use the stationary phase method in the case when the phase is given by a quadratic form (see [**12,** Lemma 7.7.3]). Since in these coordinates we have

$$|\det \|\widetilde{q}^{\pm}_{ij}(z)\|\,| = |\det \|\widetilde{q}^{\pm}_{ij}(0)\|\,| = |\det \|q^{\pm}_{ij}(0)\|\,| = |\det Q^{\pm}| \cdot \left(\frac{\partial(v,u)}{\partial z}\right) = 1,$$

Theorem 1.3 follows. □

COROLLARY 1.4. *If in the conditions of Theorem* 1.2 *for any* $(x,\theta) \in S^*X$ *the relation*

$$a(x,\omega,u) = \frac{\kappa_+}{\Omega \otimes \rho_{x,\omega}}$$

is satisfied in a neighborhood of the point $(\theta, u(x,\theta)) \in S^{n-1} \times U$, *then*

$$(-\Delta)^{(n-1)/2} R^*_{n-1} R_{n-1} f \equiv f \mod C^\infty(X)$$

for any function $f \in \mathscr{D}'(X)$.

PROOF. Let us note that for any $(x,\omega) \in S^*X$ we have

$$\frac{\Omega \otimes \rho_{x,\omega}}{\kappa_\pm}(\pm\omega, u(x,\pm\omega)) \equiv 1.$$

Therefore, in the conditions of Corollary 1.4 we have $\sigma_K(x,\xi) = 0$, so that K is an infinitely smoothing operator. □

§2. Inversion of the generalized Radon transform for a family of submanifolds of an arbitrary dimension

Let us consider a family of k-dimensional $(1 \le k \le n-2)$ manifolds in a region $X \subset \mathbb{R}^n$ defined by a mapping $\varphi\colon Y \times U \to X$, where Y and U are smooth manifolds, $\dim U = k$, and $\varphi(y,\cdot)\colon U \to X$ is an immersion for all $y \in Y$. Let $H_y = \operatorname{Im}(\varphi(y,\cdot))$. Let $R_k\colon C^\infty(X) \to C^\infty(Y)$ be the k-dimensional generalized Radon transform,

$$R_k f(y) = \int_U f(\varphi(y,u))\sigma_y(u).$$

The family of densities σ_y must satisfy the condition that σ_y have a compact support $\operatorname{supp}\sigma_y \subset U$ for each $y \in Y$.

Denote by $V \subset \mathbb{R}^{n-1-k}$ a simply connected neighborhood of the origin.

DEFINITION 2.1. We say that a family Y of k-dimensional submanifolds in a region X *satisfies the completeness condition* if there exists a smooth mapping $\Pi\colon S^*X \times V \to Y$ such that the mapping $\Phi\colon S^* \times V \times U \to X$ given by the formula $\Phi(x, \omega, v, u) = \varphi(\Pi(x, \omega, v), u)$ satisfies the following conditions for all $(x, \omega) \in S^*X$:

(1) $\Phi(x, \omega, \cdot, \cdot)\colon V \times U \to X$ is an immersion;
(2) the submanifold $H_{x,\omega}$ passes through the point x for $v = 0$ and a value of the parameter $u = u(x, \omega)$ that depends smoothly on (x, ω), and is orthogonal to ω at this point;
(3) $\operatorname{rank} d_{\omega,v,u}\Phi = n$ for $(v, u) \neq (0, u(x, \omega))$.

Let us take an auxiliary compactly supported density υ in V such that $0 \in \operatorname{supp} \upsilon$. Define the operator $T\colon C^\infty(Y) \to C^\infty(S^*X)$ by the formula

$$Tg(x, \omega) = \int_V g(\Pi(x, \omega, v))\upsilon.$$

THEOREM 2.2. *Let a family of k-dimensional $(1 \le k \le n-1)$ manifolds in a region $X \subset \mathbb{R}^n$ satisfying the completeness condition be given. Then the mapping Φ defines a complete family of hypersurfaces $H_{x,\omega} = \operatorname{Im}\Phi(x, \omega, \cdot, \cdot)$ in Y.*

Furthermore, if for each point $(x, \omega) \in S^*X$ we have $\sigma_y(u) \neq 0$ for $y = \Pi(x, \omega, 0)$, $u = u(x, \omega)$, and define

$$b(x, \omega) = \left.\frac{\rho_{x,\omega}(v, u)}{\sigma_y(u) \otimes \upsilon(v)}\right|_{v=0, u=u(x,\omega), y=\Pi(x,\omega,0)},$$

where $\rho_{x,\omega}$ is the volume element on $H_{x,\omega}$ induced by the Euclidean metric on X in a standard manner, then for any function $f \in C^\infty(X)$ we have

$$(-\Delta)^{(n-1)/2} R^*_{n-1} T R_{n-1} f = f + Kf,$$

where K is a classical pseudodifferential operator of order -1 and R^*_{n-1} is the back projection operator with weight b (see (1.1)).

PROOF. The first statement follows from the completeness of the family. To prove the second statement we apply Theorem 1.2 to the family $H_{x,\omega}$ and the Radon transform

$$R_{n-1}f = \int_{V \times U} f(\phi(\Pi(x, \omega, v), u))a(x, \omega, v, u)\rho_{x,\omega},$$

where

$$a(x, \omega, v, u) = \left.\frac{\sigma_y(u) \otimes \upsilon(v)}{\rho_{x,\omega}}\right|_{y-\Pi(x,\omega,v)}.$$

It is clear that $R_{n-1}f = TR_k f$. □

REMARK. In **[9]**, Palamodov formulated a condition for a family of lines in the space that is sufficient for the existence of a well-posed inversion of the ray transform up to an infinitely smooth function. Let $X \subset \mathbb{R}^n$, let Y be a family of curves in the region X, and let $t \in \mathbb{R}$ be a parameter along the curves. Palamodov's condition is that for any point $(x, \omega) \in S^*X$ there exist a curve $y_0 \in Y$ and a value of the parameter $t_0 \in \mathbb{R}$ such that

(1) $y_0(t_0) = x$ and $\langle \omega, \dot{y}_0)(t_0)\rangle = 0$, where $\dot{y} = dy/dt$;

(2) the jet of the mapping $P_\omega\colon Y\times\mathbb{R}\to X\times\mathbb{R}$ given by

$$P_\omega\colon (y,t)\to (y(t),\langle\omega,\dot y(t)\rangle)$$

at the point (y_0,t_0) is a diffeomorphism.

The condition in Definition 2.1 is stronger than Palamodov's condition. One can show that if Palamodov's condition is satisfied, then our completeness condition is satisfied at least locally.

§3. Inversion of the ray transform for characteristic complexes of lines in $\mathbb{R}^n$

In this section we present explicit inversion formulas for the ray transform corresponding to n-dimensional characteristic complexes of lines in $\mathbb{R}^n$. Let $\gamma\subset\mathbb{R}^n$ be a smooth curve parameterized by $\lambda\in\mathbb{R}$. Let

$$g(\lambda,\xi)=\int_0^\infty f(\gamma(\lambda)_t\xi)\,dt$$

be the ray transform of the function f. Here $\xi=(\xi^1,\dots,\xi^n)$, $\sum(\xi^i)^2=1$, is the unit director vector of the line. Let $H_{\omega,p}$ be the hyperplane $\langle x,\omega\rangle=p$ in $\mathbb{R}^n$, where $\omega=(\omega_1,\dots,\omega_n)$, $\sum(\omega_j)^2=1$, is the unit conormal vector to $H_{\omega,p}$, $p\in\mathbb{R}$.

DEFINITION 3.1. Let K be the complex of all lines in $\mathbb{R}^n$ that intersect a given curve $\gamma\subset\mathbb{R}^n$, and let B be a region in $\mathbb{R}^n$. We say that K and B *satisfy the K-T condition* if for any hyperplane $H_{\omega,p}$ such that $H_{\omega,p}\cap B\neq\varnothing$ there exists a value of the parameter $\lambda=\lambda(\omega,p)$ such that the curve γ intersect $H_{\omega,p}$ transversely at the point $\gamma(\lambda(\omega,p))$.

This condition is a straightforward generalization of the Kirillov-Tuy condition (see **[6, 21]**) for the complex of lines intersecting a given curve in $\mathbb{R}^3$.

THEOREM 3.2. *Let K be the complex of lines in $\mathbb{R}^n$ intersecting a given curve $\gamma\subset\mathbb{R}^n$, B a region in $\mathbb{R}^n$, and let the K-T condition be satisfied. Then for any function $f\in S_B(\mathbb{R}^n)=\{f\in S(\mathbb{R}^n)\mid \operatorname{supp} f\subset B\}$, where $S(\mathbb{R}^n)$ is the Schwartz space, we have the following inversion formula for the ray transform*:

a) *if $n=2k+1$, then*

$$f(x)=\frac{(-1)^{(n-1)/2}}{2(2\pi)^{n-1}}\times\int_{S^{n-1}}\Omega_{n-1}(\omega)\left(\frac{1}{\langle\omega,\gamma'_\lambda\rangle}\frac{d}{d\lambda}\int_{S^{n-1}(\omega)}\Omega_{n-2}(\xi)L^{n-2}(\omega,D)g(\lambda,\xi)\right)\Bigg|_{\lambda=\lambda(\omega,\langle\omega,x\rangle)};$$

b) *if $n=2k$, then*

$$f(x)=\frac{(-1)^{(n-2)/2}}{2(2\pi)^{n-1}}\int_{S^{n-1}}\Omega_{n-1}(\omega)\times\int_{-\infty}^{\infty}\frac{dp}{\langle\omega,x\rangle-p}\left(\frac{1}{\langle\omega,\gamma'_\lambda\rangle}\frac{d}{d\lambda}\int_{S^{n-2}(\omega)}\Omega_{n-2}(\xi)L^{n-2}(\omega,D)g(\lambda,\xi)\right)\Bigg|_{\lambda=\lambda(\omega,p)},$$

where $g(\lambda,\xi)$ is the ray transform, Ω_l is the standard volume form on the unit sphere S^l, $S^{n-2}(\omega)=\{\xi\in S^{n-1}\mid\langle\omega,\xi\rangle=0\}$, and

$$L(\omega,D)=\sum_{j=1}^n\omega_j\frac{\partial}{\partial\xi^j}.$$

REMARK. For $n = 3$ our inversion formula is contained in Grangeat's thesis [15], although in a somewhat different form.

PROOF. Consider an arbitrary hyperplane $H_{\omega,p}$ that intersects the support of f. Denote by $Rf(\omega, p)$ the classical Radon transform of the function f. Passing to spherical coordinates on the hyperplane $H_{\omega,p}$ centered at the point $\gamma(\lambda(\omega, p))$, we have

$$\begin{aligned} Rf(\omega,p) &= \int_{H_{\omega,p}} f(x)\,dS \\ &= \int_{S^{n-2}(\omega)} \Omega_{n-2}(\xi) \int_0^\infty f(\gamma(\lambda(\omega,p)) + t\xi)t^{n-2}\,dt. \end{aligned} \tag{3.1}$$

Now let us note that

$$\frac{\partial g}{\partial \xi^i} = \int_0^\infty \frac{\partial f}{\partial x^i}(\gamma(\lambda) + t\xi)t\,dt.$$

Therefore,

$$L(\omega, D) = \int_0^\infty \sum_{i=1}^n \omega_i \frac{\partial f}{\partial x^i}(\gamma(\lambda) + t\xi)t\,dt,$$

$$\frac{\partial}{\partial \lambda} g(\lambda, \xi) = \int_0^\infty \sum_{i=1}^n \frac{d\gamma^i}{d\lambda}\frac{\partial f}{\partial x^i}(\gamma(\lambda) + t\xi)t\,dt.$$

Therefore, taking into account (3.1), we get

$$\frac{d}{d\lambda}\int_{S^{n-2}(\omega)} \Omega_{n-2}(\xi)L^{n-2}(\omega, D)g(\lambda,\xi)\,|_{\lambda=\lambda(\omega,p)} = \langle \omega, \gamma'_\lambda\rangle \frac{d^{n-1}}{dp^{n-1}} Rf(\omega, p).$$

In the proof of this equality we use the following property of the Radon transform (see [3]):

$$R\left(\sum a_j \frac{\partial f}{\partial x^j}\right)(\omega, p) = \left(\sum a_j\omega_j\right)\frac{d}{dp}Rf(\omega,p).$$

Now we use the inversion formulas for the Radon transform [8]: for odd n

$$f(x) = \frac{(-1)^{(n-1)/2}}{2(2\pi)^{n-1}} \int_{S^{n-1}} \frac{d^{n-1}}{dp^{n-1}} Rf(\omega, \langle\omega, x\rangle)\Omega_{n-1}(\omega), \tag{3.2}$$

and for even n

$$f(x) = \frac{(-1)^{(n-2)/2}}{(2\pi)^n} \int_{S^{n-1}} \Omega_{n-1}(\omega) \int_{-\infty}^\infty \frac{\frac{d^{n-1}}{dp^{n-1}}Rf(\omega,p)}{\langle\omega, x\rangle - p}\,dp. \tag{3.3}$$

The theorem is proved. □

The inversion formula for the ray transform in the case of complexes of lines in $\mathbb{R}^3$ was obtained by the author together with V. P. Palamodov. In a somewhat different form this formula was published in [19].

Let $H_{\omega,p}$ be an arbitrary hyperplane that intersects a surface W transversely. Denote $\Gamma_{\omega,p} = H_{\omega,p} \cap W$; $\Gamma_{\omega,p}$ is a smooth plane curve in $\mathbb{R}^3$. Denote by s the natural parameter on the curve $\Gamma_{\omega,p}$. To the curve $\Gamma_{\omega,p}$ one can associate the Frenet frame (τ, n, β), where τ is the tangent vector, n is the normal vector, and β is the binormal vector. To $\Gamma_{\omega,p}$ we associate also the "tangent evolvent"

$$\Phi\colon \Gamma_{\omega,p} \times \mathbb{R} \to H_{\omega,p} \qquad \Phi\colon (s,t) \mapsto \Gamma_{\omega,p}(s) + \tau(s)t.$$

Denote by K the complex of all lines in $\mathbb{R}^3$ that are tangent to the surface $W \subset \mathbb{R}^3$. Let B be an arbitrary region.

DEFINITION 3.3. We say that K and B *satisfy the K-T1 condition* if for any hyperplane $H_{\omega,p}$ such that $H_{\omega,p} \cap B \neq \varnothing$ there exists an open curve $\gamma_{\omega,p} \subset \Gamma_{\omega,p}$ such that the following conditions are satisfied:

1) the mapping $\Phi\,|_{\gamma_{\omega,p}\times\mathbb{R}_+}$ is of degree $\delta \neq 0$;
2) $B \cap H_{\omega,p} \subset \operatorname{Im} \Phi\,|_{\gamma_{\omega,p}\times\mathbb{R}_+}$.

We assume that $\gamma_{\omega,p} \times \mathbb{R}_+$ is oriented via the form $ds \wedge ds$ and $\Phi\,|_{\gamma_{\omega,p}\times\mathbb{R}_+}$ is a proper mapping onto its image; the orientation of $H_{\omega,p}$ is defined by the conormal vector ω.

Let us fix ω and define local coordinates s and q on W such that $w(s,q) \in W$ and for any fixed q_0, $w(s,q_0) \in H_{\omega,p(q_0)} \cap W$, with s being the natural parameter on this curve. Then $\tau(s,q) = w'_s$ is the unit tangent vector to the curve $\Gamma_{\omega,p}$. Denote by $\upsilon(s,q)$ the unit vector that is tangent to W at the point $w(s,q)$ and orthogonal to τ. As local coordinates on K we take the parameters (s,q,φ), so that the ray transform of the function f is given by the formula

$$g(s,q,\varphi) = \int_0^\infty f\big(w(s,q) + t(\tau(s,q)\cos\varphi + \upsilon(s,q)\sin\varphi)\big)\,dt.$$

THEOREM 3.4. *Let K be the complex of lines in $\mathbb{R}^3$ tangent to a given surface $W \subset \mathbb{R}^3$, $B \subset \mathbb{R}^3$ a region such that the K-T1 condition is satisfied for K and B. Then for any function $f \in S_B(\mathbb{R}^3)$ the following formula holds*:

$$f(x) = -\frac{1}{8\pi^2\delta}\int_{S^2} \Omega_2(\omega)\frac{1}{\langle\omega, w'_q\rangle}\frac{d}{dq}\int_{\gamma_{\omega,\langle\omega,x\rangle}} \varkappa(s) Lg(s,q,0)\,ds,$$

where

$$Lg = \frac{\langle\omega,\upsilon\rangle}{1-\langle n,\upsilon\rangle^2}\left(k(s)\frac{\partial g}{\partial\varphi} - \langle n,\upsilon\rangle\frac{\partial g}{\partial s}\right);$$

$\varkappa(s) = \operatorname{sgn}\langle\omega,\beta\rangle$, *$\beta = \beta(s,q)$ is the binormal vector, $n = n(s,q)$ is the normal vector, and $k(s)$ is the curvature of the curve $\gamma_{\omega,\langle\omega,x\rangle}$.*

PROOF. Similarly to the proof of Theorem 3.2, we prove that

$$\frac{dRf}{dp}(\omega,p) = \frac{1}{\delta}\int_{\gamma_{\omega,p}} LG\cdot\varkappa(s)\,ds$$

and then use formula (3.2) for $n = 3$. □

REMARK. If the region $B \subset \mathbb{R}^n$ is bounded, then to reconstruct the function $f \in C_0^\infty(B)$ from its integral over straight lines that form an n-dimensional characteristic complex, it is sufficient to require that the condition K-T (respectively the condition K-T1) be satisfied only for a set of planes whose unit conormal vectors fill a nonempty open set $\Sigma \subset S^{n-1}$. Indeed, defining $d^{n-1}Rf(\omega,p)/dp^{n-1}$ as in the proofs of Theorems 3.2 and 3.4 and performing the Fourier transform with respect to the variable p, we reconstruct the Fourier transform of the function f in the cone $\Sigma\mathbb{R} \subset \mathbb{R}^n$. After that we can use one of the methods for the extrapolation of the Fourier transform of a compactly supported function (see **[18, 9]**). The resulting formulas will have the exponential amplification coefficient for random errors in data (see **[18, 9]**).

4. Inversion of the generalized Radon transform for the Chow complexes of geodesics

Let X be a region in $\mathbb{R}^n$ ($n \geq 3$) and $l \subset X$ a smooth curve. Let us assume that on X a smooth Riemannian metric $g = \{g_{ij}\}$ is defined. We consider the complex K consisting of geodesic curves for the metric g that intersect the curve l. We impose the following condition on the metric g: for any two points x_1, x_2, $x_1 \in l$, $x_2 \neq x_1$, there exists a unique geodesic, denoted γ_{x_1,x_2}, passing through these two points (hence, there are no points in X that are conjugate along geodesics from the complex K). In this case, for any point $a \in l$ the mapping $\exp_a$ is a diffeomorphism of a neighborhood of the origin in T_aX to X. We call K the *Chow complex* of the curve l.

Let us consider an arbitrary geodesic $\gamma = \gamma(s)$, where s is the natural parameter, $\gamma(0) = a \in l$, $\dot\gamma(0) \equiv (d/ds)\gamma(0) = \xi \in T_aX$. The exponential mapping $\exp_a$ induces a family of isomorphisms $E_s = d(\exp_a)\colon T_aX \to T_{\gamma(s)}X$. Here we use the canonical identification of $T_{s\xi}(T_aX)$ and T_aX. For a covector $\omega \in T^*_{\gamma(s)}X$ we denote $\omega_t = (E_t^*)^{-1}E_s^*\omega \in T^*_{\gamma(s)}X$ ($t \neq 0$).

The following definition can be regarded as a generalization to curves of the Kirillov-Tuy completeness condition (see **[6,19]**).

DEFINITION 4.1. Let a metric g and a curve l in a region $X \subset \mathbb{R}^n$ satisfy the above requirements. Let K be the Chow complex of the curve l and let $B \subset X$ be a subregion, $B \cap X = \varnothing$. We say that K and B *satisfy* the *condition K-T*2 if there exists a smooth mapping $p\colon S^*B \simeq B \times S^{n-1} \to l$ such that for each point $(x, \omega) \in S^*B$ the following conditions hold:

1) The geodesic $\gamma_{p(x,\omega),x}$ passing through the points $p(x,\omega)$ and x is orthogonal to ω at the point x.
2) $\operatorname{rank} d_\omega p = 1$.
3) Let the curve l be locally parameterized by a parameter $\lambda \in \mathbb{R}$, $l(0) = p(x,\omega)$, and consider a family of geodesics $\gamma_\lambda(s)$ passing through x and $l(\lambda)$, with $\gamma_0 = \gamma_{p(x,\omega),x}$. Let $\gamma_0(s_0) = x$. We require that $\langle\omega_0, \partial\gamma_\lambda/\partial\lambda\rangle \neq 0$ for $s \neq s_0$.

THEOREM 4.2. *In a region $X \subset \mathbb{R}^n$ let there be given the Chow complex K of a curve l and a subregion $B \subset X$ such that the condition K-T2 is satisfied. Then K determines a family of curves in B that satisfies the completeness condition of Definition* 2.1.

PROOF. We must construct a mapping Π that satisfies all conditions of Definition 2.1. We will specify the complex K by a mapping $\Gamma\colon l \times S^{n-1} \times U \to X$, $U \subset \mathbb{R}_+$, where $\Gamma(a, \xi, s)$ is the geodesic from the point a in the direction ξ ($|\xi| = 1$), and s is the natural parameter. Let us note that for a fixed point a we have $\Gamma(a,\xi,s) = \exp_a(s\xi)$.

Denote by $s(x,\omega)$ the distance between points x and $p(x,\omega)$. It is clear that $s(x,\omega)$ is a smooth function. Fix a point x. Let

$$\xi(x,\omega) = \gamma_{p(x,\omega),x} \in T_{p(x,\omega)}X. \tag{4.1}$$

By $\eta_1(x,\omega), \dots, \eta_{n-2}(x,\omega) \in T_{p(x,\omega)}X$ we denote an orthonormal systems of vectors that depend smoothly on x and ω, are orthogonal to $\xi(x,\omega)$, and satisfy

$$\langle E^*_{s(x,\omega)}, \eta_j(x,\omega)\rangle = 0 \quad \text{for } j = 1,\dots,n-2.$$

Let $V = (-\varepsilon,\varepsilon)^{n-2} \subset \mathbb{R}^{n-2}$ be an $(n-2)$-dimensional cube ($\varepsilon > 0$). Define a mapping $\Pi\colon S^*X \times V \to l \times S^{n-1}$ as follows:

$$\Pi\colon (x,\omega,v) \to \Gamma\left(p(x,\omega), \xi(x,\omega) + \sum_{j=1}^{n-2} v^j \eta_j(x,\omega), s\right).$$

We claim that this mapping satisfies the desired conditions. Indeed, the mapping $\Phi(x,\omega,\cdot,\cdot)\colon V \times U \to X$,

$$\begin{aligned}\Phi(x,\omega,v,u) &= \Gamma\left(p(x,\omega), \xi(x,\omega) + \sum_{j=1}^{n-2} v^j \eta_j(x,\omega), s\right)\\ &= \exp_{p(x,\omega)}\left(s\left(\xi(x,\omega) + \sum_{j=1}^{n-2} v^j \eta_j(x,\omega)\right)\right)\end{aligned}$$

is an embedding.

Condition 2) is satisfied by the construction of the mapping.

Let us verify condition 3). Since $\operatorname{rank} d_\omega p = 1$, the mapping $p(x,\cdot)\colon S^{n-1} \to l$ is a locally trivial bundle over l. Let $(x_0,\omega_0) \in S^*X$ be an arbitrary point. As local coordinates on the sphere S^{n-1} near ω_0 we take the parameter λ on the curve l and the coordinates $w^1,\dots,w^{n-2}$ in the fiber of the bundle $p(x,\cdot)$. In these coordinates the mapping Φ takes the form (for a fixed $x = x_0$)

$$\Phi(x,\omega,v,s) = \Gamma\left(a(\lambda), \xi(\lambda) + \sum_{j=1}^{n-2} v^j \eta_j(x,\omega), s\right),$$

where we do not indicate the dependence on x in order to simplify notation.

Consider the matrix

$$\left(\frac{\partial\Phi}{\partial w^j}, \frac{\partial\Phi}{\partial s}, \frac{\partial\Phi}{\partial v^i}\right) = d\exp_{a(\lambda)}\left(s\sum_{k=1}^{n-2} v^k \frac{\partial\eta_k}{\partial w^j}, \sum_{k=1}^{n-2} v^k\eta_k + \xi, s\eta_i\right)_{i,j=1,\dots,n-2}. \tag{4.3}$$

Since for any $j = 1,\dots,n-2$ and any $\omega \in S^{n-1}$ the vector $\eta_j(\omega)$ is orthogonal to ξ and $|\eta_j(\omega)| = 1$, for any $i = 1,\dots,n-2$ the vector $\partial\eta_j/\partial w^i$ is orthogonal to ζ and η_j. Therefore, for $v \neq 0$ the rank of the matrix (4.3) equals n, and hence

$$\operatorname{rank}\left(\partial\Phi/\partial(\omega,x,s)\right) = n.$$

Now let $v = 0$. In this case $\partial\Phi/\partial w = 0$. Let us consider the matrix

$$Q(s) = \left(\frac{\partial\Phi}{\partial w^j}, \frac{\partial\Phi}{\partial s}, \frac{\partial\Phi}{\partial v^i}\right)\Bigg|_{v=0}, \qquad j = 1,\dots,n-2.$$

Here $\partial\Phi/\partial s = \dot\gamma(s)$ is the tangent vector field along the geodesics $\gamma_{p(x,\omega),x}$.

Varying the parameter v^i, we obtain a one-parameter family of geodesics passing through the point $p(x,\omega)$. Therefore, $\partial\Phi/\partial v^i = J_i(s)$ is the Jacobi normal field along the geodesic $\gamma_{p(x,\omega),x}$, $J_{n-1}(s(x,\omega)) = 0$.

Varying the parameter λ, we obtain the variation of the geodesic $\gamma_{p(x,\omega),x}$ passing through the point x. To this variation corresponds the Jacobi normal field $J_{n-1}(s)$ along the geodesic $\gamma_{p(x,\omega),x}$, $J_{n-1}(s(x,\omega)) = 0$, which differs from $\partial\Phi/\partial\lambda$ by a field of the form $(as+b)\dot{\gamma}$ (see **[4]**). Therefore,

$$\operatorname{rank}(Q(s)) = \operatorname{rank}(J_1(s), \dots, J_{n-1}(s), \dot{\gamma}(s))$$

Let us assume that there exists a value $s_0 \neq s(x,\omega)$ such that $\operatorname{rank}(Q(s)) < n$. Since $J_1, \dots, J_{n-1}$ are orthogonal to $\dot{\gamma}(s)$, the vectors $J_1(s_0), \dots, J_{n-1}(s_0)$ are linearly dependent. By the conditions of the theorem, $\langle \omega_{s_0}, J_{n-1}(s_0)\rangle \neq 0$. On the other hand, $\langle \omega_{s_0}, J_j(s_0)\rangle = 0$, $j = 1, \dots, n-2$. Therefore, $J_1(s_0), \dots, J_{n-2}(s_0)$ are linearly dependent, i.e., there exist constants $c_1, \dots, c_{n-2}$ such that $\sum_{j=1}^{n-2} c_j J_j(s_0) = 0$. Since $\sum_{j=1}^{n-2} c_j J_j(0) = 0$, we come to a contradiction with the absence of conjugate points. The theorem is proved. □

Now let us define the ray transform of a function $f(x) \in C_0^\infty(B)$ by the formula

$$R_1 f(a,\xi) = \int_{\gamma_{a,\xi}} f(x)\, ds,$$

where $\gamma_{a,\xi}$ is the geodesic from the point a in the direction ξ.

We consider the Euclidean metric in the region X and denote by $x = (x^1, \dots, x^n)$ the Cartesian coordinates. Denote $\|\xi\| = \sqrt{\sum g_{ij}\xi^i\xi^j}$, where $\xi = (\xi^1, \dots, \xi^n)$ is a tangent vector. Let V be the $(n-1)$-dimensional cube $[-\varepsilon, \varepsilon]^{n-2} \subset \mathbb{R}^{n-2}$ $(\varepsilon > 0)$. Choose an auxiliary function $\psi(v) \in C^\infty(V)$, $\psi(0) = 1$.

COROLLARY 4.1. *Under the conditions of Theorem 4.2, for any function $f \in C_0^\infty(B)$ and any $x \in B$ we have*

$$\begin{aligned}\frac{(-\Delta)^{(n-1)/2}}{2(2\pi)^{n-1}} &\int_{S^{n-1}} \Omega(\omega) b(x,\omega) \\ &\times \int_V R_1 f\left(p(x,\omega), \xi(x,\omega) + \sum_{j=1}^{n-2} v^j \eta_j(x,\omega)\right) \psi(v)\, dv \\ &= f(x) + K_1 f(x),\end{aligned}$$

where K_1 is a classical pseudodifferential operator of order -1, Δ is the Euclidean Laplace operator, $p(x,\omega)$ is the mapping from Definition 4.1,

$$b(x,\omega) = \left(\sum_{i=1}^{n} D_i^2(x,\omega)\right)^{1/2} \left(\|\gamma_{p(x,\omega),\xi(x,\omega)}\|\right)^{-1} |_{s=s(x,\omega)},$$

$\xi(x,\omega)$ and $\eta_j(x,\omega)$, $j = 1, \dots, n-2$, are defined in (4.2) and (4.3),

$$D_j(x,\omega) = \det \begin{vmatrix} \dot{\gamma}^1 & \gamma_1^1 & \dots & \gamma_{n-2}^1 \\ \dot{\gamma}^2 & \gamma_1^2 & \dots & \gamma_{n-2}^2 \\ \dots & & & \\ \dot{\gamma}^n & \gamma_1^n & \dots & \gamma_{n-2}^n \end{vmatrix}, \qquad j\text{th row deleted},$$

$$\dot{\gamma}(s) = \frac{d\gamma_{a,\xi}}{ds}\, |_{a-p(x,\omega)}, \qquad \gamma_j = \frac{d}{dv}\left(\gamma_{a,\xi,v\eta_j}\right)\Big|_{v=1,a=p(x,\omega)},$$

and $s(x, \omega)$ is the value of the parameter for which the curve $\gamma_{p(x,\omega),\xi(x,\omega)}$ passes through the point x.

References

1. I. M. Gel′fand and A. B. Goncharov, *Recovery of a compactly supported function from its integrals over lines intersecting a given set of points in space*, Dokl. Akad. Nauk SSSR **290** (1986), no. 5, 1037–1040; English transl. in Soviet Math. Dokl. **34** (1987).
2. I. M. Gel′fand and M. I. Graev, *Complexes of lines in the space* $\mathbb{C}^n$, Funktsional. Anal. i Prilozhen. **2** (1968), no. 3, 39-52; English transl. in Functional Anal. Appl. **2** (1968).
3. I. M. Gel′fand, M. I. Graev, and N. Ya. Vilenkin, *Generalized functions*. Vol. 5: *Integral geometry and representation theory*, Fizmatgiz, Moscow, 1962; English transl., Academic Press, New York, 1966.
4. D. Gromoll, W. Klingenberg, and W. Meyer, *Riemannsche Geometrie im Grossen*, Lecture Notes in Math., vol. 55, Springer-Verlag, Berlin, 1968.
5. A. S. Denisyuk, *Local structure of hyperbolic complexes*, Uspekhi Mat. Nauk **45** (1990), no. 5 (275), 185–186; English transl. in Russian Math. Surveys **45** (1990).
6. A. A. Kirillov, *On a problem of I. M. Gel′fand*, Dokl. Akad. Nauk SSSR **137** (1961), no. 2, 276–277; English transl. in Soviet Math. Dokl. **2** (1961).
7. M. M. Lavrent′ev, V. G. Romanov, and S. P. Shishat·skiĭ, *Ill-posed problems in mathematical physics and analysis*, "Nauka", Moscow, 1980; English transl., Amer. Math. Soc., Providence, RI, 1986.
8. F. Natterer, *The mathematics of computerized tomography*, Teunber, Stuttgatt, and Wiley, New York, 1985.
9. V. P. Palamodov, *The problem of data completeness and the inversion of the spatial ray transform*, Fourth All-Union Sympos. Computerized Tomography, Abstracts of Papers, Part 1, Novosibirsk, 1989, pp. 30–31. (Russian)
10. ———, *Some singular problems in tomography*, Mathematical Problems in Tomography (I. M. Gel′fand and S. G. Ginkikin, eds.), Transl. Math. Monographs, vol. 81, Amer. Math. Soc., Providence, RI, 1990, pp. 123–140.
11. S. Helgason, *The Radon transform*, Birkhäuser, Basel, 1980.
12. L. Hörmander, *The analysis of linear differential operators. Vols.* I, III, Springer-Verlag, Berlin, 1983, 1985.
13. Gr. Beylkin, *The inversion problem and applications of the generalized Radon transform*, Comm. Pure Appl. Math. **37** (1984), 579–599.
14. D. V. Finch, *Cone-beam reconstruction with sources on a curve*, SIAM J. Appl. Math. **45** (1985), no. 4, 665-673.
15. P. Grangeat, *Analyse d'une système d'imagerie* 3D *par reconstruction à partir de radiographie X en géométrie conique*, Thèse de doctorat, Grenoble, 1987.
16. A. Greenleaf and G. Uhlmann, *Nonlocal inversion formulas for the X-ray transform*, Duke Math. J. **58** (1989), no. 1, 205–240.
17. V. Guillemin, *On some results of Gelfand in integral geometry*, Pseudodifferential Operators and Applications (F. Trèves, ed.), Proc. Sympos. Pure Math., vol. 43, Amer. Math. Soc., Providence, RI, 1985, pp. 149–155.
18. V. P. Palamodov and A. S. Denisjuk [Denisyuk], *Inversion de la transformation de Radon d'après des données incomplètes*, C. R. Acad. Sci. Paris Sér. I Math. 1 **307** (1988), 181–183.
19. V. P. Palamodov, *Inversion formulas for the three-dimensional ray transform*, Mathematical Methods in Tomography (Oberwolfach, 1990), Lecture Notes in Math., vol. 1497, Springer-Verlag, Berlin, 1991, pp. 53–62.
20. J. Radon, *Über die Bestimmung von Funktionen durch ihre Integralwerte längs gewisser Mannigfaltigkeiten*, Ber. Verh. Sächs. Ges. Wiss. Leipzig, Math.-Phys. Kl. **69** (1917), 262–277.
21. H. K. Tuy, *An inversion formula for cone-beam reconstruction*, SIAM J. Appl. Math. **43** (1983), 546–552.

Amer. Math. Soc. Transl.
(2) Vol. **162**, 1994

Generalized Projection and Section Theorems in Diffraction Tomography

A. N. Panchenko

ABSTRACT. Generalizations of projection and section theorems in diffraction tomography are considered. Using asymptotic expansion with respect to the distance, two version of generalized projection and section theorems (PST) are proved. A method of proving existence and uniqueness theorems is suggested, based on PST's. Existence and uniqueness of solutions of the inverse radiation problem is proved in the case when the dependence of the source on the frequency is described by a known function, whereas the dependence of the wave field on the frequency is known in a bounded interval.

§1. Introduction

In this paper, generalizations of projection and section theorems are considered. As is known [**1, 2**], theorems of this type establish relations between the restriction of a solution of the stationary wave equation

$$P(x, \mathscr{D})u = \left[\Delta + k^2(1 + \varepsilon(x))\right] u(x) = f(x), \qquad x \in \mathbb{R}^n, \quad k > 0, \tag{1}$$

to a submanifold M of dimension $n - 1$ and the restrictions of the Fourier transform of the function f or ε to a submanifold Ξ of dimension $n - 1$. The importance of this approach to inverse problems is sustained by the existence of extensive literature. We refer the reader to the papers [**3, 4**] and to the review of Devaney [**5**], which contains numerous references. Various examples of application of projection theorems have been presented by Buchstaber and Maslov [**6–8**]. Furthermore, projection theorems provide us with effective applications of the methods of multidimensional complex analysis both for proving existence and uniqueness of solutions and for obtaining explicit formulas.

One should note that, in contrast to ray tomography [**9**], projection methods in diffraction tomography are only approximate. This is related to the use of the linearized inverse problem for equation (1) (see [**6**]). Moreover, it is usually assumed that the measurements are performed far from the object.

This last assumption is the starting point of the approach developed in this paper. The main thesis is that projection and section theorems are of "asymptotic origin". This means that for compactly supported distributions f and ε the solution of (1) for large $\gamma = k|x|$ is related to the localization of $\widehat{f}$ and $\widehat{\varepsilon}$. We consider a special case when these functions allow us to write a global solution of (1) as a series of scattering theory. However, this restriction can apparently be lifted, since for large $|x|$ the symbol of the operator $P(x, \mathscr{D})$ equals $P(\xi) = -|\xi|^2 + k^2$ for any compactly supported function ε. Therefore, the asymptotic approach allows us to reveal the universal character of the projection theorems and to obtain generalizations of known theorems.

§2. Statement of the problem and main results

Let us consider equation (1) under the following assumptions:

1) f and ε are piecewise smooth functions with compact supports $\overline{\Omega}_1$ and $\overline{\Omega}_2$, respectively.

2) The solution of (1) can be expressed in the form of a convergent series

$$u(x) = G_u * \sum_{j=0}^{\infty} A^j f, \tag{2}$$

where

$$Af(x) = -k^2 \varepsilon(x) G_n * f(x)$$

and G_n is the fundamental solution of the operator $P(\mathscr{D})$.

Section 3 contains proofs of two generalized projection and section theorems.

THEOREM 1. *Let the conditions* 1) *and* 2) *be satisfied. Then the solution of the equation* (1) *admits the following asymptotic expansion as* $\gamma = k|z| \to \infty$:

$$\begin{aligned} u(x) =& (2\pi)^{-n} (4\pi/\gamma)^{(n-1)/2} e^{i\pi(n-1)/4} e^{ik|x|} \\ &\times \sum_{j=0}^{\infty} \frac{1}{j!} \left(\frac{2}{\gamma}\right)^j \left(\sum_{m=1}^{n-1} \frac{\partial^2}{\partial y_m^2}\right)^j \widehat{g}(k\theta(y'), x)\big|_{y'=0} + O(\gamma^{-\infty}), \end{aligned} \tag{3}$$

where

$$\widehat{g}(\xi, x) = \widehat{f}(\xi) a(x, \xi)$$

and $a(x, \xi)$ *is a symbol that depends on* ε *but not on* f. *Here the* y_l *are local Cartesian coordinates with origin at the point* $k\theta$, $\theta \in S^{n-1}$, S^{n-1} *being the unit sphere in* $\mathbb{R}^n$ *such that* y_n *is the normal vector to* S^{n-1} *at the point* θ.

Theorem 1 gives a local expression for the solution of the equation (1) at the point $x|\theta|$ in terms of the spectrum of the function f at the point $k\theta$ for any θ. If the solution of (1) is measured on a sphere of a sufficiently large radius d, then Theorem 1 implies the following formula:

$$\begin{aligned} u(d\theta) =& (2\pi)^{-n} (4\pi/kd)^{(n-1)/2} e^{i\pi(n-1)/4} e^{ikd} P_N(\xi, \mathscr{D}) \widehat{f}(\xi) a(d\theta, \xi)\Big|_{\xi = k\theta} \\ &+ O((kd)^{-N}) \end{aligned}$$

for any natural N, where P_N is a differential operator of order $2N$. Example 1 considered in §4 shows that for $\varepsilon \equiv 0$, $N = 1$ relation (3) yields a known **[2]** relation between the directional pattern and the section of the spectrum of f.

In analyzing inverse problems, it is often assumed that the solution of (1) is known on the tangent bundle to a sphere of a sufficiently large radius d; that is, the receiving aperture is a family of hyperplanes $M = \bigcup M_n = \{x \in \mathbb{R}^n : (x, \overline{n}) = d\}$, $\overline{n} \in S^{n-1}$. The relation between the Fourier transform of the restriction of $u(x)$ to

M_n with respect to the "internal variables" and the spectrum of f is given by the following theorem.

THEOREM 2. *Assume that conditions* 1) *and* 2) *are satisfied and the solution of* (1) *is known on the hyperplane* $M_n = \{x \in \mathbb{R}^n : (x, \overline{n}) = d\}$, $M_n \cap \overline{\Omega}_1 = \varnothing$, $M_n \cap \overline{\Omega}_2 = \varnothing$. *Then*

$$\widehat{\Gamma}(\lambda_n) = \frac{1}{2i}(\xi, \overline{n})^{-1} e^{i(\xi,\overline{n})} C\widehat{f}(\xi)\Big|_{|\xi|=k,(\xi,\overline{n})>0} + O(d^{-\infty}), \tag{4}$$

where

$$\Gamma(p) = u\left(\sum_{j=1}^{n-1} p_j \overline{n}_j + d\overline{u}\right),$$

$\overline{n}_j \in S^{n-1}$, $(\overline{n}_j, \overline{n}) = 0$ *for all* j, $(\overline{n}_j, \overline{n}_l) = 0$ *for all* j, l. *Here* C *is a linear integral operator with kernel depending on* $\widehat{\varepsilon}$:

$$C\widehat{f} = \sum_{j=0}^{\infty} \widehat{A}^j \widehat{f}, \tag{5}$$

$\widehat{\Gamma}$ *is the Fourier transform with respect to* $p = (p_1, \ldots, p_{n-1})$, *and* λ *is the corresponding spectral variable.*

If the inverse problem for ε is considered in the linear approximation, i.e., the Born approximation is used for the solution of (1), then Theorem 2 implies, in particular, projection and section theorems obtained by Buchshtaber and Maslov in **[6]** by a somewhat different method (see Example 2 in §4). Let us note that the large distance asymptotics was used in **[6]** for the derivation of the integral representation of the fundamental solution of $P(\mathscr{D})$. Theorem 2 can also be proved by using the approach suggested by Buchshtaber and Maslov.

In this paper Theorems 1 and 2 are proved using the stationary phase method. This method is applied to the integrals in the expression for the inverse operator (2).

Since the Fourier transform of a distribution with compact support is an entire function of exponential type, generalized projection theorems can be used in proving existence and uniqueness of solution of inverse problems. Using projection theorems, the proof of uniqueness can be reduced to detecting of a uniqueness set of an entire function in $\mathbb{C}^n$. This problem can be solved by methods developed in multidimensional complex analysis. To illustrate this approach we give in §5 a proof of the uniqueness and existence problem for a special case of the inverse problem for f.

Assume that we know the restriction of the solution of the stationary wave equation

$$\left[\Delta + k^2(1 + \varepsilon(k, x))\right] u(k, x) = h(k) f(x) \tag{1'}$$

to the set $M = U_x \times U_k$, where U_x is a neighborhood of the point x on a sphere of sufficiently large radius d, $U_k \subset \mathbb{R}_+$ is a neighborhood of the point k. The inverse problem we consider is formulated as follows:

Let it be known that

1) $\Gamma(d\theta, k) = u(x, k)\,|_{(x,k)\in M}$;
2) $\varepsilon(x, k)$ is a known function satisfying the conditions 1) and 2) at the beginning of this section for any k and is smooth in k;
3) $h(k)$ is a known C^∞ function with $h(k) \neq 0$ for all $k \in U_k$;

4) f satisfies the condition 1) at the beginning of this section.
We must find f.

THEOREM 3. *The solution of the above problem exists and is unique.*

§3. Proof of generalized projection and section theorems

PROOF OF THEOREM 1. By the assumptions, the solution of equation (1) can be written as

$$u(x) = (2\pi)^{-n} \int e^{ix\cdot\xi} E(\xi) \sum_{j=0}^{\infty} \widehat{A}^j \widehat{f}(\xi)\, d\xi, \tag{6}$$

where $E(\xi)$ is the distribution corresponding to the Fourier transform of the fundamental solution of the operator $P(\mathscr{D}) = \Delta + k^2$:

$$E(\xi) = \text{p.v. } (-|\xi|^2 + k^2)^{-1} + \pi i \delta(-|\xi| + k)$$

and the operator $\widehat{A}$ is defined by

$$\widehat{A}\widehat{f}(\xi) = -k^2 \int \widehat{\varepsilon}(\xi_1 - \xi) E(\xi_1) \widehat{f}(\xi_1)\, d\xi_1.$$

Using a partition of unity, one can show that the main contribution to the asymptotics of $u(x)$ as $k|x| \to +\infty$ is from a neighborhood of the set of zeros of the symbol $P(\xi)$, i.e.,

$$u(x) = I(x) + O(\gamma^{-\infty}),$$

where

$$I(x) = (2\pi)^{-n} \int e^{ix\cdot\xi} h(\xi) E(\xi) \sum_{j=0}^{\infty} \widehat{A}^j \widehat{f}(\xi)\, d\xi,$$

and the function $h(\xi) \in C_0^\infty(\mathbb{R}^n)$ equals 1 at $|\xi| = k$ and is supported in the annulus $k - c \le |\xi| \le k + c$.

Denote the jth term of the series (6) by I_j and transform it by changing the order of integration. We obtain

$$\begin{aligned} I_j(x) = &\int d\xi e^{ix\cdot\xi} \widehat{f}(\xi) E(\xi) \int d\lambda_j e^{ix\cdot\lambda_j} \widehat{\varepsilon}(\lambda_j) E(\xi + \lambda_j) \\ &\times \int d\lambda_{j-1} e^{ix\cdot\lambda_{j-1}} \widehat{\varepsilon}(\lambda_{j-1}) E(\xi + \lambda_j + \lambda_{j-1}) \\ &\times \cdots \times \int d\lambda_1 e^{ix\cdot\lambda_1} \widehat{\varepsilon}(\lambda_1) E\left(\xi + \sum_{m=1}^{j} \lambda_m\right), \end{aligned}$$

where $\lambda_m = \xi_m - \xi_{m-1}$.

Since this relation is a family of similar "imbedded" integrals, to analyze the asymptotic behavior of $I_j(x)$ it suffices to consider a "typical" integral

$$\begin{aligned} F(x) &= \int d\xi e^{ix\cdot\xi} g(\xi) h(\xi) E(\xi) \\ &= \text{p.v.} \int d\xi e^{ix\cdot\xi} \frac{gh}{-|\xi|^2 + k^2} + \pi i \int_{|\xi|=k} e^{ix\cdot\xi} gh\, dS. \end{aligned}$$

The first integral can be represented in the form

$$\text{p.v.} \int d\xi e^{ikx\cdot\xi} \frac{gh(k\xi)}{-|\xi|^2 + 1} = \text{p.v.} \int dc \frac{M_x(c,k)}{c}, \tag{7}$$

where

$$M_x(c,k) = \int_{|\xi|=\sqrt{1+c}} e^{ikx\cdot\xi} g(k\xi) h(k\xi)\, d\xi.$$

On the manifold $V_c(\xi) = \{\xi : |\xi| = \sqrt{1+c}\}$ the phase function $\varphi(x/|x|, \xi)$ has two stationary points $\xi^{\pm} = \pm(x/|x|)\sqrt{1+c}$. Using a partition of unity, one can easily show that

$$M_x(c,k) = e^{ik|x|\sqrt{1+c}} M_+(c,k) + e^{-ik|x|\sqrt{1+c}} M_-(c,k) + O(\gamma^{-\infty}), \tag{8}$$

Substituting (8) in (7) and using Lemma 2 (which will be formulated in the proof of Theorem 2, below), we obtain

$$\begin{aligned} &\text{p.v.} \int e^{ikx\cdot\xi} g(k\xi) h(k\xi) \frac{1}{-|\xi|^2 + 1}\, d\xi \\ &= \pi i \left[M_+(0,k) e^{ik|x|} - M_-(0,k) e^{-ik|x|} \right] + O(\gamma^{-\infty}). \end{aligned} \tag{9}$$

Similarly, the integral

$$\int e^{ikx\cdot\xi} \delta(-|\xi| + 1) g(\xi)\, d\xi$$

has the asymptotic expansion

$$\int_{|\xi|=1} e^{ikx\cdot\xi} g(k\xi)\, dS = \pi i \left[M_+(0,k) e^{ik|x|} - M_-(0,k) e^{-ik|x|} \right] + O(\gamma^{-\infty}). \tag{10}$$

Therefore, to find the asymptotic behavior of $F(x)$ it suffices to compute $M_+(0,k)$.

Without loss of generality we can assume that $x = (0, \dots, 0, x_n)$. Introduce local coordinates y_l near the stationary point $\xi^+ = (0, \dots, 0, 1)$ as follows:

$$y_m = \xi_m, \quad m = 1, 2, \dots n-1, \qquad y_n = \xi_n - 1.$$

In these local coordinates the manifold $|\xi| = 1$ is given by the equation

$$y_n = \frac{1}{2} \sum_{m=1}^{n-1} y_m^2 + O(y_m^3).$$

Passing to local coordinates, from (8) we obtain

$$\begin{aligned} &M_+(0,k)e^{ik|x|} \\ &= \int dy' \left(1 - \sum_{m=1}^{n-1} y_m^2\right)^{-1/2} \exp\left(-ik\left(\frac{1}{2}\sum_{m=1}^{n-1} y_m^2 - 1\right)x_n\right)\widehat{g}(k\xi(y'),x) \\ &\quad + O(\gamma^{-\infty}), \end{aligned}$$

where $y' = (y_1, \dots, y_{n-1})$.

The general theorem on the multidimensional stationary phase method **[10]** implies the following lemma.

LEMMA 1. *Let μ_j be nonzero real numbers, and let $f(x) \in C_0^\infty(\mathbb{R}^n)$. As $\gamma \to +\infty$, the following asymptotic expansion holds:*

$$\begin{aligned} &\int f(x) \exp\left(\frac{i\gamma}{2}\sum_{j=1}^n \mu_j x_j^2\right) dx \\ &= \left(\frac{2\pi}{\gamma}\right)^{n/2} \exp\left(\frac{i\pi}{4}\sum_{j=1}^n \operatorname{sgn}\mu_j\right) \sum_{l=0}^\infty \frac{\gamma^{-l}}{l!}\left(\sum_{j=1}^n \mu_j^{-1}\frac{\partial^2}{\partial x_j^2}\right)^l f(x)\Big|_{x=0} + O(\gamma^{-\infty}). \end{aligned}$$

Applying Lemma 1, we obtain that, as $\gamma \to \infty$, $M_+(0,k)$ has the following asymptotic expansion:

(11)

$$\begin{aligned} M_+(0,k)e^{ik|x|} &= \left(\frac{4\pi}{\gamma}\right)^{(n-1)/2} e^{i\pi(n-1)/4} e^{ik|x|} \sum_{j=0}^\infty \frac{1}{j!} B^j \widehat{g}(k\xi(y'),x)\,|_{y'=0} + O(\gamma^{-\infty}) \\ &= \left(\frac{4\pi}{\gamma}\right)^{(n-1)/2} e^{i\pi(n-1)/4} e^{ik|x|} e^B \widehat{g}(k\xi(y'),x)\,|_{y'=0} + O(\gamma^{-\infty}), \end{aligned}$$

where B is the following differential operator:

$$B = \frac{2}{k|x|}\sum_{m=1}^{n-1}\frac{\partial^2}{\partial y_m^2}.$$

To complete the proof of the theorem it remains to apply the relation (11) to all integrals in the expression for $u(x)$ and to combine the resulting expressions. Theorem 1 is proved. □

PROOF OF THEOREM 2. For any $x \in M_n$ the solution of (1) has the form

(12)

$$\begin{aligned} \Gamma(p) &= u(x)\,|_{x \in M_n} \\ &= (2\pi)^{-n}\int \exp\left(i\left(d\overline{n} + \sum_{m=1}^{n-1} p_m \overline{n}_m\right)\cdot\xi\right) E(\xi) C\widehat{f}(\xi)\,d\xi, \end{aligned}$$

where $\overline{n}_j \in S^{n-1}$, $(\overline{n}_j, \overline{n}) = 0$ for all j, $(\overline{n}_j, \overline{n}_l) = 0$ for all j, l, and the operator C is defined by

$$C\widehat{f} = \sum_{j=0}^\infty \widehat{A}^j \widehat{f}.$$

After we rotate the coordinate system, the relation (12) takes the form

$$\Gamma(p) = (2\pi)^{-n} \int \exp\left(i\left(d\sigma + \sum_{m=1}^{n-1} p_m\xi_m\right)\right) \times E(\sigma\overline{n} + \sum_{m=1}^{n-1} \xi_m\overline{n}_m) C\widehat{f}\left(\sigma\overline{n} + \sum_{m=1}^{n-1} \xi_m\overline{n}_m\right) d\sigma\, d\xi', \tag{13}$$

where $d\xi' = d\xi_1 \cdots d\xi_{n-1}$. Applying to both sides of (13) the Fourier transform with respect to p, we obtain

$$\widehat{\Gamma}(\lambda) = (2\pi)^{-1} \int d\sigma e^{id\sigma} E\left(\sigma\overline{n} + \sum_{m=1}^{n-1} \lambda_m\overline{n}_m\right) C\widehat{f}(\cdots). \tag{14}$$

Let us consider the integral

$$I(\lambda) = \text{p.v.} \int d\sigma e^{id\sigma} \left(k^2 - \sum_{m=1}^{n-1} \lambda_m^2 - \sigma^2\right)^{-1} g\left(\sigma\overline{n} + \sum_{m=1}^{n-1} \lambda_m\overline{n}_m\right)$$

corresponding to the first summand in the expression for E, and compute its asymptotics as $d \to +\infty$. The main contribution to this asymptotics is given by zeros of the polynomial $k^2 - \sum_{m=1}^{n-1} \lambda_m^2 - \sigma^2$, i.e., by the points $\sigma^\pm = \pm(k^2 - \sum \lambda_m^2)^{1/2}$. In the arguments based on the choice of the expression for E the contribution of the point $\sigma^- = -(k^2 - \sum \lambda_m^2)^{1/2}$ cancels in exactly the same way as in Theorem 1. Therefore, the asymptotics of the integral in (13) equals twice the contribution of the point σ^+ to the asymptotics of $I(\lambda)$. This last asymptotics is determined using the following lemma.

LEMMA 2. *Let $f(x) \in C_0^\infty(\mathbb{R}^n)$. Then, as $d \to +\infty$,*

$$\text{p.v.} \int e^{\pm idx} f(x) \frac{dx}{x} = \pm\pi i f(0) + O(d^{-\infty}).$$

The proof of this lemma can be found, for example, in the book **[11]** (Lemma 1.5 in §1 of Chapter III).

Applying Lemma 2 to $I(\lambda)$ and substituting in (14), we obtain

$$\widehat{\Gamma}(\lambda) = \frac{1}{2i\,(k^2 - \sum \lambda_m^2)^{1/2}} e^{id\sqrt{k^2 - \sum \lambda_m^2}} C\widehat{f}\left(\sigma^+\overline{n} + \sum_{m+1}^{n-1} \lambda_m\overline{n}_m\right) + O(d^{-\infty}).$$

Since $(k^2 - \sum_{m=1}^{n-1} \lambda_m^2)^{1/2} = (\xi, \overline{n})$ for $|\xi| = k$, we get the desired result. Theorem 2 is proved. □

§4. Some examples and corollaries

The theorems just proved are, in essence, versions of projection and section theorems known before. To illustrate this we consider the following example.

EXAMPLE 1. Let $k = 3$, $N = 1$. Assume that the function $\varepsilon(x)$ in the equation (1) is known, whereas the function $f(s)$ must be determined from the measurement of the field $u(x)$ on a sphere of radius R that contains the supports of ε and of f.

Applying (3) and restricting consideration to the principal term of the asymptotic expansion (this corresponds to the case $N = 1$), we obtain

$$u(\theta R) = 4\pi i \frac{e^{ikR}}{kR} \widehat{f}(k\theta) a(R\theta, k\theta) + O(1/kR), \tag{15}$$

where $a(x, \xi)$ is a function of the form

$$a(x, \xi) = 1 + \sum_{m=1}^{\infty} C_m \widehat{\varepsilon}(x, \xi)$$

and the operators C_m are defined by

$$C_m \widehat{\varepsilon} = \int d\lambda_m \widehat{\varepsilon}(\lambda_m) e^{ix\cdot\lambda_m} E(\xi + \lambda_m) \int d\lambda_{m-1} \cdots \int d\lambda_1 \widehat{\varepsilon}(\lambda_1) e^{ix\cdot\lambda_1} E\left(\xi + \sum_{l=1}^{m} \lambda_l\right).$$

For $\varepsilon \equiv 0$ we have $a(x, \xi) = 1$, and (15) gives the known relation between the directional pattern and the section of the source spectrum **[2, 8]**.

REMARK. Whenever necessary, the expression for $C_m \widehat{\varepsilon}$ can be simplified further using the approach developed in the proof of Theorem 1. The function $a(x, \xi)$ has the asymptotic expansion

$$a(R\theta, k\theta) = L_N \widehat{\varepsilon}(\theta, k) + O(\gamma^{-N}),$$

where L_N is the restriction of a nonlinear differential operator applied to $\widehat{\varepsilon}$ to the set of points $M = \{\xi = tk\theta,\ t = 0, 1, 2, \dots, N\}$.

EXAMPLE 2. Let $n = 3$. We assume that the function $\varepsilon(x)$ is unknown, and as a probe field we take the plane wave ψ_0 with the wave vector $k\overline{n}$, $\overline{n} \in S^2$. The scattered field is known at the points of the plane M_n with normal vector $\overline{n}$, at a sufficiently large distance d from the probe inhomogeneity. For any $x \in M_n$ the Born approximation for the scattered field is given by the formula

$$\Gamma(p_1, p_2) = -k^2 (2\pi)^{-3} \int d\sigma\, d\xi_1\, d\xi_2 e^{i(d\sigma + p_1\xi_1 + p_2\xi_2)} \times E(d\overline{n} + p_1\overline{n}_1 + p_2\overline{n}_2) \widehat{\varepsilon}(d\overline{n} + p_1\overline{n}_1 + p_2\overline{n}_2 - k\overline{n}).$$

Applying the Fourier transform and using Theorem 2, we obtain

$$\widehat{\Gamma}(\xi_1, \xi_2) = -k^2 \frac{e^{id(\xi, \overline{n})}}{2i(\xi, \overline{n})} \widehat{\varepsilon}(\xi - k\overline{n}) \Big|_{|\xi| = k,\ (\xi, \overline{n}) > 0} + O(d^{-\infty}). \tag{16}$$

The expression (16) coincides with the version of the projection and section theorem from **[8]**.

§5. Proof of the existence and uniqueness of the solution of the inverse radiation problem

The proof consists of two steps. First we prove that the differential equation

$$u(|x|\theta) = \sum_{j=0}^{N} \frac{1}{j} \left(\frac{1}{k|x|} B'\right)^j q(\theta), \qquad \theta \in S^{n-1}, \tag{17}$$

on the unit sphere S^{n-1} has a unique solution for each N. Here B' is the elliptic second order operator corresponding to the operator B introduced in the proof of Theorem 1. In local coordinates the equation (17) takes the form

$$\widetilde{u}(|x|,x') = \sum_{j=0}^{N} \frac{1}{j}\left(\frac{1}{k|x|}\widetilde{B}\right)^{j} \widetilde{q}(x'), \qquad x' \in \mathbb{R}^{n-1}, \tag{18}$$

where $\widetilde{B}$ is a certain elliptic operator of the second order. Therefore the equation (18) is elliptic. Using the construction of a pseudodifferential parametrix **[12]**, one can show that the equation (18) has a unique local solution for any N. Now we let N tend to ∞. It is clear that $\widetilde{u}$ becomes a solution of the Cauchy problem

$$\frac{\partial}{\partial t}\widetilde{u}(t,x') = \widetilde{B}(x',\mathscr{D})\widetilde{u}, \qquad \widetilde{u}(0,x') = \widetilde{q}(x'), \tag{19}$$

where the role of t is played by $|x|^{-1}$. Therefore, the solution of (18) is equivalent to the solution of the inverse reconstruction problem for initial data of the Cauchy problem. Let us prove that this problem has a unique solution. We use the fact that $\widetilde{B}(x',\mathscr{D})|_{x'=0} = \Delta_{x'} = \widetilde{B}_0$. Since $e^{t\widetilde{B}_0}$ is a convolution operator with a smooth kernel, the inverse Cauchy problem for $\widetilde{B}_0$ can be solved analytically. Denote by $\widetilde{L}$ the inverse operator for $e^{t\widetilde{B}_0}$. Then

$$\widetilde{L}\widetilde{u} = \widetilde{q} + R\widetilde{q}, \tag{20}$$

where R is an integral operator with a smooth kernel. Using standard ideas of the theory of elliptic operators **[13]**, we can assert that there exists a neighborhood where the norm of $R\widetilde{q}$ is less the $1/2$ and the equation (20) has a unique solution. This means that the local inverse operator L_N exists for each N.

At the second step we must prove that the spectrum of f can be determined from the inverse problem data in some neighborhood $U_\xi \subset \mathbb{R}^n$. After that it remains to use the lemma about the uniqueness of continuation in $\mathbb{C}^n$.

Applying the operator L_N to both sides of (3), we obtain that for each k

$$c_n h^{-1}(k)(kd)^{(n-1)/2} e^{-ikd} L_N u(d\theta) = \widehat{f}(k\theta), \qquad \theta \in U_\theta \subset S^{n-1},$$

where U_θ is a neighborhood on the unit sphere corresponding to the neighborhood U_x on the sphere of radius d.

If k runs over a neighborhood $U_k \subset \mathbb{R}_+$, then $\widehat{f}(k\theta)$ runs over a neighborhood $U_0 \subset U_k \times U_\theta \subset \mathbb{R}^n$. The following lemma completes the proof.

LEMMA 3. *If a holomorphic function f on $\mathbb{C}^n$ vanishes in a real neighborhood of a point $a = x^0 + iy^0 \in \mathbb{C}^n$, i.e., on a set $\{z = x + iy \in \mathbb{C}^n : |x - x^0| < r,\ y = y^0\}$, then $f = 0$ in $\mathbb{C}^n$.*

The proof can be found, for example, in **[14]**.

The conditions of Lemma 3 are satisfied, since the Fourier transform of a compactly supported distribution is an entire function of exponential type.

REMARKS. 1. An absolutely similar theorem holds for the linearized form of the inverse scattering problem under the condition that the probing is performed by a plane wave with the wave vector $k\overline{n}$, where the direction $\overline{n}$ is fixed and k runs over a neighborhood $U_k \subset \mathbb{R}^n$. In addition, we must assume that the function $\widehat{\varepsilon}$ does not depend on k, i.e., that there is no frequency dispersion.

2. The above problem shows a clear analogy with the problem of reconstruction from incomplete data in ray tomography. It was shown in [**15**] that algorithms for reconstruction from incomplete data are exponentially unstable. Presumably, a similar phenomenon should be present in our problem as well. Theorem 3 allows us to design an informative scheme of the experiment for a specific object and a specific measurement system.

We can illustrate this with the following example. It is known [**6**] that there exist two basic well-posed (in terms of the existence and uniqueness theorem) formulations of the inverse scattering problem:

(a) The probing is performed by plane waves $e^{ik\overline{n}}$, where $\overline{n}$ is fixed and k runs over the set $\mathbb{R}_+$. The receiving aperture is a plane with the normal vector $\overline{n}$.

(b) The probing is performed by plane waves with a fixed k for all $\overline{n} \in S^{n-1}$. The receiving aperture is the tangent bundle to the sphere.

Theorem 3 asserts that there exist well-posed "intermediate" formulations of the inverse scattering problem.

Acknowledgements

The author is grateful to Professors D. A. Popov and V. M. Buchstaber for useful discussions and attention to this work.

References

1. A. J. Devaney, *A filtered backprojection algorithm for diffraction tomography*, Ultrasonic Imaging **4** (1982), no. 4, 336–350.
2. ———, *Inverse source and scattering problems in ultrasonics*, IEEE Trans. Sonics and Ultrasonics **SU-30** (1983), no. 6, 355–364.
3. M. Kaveh, M. Soumekh, and J. F. Greenleaf, *Signal processing for diffraction tomography*, IEEE Trans. Sonics and Ultrasonics **SU-31** (1984), no. 4, 230–239.
4. A. J. Devaney, *Inverse scattering as a form of computed tomography*, Application of Mathematics in Modern Optics (San Diego, CA, 1982; W. H. Carter, ed.), Proc. SPIE [Soc. Photo-optical Instrumetation Engineers], vol. 358, SPIE—Internat. Soc. Optical Engrg., Bellingham, WA, 1982, pp. 10–16.
5. ———, *Reconstructive tomography with diffracting wavefields*, Inverse Problems **2** (1986), no. 2, 161–183.
6. V. M. Buchstaber and V. K. Maslov, *Methods of tomographic synthesis of wave fields and nonhomogeneous media*, Tomographic Methods in Physical and Technical Measurements, VNIIFTRI, Moscow, 1985, pp. 7–34. (Russian)
7. ———, *Projection and section theorems in emission and transmission tomography*, Tomographic Methods in Physical and Technical Measurements, VNIIFTRI, Moscow, 1988, pp. 6–22. (Russian)
8. ———, *Mathematical models and algorithms of tomographic synthesis of wave fields and inhomogeneous media*, Mathematical Problems in Tomography, Amer. Math. Soc., Providence, RI, 1990, pp. 225–267.
9. F. Natterer, *The mathematics of computerized tomography*, Wiley, New York, 1986.
10. M. F. Fedoryuk, *Stationary phase methods for multiple integrals*, Zh. Vychisl. Mat. i Mat. Fiz. **2** (1962), no. 1, 145–150; English transl. in U.S.S.R. Comput. Math. and Math. Phys. **2** (1962).
11. ———, *Asymptotics: integrals and series*, "Nauka", Moscow, 1987, (Russian).
12. F. Trèves, *Introduction to pseudodifferential and Fourier integral operators*. Vol. 1, Plenum Press, New York, 1980.
13. L. Hörmander, *The analysis of linear partial differential operators*. Vol. II, Springer-Verlag, Berlin, 1983.
14. B. V. Shabat, *Introduction to complex analysis*. Vol. 2, 3rd ed., "Nauka", Moscow, 1985; English transl., Amer. Math. Soc., Providence, RI, 1992.
15. V. P. Palamodov, *Some singular problems in tomography*, Mathematical Problems in Tomography, Amer. Math. Soc., Providence, RI, 1990, pp. 123–140.

Kharkov Polytechnical Institute, 21, Frunze Street, Kharkov, 310002 Ukraine

Amer. Math. Soc. Transl.
(2) Vol. **162**, 1994

Computation of Singular Convolutions

D. A. Popov and D. V. Sushko

Contents

INTRODUCTION

In the Introduction we present an informal description of the main subject of the paper, and formulate certain results.

§0.1. General formulation of the problem

The simplest way to introduce the notion of the *singular convolution* (SC) is to work in the context of distributions. Let L_t be the shift of a distribution L, and let u be a test function. By the *singular convolution* (SC—we use the same abbreviation for both singular and plural) we mean the function

$$Z(t) = L_t u.$$

0065-9290/94/\$1.00 + \$.25 per page

We shall write it (formally) as the integral

$$Z(t) = \int L(t - t')u(t')\,dt'. \tag{0.1}$$

The *problem of computing* an SC consists in the construction of an estimate $Z^A(t)$ of the function $Z(t)$ from samples $u_n \stackrel{\text{def}}{=} u(t_n)$ $(t_n = n\Delta t)$ of the function $u(t)$. We restrict ourself to the case when the Fourier transform $\widehat{L}(\omega)$ is a usual function. In this case instead of the symbolic formula (0.1) we have

$$Z(t) = \frac{1}{2\pi}\int d\omega e^{-i\omega t}\widehat{L}(\omega)\widehat{u}(\omega). \tag{0.2}$$

This formula defines SC for functions $u(t)$ satisfying certain smoothness conditions. Everywhere below omitted summation (or integration) limits mean that the summation (or integration) is from $-\infty$ to $+\infty$. We define the *Fourier transform* of the function $f(t)$ by the formula

$$\widehat{f}(\omega) = \int f(t)e^{i\omega t}\,dt.$$

In the Introduction we assume for simplicity that $u(t) \in C_0^\infty$. In this case all summation and integration limits are essentially finite, and the convergence problem does not come up.

In its original formulation, the problem of computing SC occurs in tomography (where $L(t) = t^{-2}$) and in certain problems of continuum mechanics and of electrodynamics (where $L(t) = t^{-1}$). A number of problems in numerical analysis also can be formulated as the computation of SC. For example, in interpolation theory we have $L(t) = \delta(t)$, and in numerical differentiation we have $L(t) = \delta^{(n)}(t)$. The *deconvolution problem*, i.e. the numerical solution of the convolution equation

$$\int K(t - t')Z(t')\,dt' = u(t) \tag{0.3}$$

also can be reduced to the computation of SC. In this case $\widehat{L}(\omega) = \widehat{K}^{-1}(\omega)$ and we assume that $\widehat{K}(\omega) \neq 0$. With this example in mind, the problem of computing SC sometimes will be called the *reconstruction* problem, the function $u(t)$ will be called the right-hand side, and L the kernel.

A method for constructing an estimate $Z^A(t)$ (result of the reconstruction) will be called an *algorithm*. So, an algorithm is a mapping

$$u_n \xrightarrow{A} Z^A(t) \quad (Z^A(t) = A(u_n)).$$

Usually we shall consider a family of algorithms depending on certain parameters that will be denoted by $\overline{\beta}$. One of this parameters is the step Δt, $\overline{\beta} = (\Delta t, \dots)$. The set of admissible values of parameters is denoted by $\mathscr{D}_{\overline{\beta}}$. The set of possible values of the argument of $Z^A(t)$ is denoted by $\mathscr{J}$. Most frequently, we have $\mathscr{J} = \mathbb{R}$ or $\mathscr{J} = \{t_n = n\Delta t,\ t = 0, \pm 1, \dots\}$. If there is no mention of the set $\mathscr{J}$ we assume that $J = \mathbb{R}$. An indication of the second possibility is the notation $Z_n^A \equiv Z^A(t_n)$ for the solution. Any other set $\mathscr{J}$ will be mentioned specifically.

The *convergence problem* for an algorithm $A(\overline{\beta})$ is the question about the behavior of the *reconstruction error*

$$\Delta Z^A(t) \stackrel{\text{def}}{=} Z^A(t) - Z(t), \qquad t \in \mathcal{J}, \tag{0.4}$$

as $\overline{\beta} \to 0$. Let us note here that if the dimension of $\mathcal{D}_{\overline{\beta}}$ is greater than 1, the behavior of the reconstruction error as $\overline{\beta} \to 0$ depends on how (along which path) the limit is taken. We assume, of course, that $\overline{0}$ is a limit point of $\mathcal{D}_{\overline{\beta}}$. Our main technical results consist in obtaining both pointwise and uniform in t estimates for the reconstruction error for various paths along which $\overline{\beta} \to 0$.

All our main results deal with so-called *RT-algorithms*, i.e., algorithms that can be written as a *discrete convolution*

$$Z^A(t) = \sum_n H^A(t - t_n) u_n \Delta t, \tag{0.5}$$

where $H^A(t)$ is a certain regularization of the distribution $L(t)$; we will call this regularization a *regularized kernel.* This means that

$$\widehat{H}^A(\omega) = \widehat{L}(\omega) R(\omega, \overline{\alpha}). \tag{0.6}$$

The family $R(\omega, \overline{\alpha})$ is called a *regularizer* **[2–4]**; $\overline{\alpha}$ is a family of parameters on which it depends. The step Δt can be one of these parameters $\overline{\alpha}$. The parameters $\overline{\alpha}$ are called *parameters of regularization.*

Let us assume that the regularization vanishes as $|\overline{\alpha}| \to 0$,

$$R(\omega, \overline{\alpha}) \to 1, \qquad |\overline{\alpha}| \to 0,$$

and for $|\overline{\alpha}| > 0$ the condition

$$\widehat{H}^A(\omega) \subset L^1 \cap L^2$$

is satisfied. Let us assume also that the regularizer satisfies certain smoothness and boundedness conditions, and $R(0, \overline{\alpha}) = 1 + O(|\overline{\alpha}|^\delta)$. Here and everywhere below δ denotes an arbitrary positive constant (different in different formulas). The RT-algorithm with the regularizer R will be denoted by $A_{RT}(R)$. The approximate solution obtained using such an algorithm will be denoted by

$$Z^{A_{RT}}(t) \stackrel{\text{def}}{=} Z^{R,T}(t),$$

and similarly for the reconstruction error (0.4):

$$\Delta Z^{A_{RT}}(t) \stackrel{\text{def}}{=} \Delta Z^{R,T}(t).$$

Let us note that if Δt is one of the regularization parameters, then the parameters $\overline{\beta}$ of the corresponding algorithm A_{RT} coincide with the regularization parameters $\overline{\alpha}$ ($\overline{\beta} = \overline{\alpha}$); if $\overline{\alpha}$ does not contain Δt, then $\overline{\beta} = (\Delta t, \overline{\alpha})$.

Given an algorithm A, one can ask whether or not it is an RT-algorithm (for an appropriate choice of the regularization). If it is, we say that the algorithm A has an *efficient regularizer*, which is denoted by $R^{\text{ef}}(A)$. For a number of algorithms the construction of efficient regularizers is easy (see below). Let us remark that (0.5) gives the most general linear operator that is invariant under a shift by Δt. Therefore the existence of an efficient regularizer for such an algorithm reduces to the question of whether the regularizer defined formally by (0.6) satisfies the necessary conditions. It seems likely that all convergent (see below) linear algorithms that are invariant under translation by Δt possess efficient regularizers, and if this is the case, such algorithms can be analyzed using the methods of the present paper. Below we give examples of the application of this approach to the analysis of algorithms that are not of the form A_{RT}.

The problem of computing an SC can be reformulated as a deconvolution problem or as a problem of the reconstruction of an unbounded operator (with kernel $\widehat{L}(\omega)$) from a finite family of linear functionals $u_n = u(n\Delta t)$. So reformulated, this problem can be included in the framework of the theory of ill-posed operators. The main technique here is the theory of operators in Banach (Hilbert) spaces, which predetermines the statements of problems and the form of results obtained. However, problems concerning pointwise convergence of even very simple and practical algorithms fit badly into this framework. In this paper we adopt a completely analytic approach, in which we use a simple form of the operator (multiplication by $\widehat{L}(\omega)$) to study the problem of pointwise convergence for a very simple, and, at the same time, sufficiently general class of linear algorithms. We think that this point of view, where the construction of efficient regularizers plays the most important role, allows us to obtain a new look at certain well-known algorithms. We want to emphasize again that it is the form of the efficient regularizer that determines the quality of the reconstruction (approximation rate).

§0.2. Examples of algorithms

We start with the analysis of RT-algorithms. The simplest and the most natural way to construct such an algorithm is to choose a regularizer $R(\omega)$ ($R(\omega, \overline{\alpha})$ satisfies the necessary conditions) and to define $H^A(t) \equiv H^R(t)$ by the formula

$$H^R(t) = \frac{1}{2\pi}\int d\omega e^{-i\omega t}\widehat{H}^R(\omega), \qquad \widehat{H}^R(\omega) = \widehat{L}(\omega)R(\omega).$$

Then we can define

$$Z^R(t) = \frac{1}{2\pi}\int d\omega e^{-i\omega t}\widehat{H}^R(\omega)\widehat{u}(\omega). \tag{0.7}$$

Since, by the convolution theorem,

$$Z^R(t) = \int H^R(t-t')u(t')\,dt', \tag{0.8}$$

to construct $Z^{R,T}(t)$ we can apply the simplest quadrature formula to the integral (0.8):

$$Z^{R,T}(t) = \sum_n H^R(t-t_n)u_n\Delta t. \tag{0.9}$$

The name of the class of algorithms (RT-algorithms) is determined by the method used to obtain them: we take the regularized (R) expression and apply to it the trapezoid (T) formula. One can easily see that

$$Z^{R,T}(t) = \frac{1}{2\pi}\int d\omega e^{-i\omega t}\widehat{H}^R(\omega)\widehat{u}^T(\omega), \tag{0.10}$$

where $\widehat{u}^T(\omega)$ is the *discrete Fourier transform* (DFT) of the function $u(t)$:

$$\widehat{u}^T(\omega) \overset{\text{def}}{=} \sum_n u_n e^{i\omega n\Delta t}\Delta t. \tag{0.11}$$

As a regularizer one usually takes an one-dimensional family $R(\omega) \equiv R(\omega, \alpha) = R_\alpha(\omega)$, $\overline{\alpha} = \alpha$. Most often used are *homogeneous regularizers*, i.e., regularizers of the form

$$R_\alpha(\omega) = S(\alpha\omega).$$

For example,

$$R_\alpha(\omega) = \frac{1}{1 + |\alpha\omega|^q}, \qquad R_\alpha(\omega) = e^{-(\alpha\omega)^2}. \tag{0.12}$$

An example of a nonhomogeneous regularizer is the so-called Wiener regularizer (in the simplest form)

$$R_\alpha(\omega) = [1 + \alpha(\omega/\omega_R)^h \exp(\omega/\omega_R)]^{-1}. \tag{0.13}$$

Since $H^R(t) \to L(t)$ as $\alpha \to 0$ and $L(t)$ is a distribution, the above algorithm clearly diverges as $\alpha \to 0$, $\Delta t = \text{const}$. This might be a reason why it was not studied in the framework of the theory of ill-posed problems [**3, 5**]. On the other hand, this algorithm is widely used in practice [**6, 7**]. The formulation of the convergence problem corresponding to the situation that occurs in practice will be considered below. Here we only remark that for homogeneous regularizers it corresponds to the choice $\alpha = \Delta t$. With this choice, the algorithm $A_{RT}(R)$ diverges for regularizers (0.12), but there are other regularizers for which the corresponding algorithm converges. One of the goals of this paper is to describe these regularizers. Together with one-parameter regularizers, one can consider regularizers depending on several parameters. The simplest way to obtain a two-parameter regularizer is to multiply two one-parameter ones.

Now we consider other algorithms. Let $u^\delta(t)$ (or $\widehat{u}^\delta(\omega)$) be an approximation of $u(t)$ (or of $\widehat{u}(\omega)$) constructed using samples $\{u_n\}$. The algorithm A_δ has the form

$$Z^{A_\delta}(t) \equiv Z^{R,\delta}(t) \stackrel{\text{def}}{=} \int H^R(t - t')u^\delta(t')\,dt', \tag{0.14}$$

or

$$Z^{A_\delta}(t) \equiv Z^{R,\delta}(t) \stackrel{\text{def}}{=} \frac{1}{2\pi} \int d\omega e^{-i\omega t} \widehat{H}^R(\omega)\overline{u}^\delta(\omega). \tag{0.15}$$

Let us note that this scheme yields the algorithm A_{RT} in the case when for $u^\delta(t)$ we take the distribution $u^\delta(t) = \sum_n u_n \delta(t - t_n)\Delta t$. Let us remark also that this algorithm depends on the choice of a regularizer R, $A_\delta \equiv A_\delta(R)$; the regularizer enters the regularized kernel H^R in (0.14) or (0.15).

Let us construct examples of algorithms A_δ. We call $\Omega = \pi/\Delta t$ the *Nyquist frequency* and the interval $[\Omega, -\Omega]$ the *Nyquist interval*. By χ_Ω we denote the characteristic function of the Nyquist interval. Take an approximation to $u(t)$ using the interpolation formula

$$u^\Omega(t) = \sum_n u_n \frac{\sin(t - t_n)\Omega}{(t - t_n)\Omega}; \tag{0.16}$$

this corresponds to an approximation of $u(t)$ by entire functions of exponential growth ($u^\Omega(t) \in W^\Omega$, see [**8**]). Denote the resulting algorithm (0.14) by A_Ω. Since

$$\widehat{u^\Omega}(\omega) = \widehat{u}^T(\omega)\chi_\Omega(\omega),$$

by comparing (0.10) and (0.15) we easily see that an efficient regularizer for the algorithm A_Ω exists and is equal to

$$R^{\text{ef}}(A_\Omega(R))(\omega) = R(\omega)\chi_\Omega(\omega).$$

We say that a regularizer R satisfies the *Nyquist condition* (NC), $R \in \mathcal{N}$, if

$$\operatorname{supp} R(\omega) \subset [-\Omega, \Omega]. \tag{0.17}$$

The efficient regularizer for A_Ω satisfies the Nyquist condition by its very construction.

Using, instead of (0.16), the approximation of $u(t)$ of the form

$$u^V(t) = \sum_n V(t - t_n)u_n\Delta t, \tag{0.18}$$

we obtain the algorithm A^V. We have

$$\widehat{u}^V(\omega) = \widehat{V}(\omega)\widehat{u}^T(\omega),$$

and, similarly to the previous case,

$$R^{\text{ef}}(A_V(R))(\omega) = R(\omega)\widehat{V}(\omega). \tag{0.19}$$

In particular, for the approximation by the B-spline of order $m-1$ we have

$$\widehat{V}_m(\omega) = \left(\frac{\sin(\omega\Delta t/2)}{\omega\Delta t/2}\right)^m, \tag{0.20}$$

obtaining the algorithm A_{V_m} with the efficient regularizer

$$R^{\text{ef}}(A_{V_m}(R))(\omega) = R_\alpha(\omega)S(\omega/\Omega),$$

where $R_\alpha(\omega)$ is the regularizer used in the construction of H^R:

$$S(\xi) = \left(\frac{\sin(\pi\xi/2)}{\pi\xi/2}\right)^m.$$

In this case $\overline{\alpha} = (\Delta t, \alpha)$. Let us remark that for a sufficiently large m in the algorithm A_{V_m} we can take $R(\omega) = 1$ (or $R(\omega) = R_\alpha(\omega)$ with $\alpha = 0$).

Formula (0.18) can be considered as a certain interpolation algorithm A ($\widehat{L}(\omega) = 1$). This formula corresponds to

$$\widehat{H}^A(\omega) = R^{\text{ef}}(A)(\omega) = \widehat{V}(\omega),$$

and in the case of linear interpolation ($m = 2$) we have, for example,

$$H^A(t) = \frac{1}{2\Delta t}\begin{cases} 1 - |t|/\Delta t, & |t| \le \Delta t, \\ 0, & |t| > \Delta t. \end{cases}$$

For this algorithm we have $\overline{\beta} = \overline{\alpha} = \Delta t$.

Let us discuss now the algorithms that are obtained when we compute the integral (0.8) using quadrature formulas other than the trapezoid rule. For example, the formula

$$Z^A(t) = \sum_n u_n \int_{t_n-\Delta t/2}^{t_n+\Delta t/2} H^R(t-t')\,dt'$$

yields an algorithm of discrete convolution type with the efficient regularizer

$$R^{\text{ef}}(\omega) = R(\omega)\frac{\sin(\omega\Delta t/2)}{\omega\Delta t/2}.$$

Now let us apply the Simpson formula. Then instead of (0.9) we have

$$Z^A(t) = \frac{4}{3}\sum_n H^R(t-t_n)u_n\Delta t - \frac{1}{3}\sum_n H^R(t-t_n)u_{2n}(2\Delta t).$$

Therefore, we obtain the superposition of two trapezoid rules with steps Δt and $2\Delta t$. Such an algorithm is not a discrete convolution type algorithm (it is not invariant under the translation by Δt, the invariance starts at the step $2\Delta t$). It can be included in the class of algorithms of the form

$$Z^A(t) = \sum_{p=1}^{P}\sum_n H_p^A(t-pt_n)u_{pn}(p\Delta t). \tag{0.21}$$

Our results about RT-algorithms can be trivially extended to algorithms of the form (0.21), which are just weighted sums of RT-algorithms. Let us remark that the class of algorithms (0.21) includes all algorithms that are obtained by applying to (0.8) a quadrature formula based on a local interpolation of the function under the integral sign by polynomials on a uniform lattice.

If, in all the examples above (except, of course, the last one), an algorithm is not of the form A_{RT}, one can easily transform it to the required form and obtain an expression for the efficient regularizer. The resulting expressions for R^{ef} are sufficiently simple, and one can easily see that R^{ef} satisfies all required conditions.

The algorithms most frequently used in practice are those that allow one to compute the values of an approximate solution at the nodes of the lattice t_n: $Z_n^A \equiv Z^A(n\Delta t)$, i.e., algorithms with $\mathcal{J} = \{t_n\}$. Such algorithms will be called *lattice* algorithms. In constructing a lattice algorithm one usually starts with a discrete analog of the problem and then takes the solution (often after regularization) of this discrete analog as an approximate solution of the initial problem. We denote lattice algorithms by $A^{\Delta t}$:

$$\{u_n\} \xrightarrow{A^{\Delta t}} \{Z_n^{A^{\Delta t}}\}.$$

Starting with a lattice algorithm $A^{\Delta t}$, one can construct a family of continuous algorithms using, for example, the interpolation V:

$$Z^A(t) = \sum_n V(t-t_n)Z_n^{A^{\Delta t}}\Delta t.$$

A regularizer $R(\omega)$ is called efficient for $A^{\Delta t}$ if the corresponding continuous algorithm coincides with the lattice algorithm at the nodes of the lattice, i.e.,

$$Z^{A_{RT}(R^{\text{ef}})}(t_n) = Z_n^{A^{\Delta t}}.$$

Let us remark that we do not claim that an efficient regularizer is unique even for continuous algorithms, let alone discrete ones.

As a rule, a discrete algorithm has the form of the discrete convolution

$$Z_n^{A^{\Delta t}} = \sum_m A_{n-m}^{\Delta t} u_m \Delta t, \tag{0.22}$$

i.e., it is a generic lattice algorithm that is linear and invariant under the translation by the step Δt of the lattice. For such an algorithm one can easily construct a (nonunique) continuous algorithm A such that

$$Z^A(t_n) = Z_n^{A^{\Delta t}}.$$

For example, one can take

$$H^A(t) = \sum_n A_n^{\Delta t} \frac{\sin(t - t_n)\Omega}{(t - t_n)\Omega},$$

and respectively

$$\widehat{H}^A(\omega) = \sum_n A_n^{\Delta t} e^{i\omega n\Delta t} \chi_\Omega(\omega)\Delta t. \tag{0.23}$$

The construction of an efficient regularizer for such an algorithm reduces to the question of whether the function $R(\omega)$ defined by

$$\widehat{H}^A(\omega) = \widehat{L}(\omega)R(\omega)$$

is a regularizer (i.e., whether it satisfies certain conditions). To answer this question is not always an easy task. Let us remark, however, that if $R(\omega)$ is a regularizer, then, by (0.23), it satisfies the Nyquist condition (0.17), i.e., $R(\omega) \in \mathscr{N}$. It is likely that in the analysis of lattice algorithms it is sufficient to consider only efficient regularizers satisfying the Nyquist conditions.

As the simplest example of a lattice algorithm let us consider the following algorithm A of numerical differentiation:

$$z_n^A = \frac{u_{n+1} - u_{n-1}}{2\Delta t}.$$

This algorithm has the form of discrete convolution (0.22) with

$$A_n = \begin{cases} \pm(2\Delta t^2)^{-1}, & n = \pm 1, \\ 0, & n \neq \pm 1. \end{cases}$$

Formula (0.23) gives

$$\widehat{H}^A(\omega) = i\omega \frac{\sin \omega\Delta t}{\omega\Delta t} \chi_\Omega(\omega).$$

Since in this case $\widehat{L}(\omega) = i\omega$, we get

$$R^{\text{ef}}(A)(\omega) = \frac{\sin \omega\Delta t}{\omega\Delta t} \chi_\Omega(\omega).$$

As the last example, we consider the lattice algorithm $A_T \subset \{A^{\Delta t}\}$ that was suggested in **[5]** for solving convolution equations. This algorithm will be considered in §3.3 below, where it is called the Tikhonov algorithm. Let us describe briefly a general approach to the solution of Fredholm equations of the first kind that is used in the theory of ill-posed problems **[2, 3]**. We begin with the continuous case. Let an operator K with the kernel $K(t,t')$ act from a Hilbert space H_1 to a Hilbert space H_2:

$$H_1 \xrightarrow{K} H_2; \qquad (KZ)(t) = \int K(t,t')Z(t')\,dt'.$$

As an approximation to a normal solution $\widetilde{Z}$ (see **[3]**) of the equation $KZ = u$ we choose the function Z_{α_T} that minimizes the Tikhonov functional **[2]**

$$M_{\alpha_T}[Z] = \| KZ - u \|^2_{H_2} + \alpha_T \Omega[Z]. \tag{0.24}$$

The term $\Omega[Z]$ is called the *stabilizing functional*, α_T is the regularization parameter (the index T reminds us of its origin). Most frequently one takes $H_2 = L^2$ and $\Omega[Z] = \| Z \|^2_{H_1}$. For the generic convolution equation a natural choice is

$$\Omega[Z] = \frac{1}{2\pi}\int M(\omega)|\widehat{Z}(\omega)|^2\,d\omega, \tag{0.25}$$

where the *stabilizing factor* $M(\omega)$ is a real even nonnegative function such that $M(\omega) > C$ for sufficiently large ω and $M(\omega) \neq 0$ for $\omega \neq 0$. Here and later C denotes a positive constant, different in different formulas. In particular, for

$$M(\omega) = \sum_{n=0}^{r} q_n\omega^{2n}, \qquad q_n \geq 0, \quad q_r > 0, \tag{0.26}$$

we have

$$\Omega[Z] = \sum_{n=0}^{r} q_n \int |Z^{(n)}(t)|^2\,dt,$$

and if $r \geq 1$, $q_0 > 0$, then the functional $\Omega[Z]$ defines a norm $\|\cdot\|$, which is equivalent to the norm in the Sobolev space W_2^r, which, in turn, majorizes the uniform norm. In this case one can obtain uniform bounds for $|Z_{\alpha_T} - \widehat{Z}|$ in the framework of the theory of ill-posed problems. One can easily see that in the case (0.25) we have

$$Z_{\alpha_T}(t) \equiv Z^R(t), \tag{0.27}$$

where $Z^R(t)$ is defined in (0.7) and

$$R(\omega) = \frac{|\widehat{K}(\omega)|^2}{|\widehat{K}(\omega)|^2 + \alpha_T M(\omega)} = \left[1 + \alpha_T\frac{M(\omega)}{|\widehat{K}(\omega)|^2}\right]^{-1}. \tag{0.28}$$

If $M(\omega)$ is of the form (0.26), the regularizer (0.28) is called a *Tikhonov regularizer.* Let us note that in the analysis of the convergence for small α_T one can replace $\widehat{L}(\omega)$ and $M(\omega)$ by the corresponding leading asymptotic terms as $|\omega| \to \infty$. In particular, if $\widehat{L}(\omega)$ is of polynomial growth, it suffices to consider the cases

$$\widehat{L}(\omega) = C|\omega|^p, \qquad M(\omega) = C\omega^{2r}.$$

Then the regularizer (0.28) becomes homogeneous:

$$R(\omega) = [1 + |\alpha\omega|^{2(r+p)}]^{-1}, \qquad \alpha = \alpha_T^{1/2(r+p)}. \tag{0.29}$$

In the case we are interested in, only samples u_n are given, and a discrete analog of the above approach was considered in **[5]**. Equation (0.5) is replaced by its discrete analog

$$\sum_m K_{n-m} Z_m \Delta t = u_n \qquad (K_n \equiv K(t_n)),$$

and we look for Z_n^A as the minimum of the functional

$$\widetilde{M}_{\alpha_T}[Z] = \sum_n \left| \sum_m K_{n-m} Z_m \Delta t - u_n \right|^2 \Delta t + \alpha_T \widetilde{\Omega}[Z_n],$$

where $\widehat{\Omega}[Z_n]$ is a certain discrete approximation of $\Omega[Z_n]$. This problem can be solved explicitly using the discrete Fourier transform, and the solution is of the form of discrete convolution (0.22). This solution is taken as an approximation in the algorithm that will be denoted below by A_T (the discrete Tikhonov algorithm for the solution of convolution equations). The algorithm contains an additional parameter N^{-1}, where the integer N essentially determines the discretization step in ω according to the formula $\Delta t \Delta \omega = 2\pi/N$. Therefore, the algorithm A_T depends on the parameters $\overline{\beta} = (\Delta t, N^{-1}, \alpha_T)$. Later we will prove the convergence of this algorithm and the existence of an efficient regularizer

$$R^{\text{ef}}(A_T)(\omega) \simeq \frac{\widehat{K}(\omega)}{\widehat{K}^T(\omega)} \frac{1}{1 + \alpha_T M(\omega)/|\widehat{K}^T(\omega)|^2} \chi_\Omega(\omega). \tag{0.30}$$

The comparison of the efficient regularizer (0.30) with the initial continuous regularizer (0.28) reveals that they are of rather different forms. In particular, $R^{\text{ef}}(A_T) \in \mathcal{N}$, and from the point of view adopted in this paper this fact explains the convergence of the suggested algorithm. The efficient regularizer constructed above will allow us not only to prove the convergence of the algorithm A_T, but also to analyze the dependence of the resulting approximation on the parameters Δt and α_T.

§0.3. Convergence problems and the choice of regularization parameters

Let us consider an algorithm A depending on parameters $\overline{\beta} = (\Delta t, \dots)$. As an example, one can always keep in mind the algorithm A_{RT} with a one-parameter regularizer $R_\alpha(\omega)$, $\overline{\beta} = (\Delta t, \alpha)$. Our problem is to analyze the behavior of the reconstruction error $\Delta Z^A(t)$ (denoted $\Delta Z^{R,T}(t)$ for the algorithm A_{RT}) (see (0.4)) as $|\overline{\beta}| \to 0$ in various possible ways (for the algorithm A_{RT}, $\Delta t \to 0$, $\alpha \to 0$, along various paths on the plane $(\Delta t, \alpha)$).

Earlier we have assumed that the samples u_n are known explicitly. This corresponds to the so-called *noiseless problem*. In the *problem with noise* one assumes that only the numbers

$$u_n^\sigma = u_n + v_n \tag{0.31}$$

are known, where v_n is a sequence of independent random variables such that

$$\mathbb{E}[v_n] = 0, \qquad \mathbb{E}[v_n, v_{n'}^*] = \sigma_u^2 \delta_{n,n'}, \tag{0.32}$$

where $\mathbb{E}[x]$ is the expectation of a random variable x, and * here and later denotes complex conjugation. Let us remark that in practice σ_u^2 may depend on Δt. It is assumed that the algorithm

$$A : \{u_n^\sigma\} \xrightarrow{A} Z^{A,\sigma}(t)$$

for the problem with noise has the same form as before. For example, this can be the RT-algorithm

$$Z^{A,\sigma}(t) \equiv Z^{R,T,\sigma}(t) \doteq \sum_n H^R(t - t_n) u_n^\sigma \Delta t.$$

The *complete reconstruction error*

$$\Delta Z^{A,\sigma}(t) \stackrel{\text{def}}{=} Z^{A,\sigma}(t) - Z(t)$$

in a problem with noise is the sum of the *statistical error* associated to noise

$$\Delta Z^\sigma(t) \stackrel{\text{def}}{=} Z^{A,\sigma}(t) - Z^A(t)$$

and the *error of the algorithm* $\Delta Z^A(t)$ (0.4) in the absence of noise. Since we consider linear algorithms,

$$\Delta Z^\sigma(t) = A(\{v_n\}),$$

and, for example, in the case of the RT-algorithm we have

$$\Delta Z^\sigma(t) = \sum_n H^R(t - t_n) v_n \Delta t.$$

Let us note that the error $\Delta Z^{R,T}$ of the RT-algorithm can, in turn, be represented as the sum $\Delta Z^{R,T} = \Delta Z^R + \Delta Z^T$ of the *regularization* error and the *discretization* error:

$$\Delta Z^R(t) \equiv Z^R(t) - Z(t), \tag{0.33}$$

where $Z^R(t)$ is determined by (0.7) or (0.8), and

$$\Delta Z^T(t) \equiv Z^{R,T} - Z^R(t). \tag{0.34}$$

Let us remark that for any algorithm involving the regularization $\widehat{L}(\omega)$ (i.e., the regularized kernel $H^R(t)$) one can define $Z^R(t)$ using one of the formulas (0.7) or (0.8). Such algorithms will be called *R-algorithms*; they have the property that the error can be broken into the regularization error and the discretization error. The error of the algorithm $\Delta Z^A(t)$ (and the corresponding regularization and discretization errors $\Delta Z^R(t)$ and $\Delta Z^T(t)$) admits pointwise and/or uniform estimates. In analyzing these estimates the following notation is used:

$$\Delta Z^A \stackrel{\text{def}}{=} \sup_t |\Delta Z^A(t)|, \quad \Delta Z^R \stackrel{\text{def}}{=} \sup_t |\Delta Z^R(t)|, \quad \Delta Z^T \stackrel{\text{def}}{=} \sup_t |\Delta Z^T(t)|, \qquad t \in \mathscr{J}.$$

For the statistical error we have $\mathbb{E}(\Delta Z^\sigma(t)) = 0$, and as a measure of the statistical error we take either its variance

$$\sigma_Z^2(t) \stackrel{\text{def}}{=} \mathbb{E}[|\Delta Z^\sigma(t)|^2],$$

or the parameter

$$\sigma_Z^2 \stackrel{\text{def}}{=} \sup_t \sigma_Z^2(t), \qquad t \in \mathscr{J}.$$

Since our algorithms are linear, it is clear that

$$\sigma_Z^2 = \sigma_u^2 f(\overline{\beta}) \qquad (= \sigma_u^2 f(\Delta t, \alpha)). \tag{0.35}$$

Let us discuss convergence problems on an informal level, postponing precise definitions until Chapter 1. Let an algorithm A depend on $\overline{\beta} \in \mathbb{R}_m^+$, $\overline{\beta} = (\beta_1 = \Delta t, \beta_2, \ldots, \beta_m \geq 0)$. We say *the algorithm A converges with respect to the set* $\mathscr{D} \equiv \mathscr{D}_{\overline{\beta}} \subset \mathbb{R}_m^+$ (or simply *converges in* $\mathscr{D}$) if

$$\Delta Z^A(t) \to 0 \qquad \text{for } |\overline{\beta}| \to 0, \; \overline{\beta} \in \mathscr{D}.$$

Here we assume that $\overline{0}$ is a limit point of $\mathscr{D}$. It is clear that in this definition one can consider an arbitrary small neighborhood of the point $\overline{\beta} = \overline{0}$. Let us remark that the convergence depends on the class of kernels $\{L\}$, on the class of right-hand sides $\{u\}$, and, for RT-algorithms, on the class of regularizers $\{R\}$. The necessity of such a definition can be seen on the example of the algorithm A_{RT} with $\overline{\beta} = (\Delta t, \alpha)$ and $R_\alpha(\omega)$, $\hat{L}(\omega) = |\omega|^\rho$, $\rho > 0$. Direct verification shows that $\Delta Z^A \equiv \Delta Z^{R,T}$ converges when $|\overline{\beta}| \to 0$ along the axis $\Delta t = 0$ and diverges when $|\overline{\beta}| \to 0$ along the axis $\alpha = 0$.

The general convergence problem consists in determining, for given $\{L\}$ and $\{u\}$ (and $\{R\}$), the convergence region $\mathscr{D}_{\overline{\beta}}$, and in determining, for $\overline{\beta} \in \mathscr{D}_{\overline{\beta}}$, the asymptotic behavior of various errors as $|\overline{\beta}| \to 0$. In another formulation, given $\{L\}$, one looks for conditions (for example, on the class of regularizes $\{R\}$) that guarantee convergence in a given region $\mathscr{D}_{\overline{\beta}} \subset \mathbb{R}_m^+$. Since the notion of convergence involves only the behavior of ΔZ^A as $|\overline{\beta}| \to 0$, one actually classifies (in the case $\overline{\beta} = (\Delta t, \alpha)$) paths $\alpha = \alpha(\Delta t)$, $\Delta t \to 0$, from the point of view of convergence. In the theory of ill-posed problems similar problems occur when one introduces the notion of regularity [3, 4] (see below).

We do not claim that we can solve the convergence problem completely in the most general case, although in certain cases (for some classes of kernels and of right-hand sides) the complete solution will be given. Let us emphasize that our definition of convergence does not involve any conditions on the behavior of the noise $\sigma_Z^2(\overline{\beta})$ of solution as $|\overline{\beta}| \to 0$; in particular, we do not require $f(\overline{\beta})$ to be bounded (see (0.35)). This is an essential difference between our formulation and the one adopted in the theory of ill-posed problems.

Since the Tikhonov regularizers (0.26), (0.28) are somewhat distinguished, and since for these regulaizers the convergence problem for RT-algorithms can be solved completely in the most general setting, we consider convergence results obtained in the main body of the paper on the example of these algorithms. Let us begin with kernels of exponential growth $\hat{L}(\omega) \sim e^{|\omega/\omega_L|^\rho}$, $\rho > 0$. In this case the Tikhonov regularizer belongs to the class of regularizers of Wiener type with $q_0 = 2\rho$ (of type (0.13); see the exact definitions in §1.1). The regularization error ΔZ^R, which depends on one parameter α_T, tends to zero as $\alpha_T \to 0$ (by Proposition 1.4, under rather general assumptions the regularization error tends to zero as regularization disappears). Therefore, the convergence of the algorithm is determined by the discretization error. Using results from §§2.1 and 2.3, and, in particular, Remark 2 to Proposition 2.7, we obtain conditions for convergence of $\mathscr{D}$ inside $\mathbb{R}_2^+ = \{\Delta t, \alpha_T\}$ in the form

$$(\log(1/\alpha_T))^{1/2\rho} < \frac{\Omega}{\omega_L}(1+\delta). \tag{0.36}$$

The same results also imply that the algorithm diverges as $|\overline{\beta}| \to 0$ in such a way that

$$(\log(1/\alpha_T))^{1/2\rho} > \frac{\Omega}{\omega_L}(1+\delta).$$

Now let us consider a polynomial kernel $\widehat{L}(\omega) \sim |\omega|^{\rho}$, $\rho > 0$. In this case the Tikhonov regularizer belongs to the class of *generalized Tikhonov regularizers* with $q_0 = 2(\rho + r)$ (see the definition in §1.1). Again, convergence is determined by the behavior of the discretization error. We will prove (see Proposition 2.14) that the largest convergence region is determined by the condition

$$\alpha_T^{-1}\Omega^{-\rho-2r} \to 0. \tag{0.37}$$

Let us mention also the case of polynomial kernels (of the form $\widehat{L}(\omega) \sim |\omega|^{\rho}$) and smooth homogeneous regularizers. In this case the convergence region of the algorithm is also completely described; see the result at the end of §2.4.

Let us discuss now the place of this problem in the framework of the theory of ill-posed problems, and, in particular, in the framework of various methods for solving Fredholm equations of the first kind. First of all, let us note that the above algorithms fit badly into the theory of projection operators, since they correspond to the decomposition of a solution with respect to translations of the function $H^R(t)$, which has a singularity as $\alpha \to 0$. Using the algorithm A_δ as an example, let us compare out results with those obtained from the theory of ill-posed problems. Assume we know that

$$\| u^\delta - u \|_{H_2} \leq \delta. \tag{0.38}$$

Then the convergence problem for the algorithm A_δ is the regularity (stability) problem of the regularization method, and the regularity condition is **[3, 4]**

$$\| Z^{R,\delta} - Z \|_{H_1} \to 0 \quad \text{for } \alpha = \alpha(\delta),\ \delta \to 0.$$

A sufficient condition for regularity of the Tikhonov regularization (0.24)–(0.28) has the form

$$\limsup_{\delta \to 0} \frac{\delta^2}{\alpha_T(\delta)} = 0. \tag{0.39}$$

If we require regularity in the class of all function u^δ satisfying (0.38), then this condition is also sufficient. If we have the condition (0.38) with the dependence $\delta = \delta(\Delta t)$, then the condition (0.39) singles out the convergence region $\mathscr{D}$ in the class of all Tikhonov regularizers (0.26), (0.28). In particular, for the algorithm A_{V_m} (here $u^\delta = u^V$, where u^V is determined by (0.18) with V from (0.20)), B-spline approximation theory gives $\delta = C(u)\Delta t^m$. The regularity condition takes the form

$$\Delta t^{2m}\alpha_T^{-1} \to 0, \tag{0.40}$$

and determines a divergence region $\mathscr{D}^m$ for the algorithm A_{V_m} ($\overline{\beta} = (\Delta t, \alpha_T)$). It might be interesting to compare this result with a similar result obtained below. According to (0.19) and (0.20), an efficient regularizer for the algorithm A_{V_m} has the form

$$R^{\text{ef}}(\omega) = \left(\frac{\sin(\omega\Delta t/2)}{\omega\Delta t/2}\right)^m \frac{1}{1+\alpha_T M(\omega)/|R(\omega)|^2}, \tag{0.41}$$

and $M(\omega)$ is of the form (0.26).

Let us start with kernels of exponential (fast) growth

$$\widehat{L}(\omega) \sim \exp|\omega/\omega_L|^\rho, \qquad \rho > 0.$$

In this case the regularizer (0.41) is the product of a homogeneous and a Wiener regularizer, $q_0 = 2\rho$. The sufficient convergence condition again takes the form (0.36). Let us rewrite this condition, which is an analog of (0.40), in the form

$$\Delta t(\log(1/\alpha_T))^{1/2\rho} < \frac{\Omega}{\omega_L}(1+\delta). \tag{0.42}$$

The convergence region $\widetilde{\mathcal{D}}$ described by (0.42) is considerably larger than the region $\mathcal{D}^m$ described by (0.40). Actually, $\widetilde{\mathcal{D}}$ is very close to the maximal possible region.

Let us consider now the kernel of polynomial growth $\widehat{L}(\omega) \sim |\omega|^\rho$, $\rho > 0$. In this case the regularizer (0.41) is the product of a homogeneous regularizer and a generalized Tikhonov regularizer with $q_0 = 2(\rho + r)$. We will show in Chapter 2 (Propositions 2.15, 2.16) that for $m \geq [\rho] + 1$ ($[\cdot]$ is the integral part) the algorithm converges in $\mathbb{R}_2^+$ (no conditions), and for $m \geq [\rho]$ the algorithm converges in the region $\widetilde{\mathcal{D}}^m$ defined by

$$\Delta t^{\rho+m+2r}\alpha_T^{-1} \to 0. \tag{0.43}$$

For each m the region $\widetilde{\mathcal{D}}^m$ determined by (0.43) is wider than the region $\widetilde{\mathcal{D}}$ determined by (0.40) and is again close to the maximal possible region. Therefore, in all cases our results are stronger than those obtained in the theory of ill-posed problems. Let us remark that in our approach the condition (0.40) is of course not necessary, since we consider the problem not for the entire class of functions u^δ satisfying (0.38), but for a function u^δ of special form ($u^\delta = u^{V_m}$).

We have discussed two examples where a practically complete solution of the convergence problem in the general setting is possible. When such results are difficult to obtain, it might be reasonable to consider from the very beginning a smaller region, which is most interesting from the practical point of view. This approach is related to the problem of the *choice of the regulaization parameter* α, which we will now discuss. Let us assume that we are dealing with an RT-algorithm with an one-parameter regularizer.

The recommendation of the theory of ill-posed problems is that we must choose α according to the residual principle [**2, 5**]. Let δ characterize the precision of samples u_n and let $\|\cdot\|_{\Delta t}$ be a norm in the space of sequences $\{u_n\}$ that characterizes the norm in H_2. Then the residual principle says that α_T should be determined from the *residual equation*

$$\| (KZ^{A,\delta})(t_n) - u_n^\delta \|_{\Delta t}^2 = \delta^2, \qquad Z^{A,\delta} = A(\{u_n^\delta\}).$$

For a problem with noise ($u_n^\delta = u_n^\sigma$, (0.31)), the constructive formulation of this principle has the form

$$\| (KZ^{A,\sigma})(t_n) - u_n^\sigma \|_{\Delta t}^2 = \delta^2. \tag{0.44}$$

In the analysis of theoretical bounds one usually considers the continuous analog of the residual equation, which, for $H_2 = L^2$, has the form

$$\| KZ^R - u \|_{L^2}^2 = \delta^2. \tag{0.45}$$

If T is the a priori size of the support of $u(t)$, then for δ^2 one takes

$$\delta^2 = T\sigma_u^2 = \sum_n \sigma^2(v_n)\Delta t. \tag{0.46}$$

Then for the Tikhonov regularize we have

$$\| KZ^R - u \|_{L^2}^2 \sim C \| u \|_{L^2}^2 \alpha_T^2, \qquad \alpha_t \to 0,$$

and, using the condition that the noise is small, $\sigma_u^2 < T^{-1} \| u \|_{L^2}^2$, we obtain from (0.45)

$$\alpha_T = C(u)\sigma_u. \tag{0.47}$$

A similar answer can be obtained from (0.44) for the lattice Tikhonov algorithm A_T as well, if the norm $\|\cdot\|$ is taken in the form

$$\| \{u_n\} \|_{\Delta t}^2 = \sum_n |u_n|^2 \Delta t$$

and the noise is assumed to be small. Let us remark that (0.46) and (0.47) imply the regularity condition (0.39). We refer to the case when δ^2 is defined according to (0.46) as *regularity conditions with respect to noise.* The condition of regularity with respect to noise, which at least assumes that

$$\sigma_u^2/\alpha_T \to 0, \qquad \sigma_u \to 0, \qquad \alpha_T \to 0, \tag{0.48}$$

is usually considered as the main condition in the theory of ill-posed problems. As we have seen, it is definitely satisfied for low noise if α_T is chosen using the residual. The regularity condition with respect to noise guarantees that the noise of the solution is small provided that the noise of initial data is small ($\sigma_Z^2 \to 0$ if $\sigma_u^2 \to 0$). Let us show that this is the case for a polynomial kernel $\widehat{L}(\omega) \sim |\omega|^p$ and one of the simplest Tikhonov regularizers corresponding to $M(\omega) = \omega^{2r}$ ($r = 1, 2, \dots$). In this case the Tikhonov regularizer (0.28) is homogeneous (0.29), $\alpha = \alpha_T^{1/2(p+r)}$. The variance σ_Z^2 for homogeneous RT-algorithms is estimated below (see (1.3)), and under the condition $\alpha\Omega \geq C$ we have

$$\sigma_Z^2 \sim C \frac{\sigma_u^2 \Delta t}{\alpha_{2p+1}} = C \frac{\sigma_u^2 \Delta t}{\alpha_T^{(2p+1)/2(r+p)}}. \tag{0.49}$$

If the conditions (0.48) are satisfied, then (0.49) immediately implies that $\sigma_Z^2 \to 0$ provided $\sigma_u^2 \to 0$. In the theory of ill-posed problems the last property is essentially the basic one in the definition of *Tikhonov convergence.* The regularity condition, and, in particular, the choice of the regularization parameter using the residual method, guarantees *just this* type of convergence. The regularity condition with respect to noise implies, of course, that $\sigma_Z^2 \to 0$ provided $\sigma_u^2 \to 0$, $|\overline{\beta}| \to 0$, but it does not guarantee convergence.

If α_T is chosen using the residual method, one must consider the convergence with respect to regions at the $(\Delta t, \sigma_u)$-plane. Given certain results about the convergence with respect to regions inside $(\Delta t, \alpha_T)$, this is an easy task. In particular, the condition (0.37) together with (0.47) implies that an RT-algorithm with the Tikhonov regularizer diverges if $\sigma_u \leq C\Delta t^{2r+p}$.

Let us consider now a different method for the choice of regularization parameters, using a homogeneous regularizer as an example. In this method α is chosen according to the condition

$$\alpha = C/\Omega \qquad (\alpha = C\Delta t). \tag{0.50}$$

Using, if necessary, the substitution $\alpha \to C\alpha$, one can assume that $\alpha = \Omega^{-1}$. For the simplest Tikhonov regularizer this means that $\alpha_T = C(\Delta t)^{2(r+p)}$. Let us remark that for

$$\Delta t < C\sigma_u^{1/p} \tag{0.51}$$

this choice of α_T contradicts the regularity condition with respect to noise, since in this case $\sigma_u^2/\alpha_T \geq C\sigma_u^{-2r/p}$, and the condition (0.48) is clearly violated. Similarly, for an arbitrary homogeneous regularizer we have

$$R_\alpha(\omega) = S(\omega/\Sigma), \tag{0.52}$$

and according to (0.49) (with $\widehat{L}(\omega) = |\omega|^p$) we have

$$\sigma_Z^2 = C\sigma_u^2/(\Delta t)^{2p},$$

so in the case (0.51) the noise of the solution tends to zero, indicating (indirectly) the violation of the regularity condition with respect to noise. Nevertheless, algorithms corresponding to (0.50) (with $\alpha = \Omega^{-1}$) attract the most interest and are widely used. First of all, let us remark that in the above examples of practical algorithms of interpolation and numerical differentiation the regularizers are of the form (0.52). In this case samples are known exactly and all problems related to noise disappear. Regulaizers of the form

$$R(\omega) = \begin{cases} 1, & |\omega| \leq \Omega, \\ 0, & |\omega| > \Omega, \end{cases} \qquad R(\omega) = \begin{cases} \frac{\sin(\pi\omega/2\Omega)}{\pi\omega/2\Omega}, & |\omega| \leq \Omega, \\ 0, & |\omega| > \Omega, \end{cases}$$

that are used in tomography **[6]**, also are of the form (0.52), and the regularity condition is ignored. Although in this case $\sigma_Z^2 \to \infty$ as $\Delta t \to 0$, for small σ_u^2 and realistic Δt, the solution noise is small.

To understand the meaning of the choice (0.50) $\alpha = C/\Omega = C'\Delta t$, let us introduce the notion of the *resolution* h_R *of a regularization*. We will not require homogeneity and consider a general regularizer $R(\omega, \overline{\alpha})$. Let us consider $Z^R(t)$ (see (0.7), (0.8)) for $Z(t) = \theta(t)$ and $Z(t) = \delta(t)$. By definition,

$$\delta^R(t) = \frac{1}{2\pi}\int d\omega\, e^{-i\omega t} R(\omega),$$

so that

$$R(\omega) = \int \delta^R(t) e^{i\omega t}\, dt. \tag{0.53}$$

Since our regularizers satisfy the condition

$$R(0, \overline{\alpha}) = 1 + O(|\overline{\alpha}|^\delta), \qquad |\overline{\alpha}| \to 0,$$

we have

$$\int \delta^R(t)\, dt = 1 + O(|\overline{\alpha}|^\delta). \tag{0.54}$$

We note that in the general case

$$Z^R(t) = \int Z(t - t')\delta^R(t')\,dt'.$$

This implies that

$$\frac{d}{dt}\theta^R(t)|_{t=0} = \delta^R(0) = \frac{1}{2\pi}\int R(\omega)\,d\omega.$$

Now we define the resolution of a regularization by either of two equivalent formulas:

$$h_R = \frac{d}{dt}\theta^R(t)|_{t=0}; \qquad h^R\delta^R(0) = 1. \tag{0.55}$$

Then

$$h_R = \left[\frac{1}{2\pi}\int R(\omega)\,d\omega\right]^{-1}. \tag{0.56}$$

Formulas (0.54) and (0.55) reveal the geometric meaning of h^R. Namely, it determines the efficient size (in t) of the support of $\delta^R(t)$ and the width of the smearing of a step function that is caused by regularization.

For homogeneous regularizers we have

$$h_R = C_R\alpha, \qquad C_R = 2\pi/\int S(\xi)\,d\xi.$$

Therefore, for homogeneous regularizes the choice of α from the condition $\alpha = C\Delta t$ means that

$$h_R = C\Delta t. \tag{0.57}$$

Similarly, in the general case a regularization satisfying (0.57) will be called a *high-resolution regularization*, and the corresponding algorithm will be called a *high-resolution algorithm*. For regularizes of the form $R_\alpha(\omega)$ (one-parameter) or $R(\omega, \Delta t, \alpha)$, formula (0.57) can be considered as an equation that determines a dependence $\alpha = \alpha(\Delta t)$. It gives another (in addition to the resudial) method for the choice of α, called the *resolution method*. High-resolution regularizations are especially interesting from the practical point of view. The high-resolution requirement can be considered as the condition of minimality for the number of measurements: if the measurement step equals Δt, then the algorithm must ensure the reconstruction of details of size Δt. The high-resolution condition

$$h_R(\alpha, \Delta t) = C\Delta t \tag{0.58}$$

naturally defines a subset (curve) $\mathcal{D} \subset \mathbb{R}_2^+$, and it is very interesting to analyze the convergence with respect to this curve. The formulation of the convergence problem for high-resolution algorithms is quite natural: we require that $Z^A(t) \to Z(t)$ as $\Delta t \to 0$ and for $\alpha = \alpha(\Delta t)$ as defined by (0.58). Although, as we mentioned earlier, the majority of algorithms used in practice are high-resolution algorithms, the precise definition was, we believe, first given in [**9**]. In the same paper the existence of convergent high-resolution algorithms was proved, and a convergence criterion for high-resolution algorithms was obtained in the case of polynomial kernels and smooth homogeneous regularizers. Let us remark that the last result is essentially contained in [**10**]. In the present paper we give a complete exposition and proofs of results from [**9, 10**].

A problem occurs about the existence of convergent *superhigh-resolution* algorithms, i.e., of algorithms with $h_R \lesssim C\Delta t^{1+\delta}$. Results presented in this paper imply that for fast-increasing kernels $(\widehat{L}(\omega) \sim \exp|\omega_1/\omega_2|^p)$ such algorithms do not exist. They do not exist also in the polynomial case for RT-algorithms with homogeneous or Wiener regularizers. However, in general it is quite easy to the construct an RT-algorithm with a superhigh-resolution regularization that converges for sufficiently smooth right-hand sides. Consider a regularizer of the form

$$R(\omega) = \begin{cases} 0, & |\omega - 2k\Omega| \le a\Omega, 0 < a < 1,\ k = \pm 1, \pm 2, \dots, \pm K, \\ 0, & |\omega| \ge K\Omega, \\ 1 & \text{otherwise.} \end{cases}$$

Proposition 2.1 implies that if $K \sim C\omega^\beta$, $\beta > 0$, and $u(t) \in C^m(\mathbb{R})$ with $m \ge p + 2\beta + \delta$, then the corresponding RT-algorithm converges. It is also clear that for the regularizer $R(\omega)$ we have $h_R \le C\Delta t^{1+\beta}$.

Let us note here that one must distinguish between the above notion of the resolution of an algorithm and the actual resolution of this algorithm. In this paper we mostly restrict ourselves to smooth functions, so that resolution problems that require the consideration of discontinuous functions similar to characteristic functions of sets are not discussed in the main part of the paper. However, let us discuss them briefly here. Define functions $\theta^A(t)$ and $\delta^A(t)$ similarly to $\theta^R(t)$ and $\delta^R(t)$, and then define h_A^θ and h_A^δ by (0.55) with θ^R and δ^R replaced by θ^A and δ^A. Unlike to h_R, $\theta^A(t)$ and $\delta^A(t)$ can fail to be appropriate characteristics of the resolution of an algorithm. This can be seen from explicit formulas for $A = A_{RT}$:

$$h_A^\theta = 2\pi \left[\int d\omega\, \omega \widehat{L}(\omega) R(\omega) \sum_n \frac{1}{\widehat{L}(\omega + 2n\Omega)(\omega + 2n\Omega)} \right]^{-1},$$

$$h_A^\delta = 2\pi \left[\int d\omega\, \widehat{L}(\omega) R(\omega) \sum_n \frac{1}{\widehat{L}(\omega + 2n\Omega)} \right]^{-1},$$

which can be easily obtained formally; they hold when the corresponding series and integrals converge. In particular, h_A^θ and h_A^δ can differ substantially, and even become negative. The following definition of the resolution at the level $\gamma < 1$ is more adequate. First of all, let us remark that $Z^A(t)$, contrary to $Z^R(t)$, is not translation invariant (it is invariant only under translations by multiples of Δt). Therefore we can consider the functions $\theta^A(t,\tau)$ and $\delta^A(t,\tau)$ that are the reconstructions of $\theta(t-\tau)$ and of $\delta(t-\tau)$ respectively. We call $h_{A,\gamma}^\theta$ a *resolution at the level* $\gamma < 1$ if

$$|\theta^A(t,\tau)| \le \gamma \quad \text{for } t < \tau - h_{A,\gamma}^\theta,$$

$$|\theta^A(t,\tau) - 1| \le \gamma \quad \text{for } t > \tau + h_{A,\gamma}^\theta,$$

for all τ, $0 \le \tau < \Delta t$. Similarly, $h_{A,\gamma}^\delta$ is defined by the requirement that

$$|\delta^A(t,\tau)| \le \gamma |\delta^A(\tau,\tau)| \qquad \text{for } |t-\tau| > h_{A,\gamma}^\delta,$$

for all τ. In the majority of practically interesting cases one can prove that a convergent RT-algorithm that has high-resolution in the sense of high-resolution regularization gives high real resolution $h_{A,\gamma}^{\theta,\delta} \le C\Delta t$ in the sense of each of the above definitions. One can formulate the following main conjecture: there exist no convergent superhigh-resolution algorithms at the level $\gamma < 0.5$ (here we mean not only RT-algorithms, but arbitrary ones).

§0.4. The method and certain results

A method used in this paper for the analysis of RT-algorithms consists in derivation of pointwise estimates for each of the components $\Delta Z^R(t)$, $\Delta Z^T(t)$, $\sigma_Z^2(t)$ of the reconstruction error. The analysis of $\Delta Z^R(t)$ is easy, and the corresponding estimates are presented in §1.3. Here we remark only that $|\Delta Z^R(t)| \to 0$ as $|\overline{\alpha}| \to 0$, uniformly with respect to t. Therefore, the regularization error converges uniformly in each region as $|\overline{\beta}| \to 0$. General formulas for $\sigma_Z^2(t)$ are obtained in §1.3. Since our definition of convergence does not involve the behavior of the statistical error $\sigma_Z^2(t)$, it suffices to use these general formulas to obtain the corresponding estimates. The main technical part of this paper is devoted to the analysis of the discretization error $\Delta Z^T(t)$ for RT-algorithms. As we already mentioned, the analysis of other algorithms reduces to the analysis of RT-algorithms (Chapter 3). Since the behavior of the discretization error determines the convergence region of a given algorithm, its analysis is of primary interest.

Our approach to the analysis of the discretization error is based on the estimation of $\Delta Z^T(t)$ by *estimating the precision of the quadrature formula* (0.9) *for the integral* (0.8). The difficulty here is that the function $H^R(t)$ under the integral sign can depend on the discretization step Δt in a singular manner (since $H^R(t)$ depends singularly on α and we are interested in the situation when α and Δt tend to 0 in a compatible way). The usual methods fail in this situation, and a new approach is necessary. Our method is based on an explicit formula for the error $\Delta Z^T(t)$ obtained from the Poisson summation formula. We illustrate this method with a simple example. Let us consider the integral

$$J = \int f(t)\,dt$$

and the simplest quadrature formula

$$J_{\Delta t} = \sum_n f_n \Delta t.$$

We can rewrite J and $J_{\Delta t}$ in the form

$$J = \widehat{f}(0), \qquad J_{\Delta t} = \widehat{f}^T(0).$$

The required Poisson formula has the form

$$\widehat{f}^T(\omega) = \sum_n \widehat{f}(\omega + 2\pi\Omega). \tag{0.59}$$

Using this formula, we easily get the following expression for the error:

$$J_{\Delta t} - J = \sum_{n \neq 0} \widehat{f}(2n\Omega).$$

Let us remark that the idea of using the Poisson formula to estimate the precision of a quadrature formula is not quite new. At the very least, it is explicitly used in some problems in number theory (similar to the problem about the number of integral points in a disk, [11, 12]). In our case the application of the formula (0.59) for $\widehat{u}^T(\omega)$ in the expression (0.10) for $Z^{A_{RT}} = Z^{R,T}$ yields

$$\Delta Z^T(t) = \frac{1}{2\pi} \sum_{n \neq 0} \int d\omega\, e^{-i\omega t} \widehat{H}^R(\omega) \widehat{u}(\omega + 2n\Omega).$$

This approach was first used in **[10]**, where it formed the basis for the main results about polynomial kernels and homogeneous regularizers. The paper **[9]** was devoted to certain generalizations of these results. All principal results of these papers, as well as some new results, will be presented here.

We conclude this Introduction with the formulation (not always rigorous) of the main results of the paper. In the precise formulations these results are given together with efficient numerical estimates of reconstruction errors. All results are formulated under smoothness assumptions for the right-hand sides.

1. A sufficient condition for the convergence of an algorithm $A_{RT}(R)$ in a region $\mathscr{D} \subset \mathbb{R}^+_m$ is that for any $\overline{\beta}$ the Nyquist condition is satisfied (i.e., $R \in \mathscr{N}$).

2. For *slowly growing kernels* $\widehat{L}(\omega) = O(|\omega|^{\overline{p}})$ and so-called *quasifinite regularizations*, the algorithm $A_{RT}(R)$ converges in the quasifiniteness region under the condition

$$R_\alpha(\omega) = 0, \qquad |\omega - 2n\Omega| < a\Omega, \quad 0 < a \leq 1, n = \pm 1, \pm 2, \dots. \tag{0.60}$$

A regularization as said to be *quasifinite* in a region $\mathscr{D}$ if for any $(\Delta t, \alpha) \in \mathscr{D}$ and for some $\kappa > 0$ we have

$$|R_\alpha(\omega)| \leq C|\omega|^{-\overline{p}-1-\delta} \qquad \text{as } |\omega| > \kappa\Omega.$$

For homogeneous regulaizers condition (0.60) implies convergence even with the quasifiniteness assumption.

3. For *kernels of polynomial growth*, i. e., those satisfying the condition

$$\widehat{L}(\omega) = |\omega|^p + O(|\omega|^{p-\delta}), \qquad |\omega| \to \infty,$$

the conditions

$$\Omega^p R_\alpha(\pm 2(1 - C)\Omega) \to 0, \qquad |\overline{\beta}| \to 0, \quad 0 < C < 1,$$

are sufficient, and the conditions

$$\Omega^p R_\alpha(\pm 2\Omega) \to 0, \qquad |\overline{\beta}| \to 0, \quad \overline{\beta} = (\Delta t, \alpha),$$

are necessary for the convergence in the class of *monotone regularizations* (i.e., those that are monotone decreasing (increasing) as $\omega \geq \omega_m$ $(\omega \leq -\omega_m)$ for sufficiently small α).

4. For kernels of polynomial growth and Wiener regularizers (of the form (0.13)) algorithms A_{RT} converge when

$$(\log(1/\alpha))^{1/q} \leq r_v(\Omega/\omega_R), \qquad r_v < 2,$$

and diverge when

$$(\log(1/\alpha))^{1/q} \geq r_v(\Omega/\omega_R), \qquad r_v > 2.$$

High-resolution algorithms correspond to the choice

$$(\log(1/\alpha))^{1/q} = k_V(\Omega/\omega_R).$$

These algorithms converge for $k_V < 2$ (this corresponds to $h_R > \Delta t/2$) and diverge for $k_V \geq 2$ (this corresponds to $h_R \leq \Delta t/2$). This solves the convergence problem completely.

5. For *purely polynomial kernels*, i.e., kernels of the form

$$\widehat{L}(\omega) = \sum_{i=0}^{I} b_i|\omega|^{\pi_i} + O(|\omega|^{-1-\delta}), \qquad |\omega| \to \infty, \quad \rho_0 > \cdots > \rho_I,$$

and smooth homogeneous regularizers the convergence region is described completely. For high-resolution algorithms (that are characterized in this case by the condition $\alpha\Omega = \varepsilon_S = \text{const}$) necessary and sufficient conditions take the form

$$R_\alpha^{(m)}(2n\Omega) = 0, \qquad m = 0, 1, \ldots, [\rho_0], \quad n = \pm 1, \pm 2, \ldots. \tag{0.61}$$

The convergence region for the same class of kernels and RT-algorithms with the so-called *generalized Tikhonov regularizers*, i.e., regularizers of the form

$$R_{\alpha_T}(\omega) = \left(1 + \alpha_T \sum_{i=0}^{I} C_i|\omega/\omega_R|^{q_i}\right)^{-1}, \qquad q_0 > \cdots > q_I \geq 0,$$

is also completely described. Namely, an algorithm converges in $\mathscr{D} = \mathscr{D}_{\overline{\beta}}$, $\overline{\beta} = (\Delta t, \alpha_T)$, if and only if

$$\alpha_T^{-1}\Omega^{\rho_0 - q_0} \to 0, \qquad |\overline{\beta}| \to 0.$$

6. In the class of purely polynomial kernels and homogeneous smooth regularizers an explicit formula for the divergent part of the discretization error is obtained (in a region larger than the convergence region). Using this formula, the so-called *algorithm with renormalization* is constructed and its convergence is proved.

7. The convergence of the Tikhonov algorithm A_T for large N (when $N \sim \Delta t^{\beta}$ with a sufficiently large β) is proved, and its efficient regularizer is computed.

Let us note that conditions (0.61) were earlier obtained in interpolation theory in attempts to determine when a function from the Sobolev space W_2^{p+1} has a good approximation by translations of a compactly supported function from W_2^p **[13]**.

We say a few words about the structure of the paper. It contains this Introduction and three chapters divided into sections. In the first two chapters algorithms of the form A_{RT} are considered. In particular, the analysis of the convergence of quadrature formulas is relegated to Chapter 2, and it is this chapter that contains our main results. Chapter 3 is devoted to the analysis of the convergence of two versions of the lattice Tikhonov algorithm. The enumeration of formulas, definitions, theorems, and propositions is separate inside each chapter: the first number is the chapter number

(0 means the Introduction), and the second number is the number inside the given chapter. Numbers of formulas are given in parenthesis, those of sections without parenthesis. The end of a proof is indicated by the Halmos symbol □.

CHAPTER 1. THE ALGORITHM A_{RT}, MAIN DEFINITIONS AND PROPERTIES

§1.1. Main definitions and functional classes

In this section we collect the main definitions used latter in the paper. After some preliminary remarks we define the classes of kernels and of right-hand sides for RT-algorithms and the classes of regularizers. The notion of a regularization is introduced. Definitions of the convergence of an algorithm and of the convergence of the discretization error for an A_{RT}-algorithm are given.

Functions are assumed to be complex-valued or real-valued (the later case is always mentioned explicitly) and defined in a classical way (so that one can consider the value of a function at a point). Whenever the domain of a function is not specified, it is assumed that the function is defined on the real line $\mathbb{R}$. All functions are assumed to be piecewise continuous, i.e., to possess a finite number of discontinuity points (in fact, one can consider even piecewise smooth functions). It is assumed that at each discontinuity point of the first kind the condition

$$f(x) = \tfrac{1}{2}(f(x+0) + f(x-0))$$

is satisfied. Unless mentioned otherwise, all conditions imposed on a function (boundedness, boundedness of variation, differentiability, etc.) are assumed to be satisfied on the entire real line.

A function is said to be piecewise smooth if it has continuous derivatives of all orders everywhere except a finite number of points. At these points the function itself and its derivatives can have discontinuities of the first kind. Integrals are assumed to be Riemann integrals

$$\int f(x)\,dx \equiv \int_{-\infty}^{+\infty} f(x)\,dx \stackrel{\text{def}}{=} \lim_{A\to+\infty} \int_{-A}^{+A} f(x)\,dx.$$

Similarly for sums we assume

$$\sum_n f_n \equiv \sum_{n=-\infty}^{+\infty} f_n \stackrel{\text{def}}{=} \lim_{N\to+\infty} \sum_{n=-N}^{+N} f_n.$$

Conditions of type $f \in L^1$ mean that f is absolutely integrable on the entire line $\mathbb{R}$ (i.e., $\int |f|\,dx < \infty$).

All asymptotic estimates are efficient, i.e. the formula $g(x) = O(f(x))$, $|x| \to \infty$, means not only that $|g(x)| \le C(x_0)f(x)$ for $|x| > x_0$, but also that x_0 and $C(x_0)$ can be efficiently computed. If g depends on an additional parameter α, then x_0 and $C(x_0)$ can depend on α. If one can find x_0 and $C(x_0)$ that serve all α, the estimate is said to be *uniform with respect to* α.

Let us consider classes of kernels. We assume that the kernel of an SC is given by a classical function $\widehat{L}(\omega)$ in the frequency domain. Therefore, in the formulation of the problem we will start with the formula (0.2) (rather than with (0.1)).

Let us describe the classes of kernels we are interested in. Let $\widehat{L}(\omega)$ be a complex-valued piecewise continuous function with a finite number of discontinuity points of the first kind. The most general class of kernels—the class of kernels with an arbitrary rate of growth—is defined as follows. Let $\Lambda(\omega)$ be a real piecewise continuous (with discontinuities of the first kind) even function that is monotone nondecreasing for $\omega \geq 0$, takes nonnegative values, and is not identically zero. Then the class of kernels that grows not faster than Λ consists of all kernels such that

$$|\widehat{L}(\omega)| \leq \Lambda(\omega);$$

it is denoted by $\mathscr{L}(\Lambda)$. If

$$\Lambda(\omega) = \begin{cases} \widetilde{L}, & |\omega| \leq \omega_L \\ \widetilde{L}|\omega/\omega_L|^{\overline{\rho}}, & |\omega| \geq \omega_L, \end{cases} \tag{1.1}$$

$\widetilde{L}, \omega_L > 0$, $\overline{\rho} \geq 0$, we obtain the class of *slowly growing functions.*

Now we describe the class of *kernels of polynomial growth* $\mathscr{L}(\rho^{\pm})$. It consists of all kernels from $\mathscr{L}(\overline{\rho})$ satisfying the additional condition

$$\widehat{L}(\omega) = \left\{ \begin{matrix} \widetilde{L}^{+}|\omega/\omega_L|^{\rho^{+}}, & \omega \geq \omega_L \\ \widetilde{L}^{-}|\omega/\omega_L|^{\rho^{-}}, & \omega \leq -\omega_L \end{matrix} \right\} + \Delta\widehat{L}(\omega), \tag{1.2}$$

where $\widehat{L}^{\pm}$ are complex constants, $\rho^{\pm}$ are real constants, and $\Delta\widehat{L}$ satisfies

$$|\Delta\widehat{L}(\omega)| \leq \begin{cases} C^{+}|\omega|^{\rho^{+}-\delta^{+}}, & \omega \geq \omega_L, \\ C^{-}|\omega|^{\rho^{-}-\delta^{-}}, & \omega \leq -\omega_L, \end{cases} \tag{1.3}$$

$\delta^{\pm} > 0$. Let us note that we can take $\overline{\rho} = \max\{0, \rho^{+}, \rho^{-}\}$.

Finally, let us consider the class of *polynomial kernels* $\mathscr{L}_0(\rho_0^{\pm})$. It consists of kernels of the form

$$\widehat{L}(\omega) = \sum_{i=0}^{I^{\pm}} l_i^{\pm}|\omega/\omega_L|^{\rho_i^{\pm}} + \Delta\widehat{L_0}(\omega), \tag{1.4}$$

where $+$ is taken for $\omega \geq \omega_L$ and $-$ for $\omega \leq -\omega_L$, $l_i^{\pm}$ are complex constants, $\rho_0^{+} > \rho_1^{+} > \cdots > \rho_{I^{+}}^{+}$ and $\rho_0^{-} > \rho_1^{-} > \cdots > \rho_{I^{-}}^{-}$ are real constants, and, finally,

$$|\Delta\widehat{L_0}(\omega)| \leq \begin{cases} C, & |\omega| \leq \omega_L, \\ C|\omega/\omega_L|^{-1-\delta}, & |\omega| \geq \omega_L, \end{cases} \tag{1.5}$$

$C > 0$, $\delta > 0$. It is clear that if $\rho_0^{\pm} = \rho^{\pm}$, $\overline{\rho} = \max\{0, \rho^{+}, \rho^{-}\}$, and $\Lambda(\omega)$ grows sufficiently slow, we have the following inclusions:

$$\mathscr{L}_0(\rho_0^{\pm}) \subset \mathscr{L}(\rho^{\pm}) \subset \mathscr{L}(\overline{\rho}) \subset \mathscr{L}(\Lambda).$$

Let us give some examples of kernels. Kernels with slow growth

$$\widehat{L}(\omega) = (i\omega)^n, \qquad \widehat{L}(\omega) = |\omega|^{\rho}, \qquad \widehat{L}(\omega) = 1 + |\omega|^{\rho}, \qquad \rho \geq 0,$$

are polynomial kernels (with $\Delta\widehat{L}_0 \equiv 0$). The class of polynomial kernels contains also the kernels

$$\widehat{L}(\omega) = \left(\sum_{n=1}^{n_1} a_n \omega^{\alpha_n}\right)\left(\sum_{n=1}^{n_2} b_n \omega^{\beta_n}\right)^{-1}, \qquad \sum_{n=1}^{n_2} b_n \omega^{\beta_n} \neq 0,$$

but now $\Delta\widehat{L}_0 \not\equiv 0$. A typical fast-growing kernel (such that $L \notin \mathscr{L}(\overline{p})$ for each $\overline{p}$) is the kernel $\widehat{L}(\omega) = \exp\{|\omega/\omega_L|^\rho\}$, $\omega_L > 0$, $\rho > 0$. Finally, an example of a kernel of slow growth that is not a kernel of polynomial growth ($L \in \mathscr{L}(\overline{p})$, $L \notin \mathscr{L}(\overline{p^{\pm}})$) is the kernel

$$\widehat{L}(\omega) = |\omega/\omega_L|^\rho \sin(e^{|\omega/\omega_L|^{\rho'}}), \qquad \omega_L, \rho, \rho' > 0.$$

Now let us discuss classes of right-hand sides u. We assume u takes complex values. We say that u belongs to the *class of admissible rigth-hand sides* for a given kernel (or for a given class of kernels) if

1) $u(t)$ is a piecewise continuous function with discontinuities of the first kind;
2) $u(t) \in L^1$ and has bounded variation; and
3) for the given kernel L (for each kernel from the given class $\{L\}$) formula (0.2) can be used to define $Z(t)$.

The first condition guarantees the existence of samples. The second condition ensures the existence of the Fourier transform $\widehat{u}(\omega)$ that is necessary for (0.2) to make sense. The last condition guarantees that the exact solution of the problem, whose approximations we are going to construct using samples, indeed exists.

The fact that $u(t)$ belongs to the class of right-hand sides that are admissible for a given kernel (or for a given class of kernels) will be denoted by $u \in \mathscr{U}(L)$ (or $u \in \mathscr{U}(\{L\})$). Let us introduce the narrower class of *admissible smooth* (or M-smooth) right-hand sides ($u \in \mathscr{U}_M(L)$ or $u \in \mathscr{U}_M(\{L\})$). We say that $u \in \mathscr{U}_M(L)$ if $u \in \mathscr{U}(L)$ and

$$\widehat{L}(\omega)\widehat{u}(\omega) \equiv \widehat{Z}(\omega) = O(|\omega|^{-M_Z}), \qquad |\omega| \to \infty; \tag{1.6}$$

$$\widehat{u}(\omega) = O(|\omega|^{-M_u}), \qquad |\omega| \to \infty, \tag{1.7}$$

with $M_Z, M_u \geq 1+\delta$. The condition $u \in \mathscr{U}_M(\{L\})$ means that (1.6) is satisfied for all kernels $L \in \{L\}$. For $\{L\} = \mathscr{L}(\Lambda)$ it suffices to verify (1.6) for the function $\Lambda(\omega)$ only. For $\{L\} = \mathscr{L}(\Lambda)$ or $\{L\} = \mathscr{L}(\overline{p})$ we denote the corresponding classes of admissible right-hand sides by $\mathscr{U}(\{L\}) = \mathscr{U}(\Lambda)$ and $\mathscr{U}(\{L\}) = \mathscr{U}(\overline{p})$ respectively. Similarly, for smooth admissible right-hand sides we use the notation $\mathscr{U}_M(\Lambda)$ and $\mathscr{U}_M(\overline{p})$, respectively. Let us note that (1.6) and (1.7) can be rewritten in the following form:

$$|\widehat{Z}(\omega)| \leq \widetilde{Z}|\omega|^{-M_Z}, \tag{1.8}$$

$$|\widehat{u}(\omega)| \leq \widetilde{u}|\omega|^{-M_u}, \tag{1.9}$$

with some constants $\widetilde{Z}$, $\widetilde{u}$. Let us remark also that if the kernel does not decrease at infinity, then (1.6) implies (1.7). For example, for kernels from the class $\mathscr{U}(\overline{p})$ (recall that $\overline{p} \geq 0$), (1.6) implies (1.7) with $M_u = M_Z + \overline{p}$. For fast-growing kernels, (1.6) implies (1.7) with $M_u = \infty$. Indeed, if, for example, $\widehat{L}(\omega) \sim \exp|\omega|^\rho$, $|\omega| \to \infty$, then $\widehat{u}(\omega) \sim |\omega|^{-M_Z}\exp(-|\omega|^\rho)$, $|\omega| \to \infty$. We do not restrict ourselves to condition (1.6) only, since, although we are interested in increasing kernels, we do not want to exclude decreasing kernels.

Let us remark that the analysis of problems in the class of smooth admissible right-hand sides $\mathscr{U}_M$ corresponds to the existence of a certain a priori information about the smoothness of the exact solution $Z(t)$: the increase of smoothness corresponds to the faster decrease of $\widehat{u}(\omega)$ (in the case of kernels $\mathscr{L}(\overline{\rho})$ the increase of the a priori smoothness increases M).

Now let us consider classes of regularizers. Below by a regularizer we understand both an $\overline{\alpha}$-parametric family of functions $R(\omega, \overline{\alpha})$ and a function from this family. Unlike the choice of a kernel and of a right-hand side, the choice of a regularizer is completely at our disposal. The most general requirements for the family $R(\omega, \overline{\alpha})$ are that each function from the family decreases fast enough so that $\widehat{H}^R(\omega) \in L^1 \cap L^2$, and for $|\overline{\alpha}| \to 0$ the regularization disappears (i.e. $R(\omega, \overline{\alpha}) \to 1$). Accordingly, introduce the class of *admissible regularizers* for a given kernel (for a class of kernels) $\mathscr{R}(L)$ (or $\mathscr{R}(\{L\})$). Let us assume that α is an one-dimensional parameter; the generalization to the multidimensional case is easy. We say that $R_\alpha(\omega) \in \mathscr{R}(L)$ if the following conditions are satisfied:

$$
(1.10) \qquad \begin{cases} \text{a) } \forall \alpha, R_\alpha(\omega) \text{ is a piecewise smooth function;} \\ \text{b) } \forall \alpha, R_\alpha(\omega) = O(|\omega|^{-1-\delta}), \ |\omega| \to \infty; \\ \text{c) } \forall \alpha, \widehat{H}^R(\omega) \overset{\text{def}}{=} \widehat{L}(\omega) R_\alpha(\omega) = O(|\omega|)^{-1-\delta}, \ |\omega| \to \infty; \\ \text{d) } |R_\alpha(\omega)| \geq \widetilde{R} \text{ simulteneously for all } \alpha; \\ \text{e) } R_\alpha(\omega) \to 1 \text{ as } \alpha \to 0 \text{ uniformly on any compact set in } \mathbb{R}. \end{cases}
$$

If (1.10) is satisfied for all $L \in \{L\}$, then $R_\alpha \in \mathscr{R}(\{L\})$. Classes of admissible regularizers for the classes of kernels $\mathscr{L}(\Lambda)$, $\mathscr{L}(\overline{p})$ are denoted $\mathscr{R}(\Lambda)$, $\mathscr{R}(\overline{p})$. The conditions (1.10b), (1.10c) for kernels from the class $\mathscr{L}(\Lambda)$ follow from the condition (1.10c) for $\Lambda(\omega)$. In this case the conditions (1.10b), (1.10c) can be combined into one condition

$$
\forall \alpha \quad R_\alpha(\omega) = \frac{1}{\Lambda(\omega)} O(|\omega|^{-1-\delta}), \qquad |\omega| \to \infty.
$$

Similarly, for kernels from the class $\mathscr{L}(\overline{p})$ we have

$$
\forall \alpha \quad R_\alpha(\omega) = O(|\omega|^{-\overline{p}-1-\delta}).
$$

We introduce the notion of a regularizer admitting a high-resolution algorithm (*high-resolution regularizer* for short) as a regularizer $R_\alpha \in \mathscr{R}$ which is one-parameter, real, and satisfies the condition that the function $h_R(\alpha)$ is continuous, monotone increasing, and $h_R(\alpha) \to 0$ as $\alpha \to 0$.

Let us give some examples. A regularizer is said to be *homogeneous* if $R_\alpha(\omega) = S(\alpha\omega)$ and the function $S(\xi)$ satisfies the following conditions:

$$
(1.11) \qquad \begin{cases} \text{a) } S(\xi) \text{ is a piecewise smooth function,} \\ \quad \text{continuous at } \xi = 0, \text{ with } S(0) = 1; \\ \text{b) } S(\xi) \text{ increases sufficiently fast as } |\xi| \to \infty, \\ \quad \text{so that (1.10b) and (1.10c) hold for } L \in \mathscr{L}(\overline{p}), \\ \quad S(\xi) = O(|\xi|^{-\overline{p}-1-\delta}) \text{ as } |\xi| \to \infty; \\ \text{c) } S(\xi) \leq \widetilde{S} \text{ (this follows from a) and b));} \\ \text{d) } S(\xi) \text{ is a real function with } \int S(\xi)\, d\xi > 0. \end{cases}
$$

Homogeneous regularizers admit high-resolution algorithms. For these regularizes we have

$$
h_R(\alpha) = \left[\frac{1}{2\pi} \int S(\xi)\, d\xi \right]^{-1} \alpha,
$$

and high-resolution algorithms correspond to the choice of α as in (0.57). Below we will write (0.57) for homogeneous regularizers in the form

$$\alpha\Omega = \varepsilon_S = \text{const}. \tag{1.12}$$

A regularizer of the form

$$R_{\alpha_T}(\omega) = [1 + \alpha_T Q(\omega/\omega_L)]^{-1}, \qquad \omega_R > 0, \tag{1.13}$$

where $Q(\xi)$ is a quasipolynomial, i.e., a function of the form

$$Q(\xi) = \sum_{i=0}^{I} C_i |\xi|^{q_i}, \qquad q_0 > \dots > q_I \geq 0, \quad C_0 > 0,$$

is called a *generalized Tikhonov regularizer.* One can assume that $C_0 = 1$. It is clear that for sufficiently small α_T the denominator does not vanish and $R_{\alpha_T} \in \mathscr{R}(\overline{p})$ $(q_0 \geq \overline{p} + 1 + \delta)$. A generalized Tikhonov regularizer with $C_1 = \dots = C_I = 0$ is homogeneous (the substitution $\alpha_T \to (\alpha\omega_k)^{q_0}$).

Formula (0.13) defines a Wiener regularizer. Its generalization is a *Wiener type regularizer*

$$R_\alpha(\omega) = [1 + \alpha H(\omega/\omega_R) \exp Q(\omega/\omega_R)]^{-1}, \tag{1.14}$$

where H and Q are quasipolynomials (with the leading coefficient 1).

All the above regularizers are real, even, and admit high-resolution algorithms. The reality assumption could have been included into the list (1.10) from the very beginning. We do not do that, since most of our results hold without this assumption.

Now we introduce the notion of a *regularization.* We say that a regularization $\operatorname{Reg}(R, \mathscr{D}_{\overline{\beta}})$ $(\overline{\beta} = (\Delta t, \alpha))$ is defined if we are given a family of regularizers $R_\alpha(\omega)$ and a region of admissible values of parameters $\overline{\beta} \in \mathscr{D}_{\overline{\beta}}$. It is clear that $\mathscr{D}_{\overline{\beta}} \subset \mathscr{D}_{\Delta t} \times \mathscr{D}_\alpha$, where $\mathscr{D}_{\Delta t}$ and $\mathscr{D}_\alpha$ are the ranges of the parameters Δt and α (for example, $\mathscr{D}_{\Delta t} = (0, \Delta t_0]$, $\mathscr{D}_\alpha = (0; \alpha_0]$); however, it might of course happen that $\mathscr{D}_{\overline{\beta}} \neq \mathscr{D}_{\Delta t} \times \mathscr{D}_\alpha$.

Let us give some clarifying examples. Let all functions $R_\alpha(\omega)$ in a family of regularizes be compactly supported. Let $\mathscr{D}_{\overline{\beta}}$ be chosen in such a way that the Nyquist condition (0.17), which we rewrite here in the form

$$R_\alpha(\omega) = 0 \quad \text{for } |\omega| > \Lambda, \quad (\Delta t, \alpha) \in \mathscr{D}_{\overline{\beta}},$$

is satisfied. Such a regularization is said to be *compactly suported.* Let a homogeneous regularizer $S(\xi)$ be given, $\operatorname{supp} S \subset [1, -1]$. In this case the regularization is compactly supported whenever

$$\mathscr{D}_{\overline{\beta}} = \{(\Delta t, \alpha) : \alpha > (1/\pi)\Delta t\}.$$

Let a regularizer admitting a high-resolution algorithm be given. A regularization $\operatorname{Reg}(R_\alpha, \mathscr{D}_{\overline{\beta}})$ with

$$\mathscr{D}_{\overline{\beta}} = \{(\Delta t, \alpha) : \ h_R(\alpha) = \Delta t/k\},$$

k a constant, is called a *high-resolution regularization.* Such a regularization corresponds to high-resolution algorithms (the choice $\alpha = \alpha_k(\Delta t)$ according to (0.58)). For homogeneous regularizers a high-resolution regularization corresponds to (1.12).

Now let us introduce an important notion of the convergence of an algorithm. Let there be given an algorithm $A(\overline{\beta})$, where $\overline{\beta} = (\Delta t, \dots)$ are the parameters of the algorithm, and a set $\mathcal{J}$ where the solution is constructed.

DEFINITION 1.1. An algorithm $A(\overline{\beta})$ is said to be:
1) convergent,
2) uniformly convergent,
3) rapidly convergent, or
4) uniformly rapidly convergent,

on the class $\{u\}$ of right-hand sides inside the set $\mathcal{D}$ of admissible values of parameters whenever, respectively, as $|\overline{\beta}| \to 0$ inside $\mathcal{D}$,
1) $\Delta Z^A(t) \to 0$ for each $t \in \mathcal{J}$,
2) $\Delta Z^A(t) \to 0$ uniformly with respect to $t \in \mathcal{J}$,
3) $\Delta Z^A(t) = O(\Delta t^\delta)$ for each $t \in \mathcal{J}$ uniformly in all other parameters,
4) $\Delta Z^A(t) = O(\Delta t^\delta)$ uniformly with respect to $t \in \mathcal{J}$ and all other parameters.

Here the algorithm error $\Delta Z^A(t)$ is defined by (0.4).

Now we consider the RT-algorithm. In this case formula (0.34) defines the discretization error $\Delta Z^T(t)$.

DEFINITION 1.2. The discretization error $\Delta Z^T(t)$ is said to be *convergent* on a class $\{u\}$ of right-hand sides inside the set $\mathcal{D}$ (with $\overline{\beta} = (\Delta t, \alpha)$) of admissible values of parameters if for any $u \in \{u\}$ and any t we have $\Delta Z^T(t) \to 0$ as $|\overline{\beta}| \to 0$, $\overline{\beta} \in \mathcal{D}$. Similarly one defines rapid, uniform, and rapid uniform convergence.

In conclusion, let us note that for high-resolution algorithms, i.e., for algorithms A_{RT} with high-resolution regularization, the admissible parameter set $\mathcal{D}_{(\Delta t, \alpha)}$ is the curve $\alpha = \alpha(\Delta t)$ in the $(\Delta t, \alpha)$-plane. In this case convergence means convergence to 0 as $\Delta t \to 0$ and $\alpha = \alpha(\Delta t)$ (clearly, $\alpha(\Delta t) \to 0$ as $\Delta t \to 0$).

§1.2. Properties of the definition of the algorithm A_{RT} and expressions for errors

In this section we formulate the conditions that ensure that algorithms of the form A_{RT} are well defined. Also, we obtain expressions for errors, which will form the basis of the further analysis. Proposition 1.1 below shows that under certain weak assumptions $Z^A(t)$ and $Z^R(t)$ are well defined, so that the algorithm itself and the regularization and discretization errors are also well defined. At the same time, the proposition gives other expressions for Z^A and Z^R.

PROPOSITION 1.1. *Let $u(t)$ be a piecewise continuous function with possible discontinuities of the first kind only. Assume also that $u(t) \in L^1$ and $u(t)$ has a bounded variation. Let $\widehat{H}^R(\omega) \in L^1$. Then*:
1) *Formula* (0.7) *defines $Z^R(t)$, i.e., the integral on the right-hand side converges absolutely and uniformly, and* (0.7) *holds.*
2) *Formula* (0.9) *defines $Z^A(t) \equiv Z^{R,T}(t)$, i.e., the series on the right-hand side converges absolutely and uniformly.*
3) *The DFT $\widehat{u}^T(\omega)$ is defined by* (0.11), *the series on the right-hand side converges absolutely and uniformly, and the Poisson formula holds*:

$$\widehat{u}^T(\omega) = \sum_n \widehat{u}(\omega + 2\pi\Omega), \qquad \Omega = \pi/\Delta t.$$

4) *Formula* (0.10) *holds.*

PROOF. 1) Since $u(t) \in L^1$, we have $|\widehat{u}(\omega)| < \int |u(t)|\,dt < \infty$. Therefore

$$|Z^R(t)| \le \frac{1}{2\pi} \int |\widehat{u}(\omega)|\, |\widehat{H}^R(\omega)|\, d\omega \le C \int |\widehat{H}^R(\omega)|\, d\omega < \infty;$$

the last inequality follows from $\widehat{H}^R(\omega) \in L^1$. Since $u(t) \in L^1$, and $\widehat{H}^R(\omega) \in L^1$, the second assertion in 1) is the convolution theorem in L^1 (see, for example, **[14]**).

2) The condition $\widehat{H}^R(\omega) \in L^1$ implies $|H^R(t)| \le \overline{H}^R < \infty$. Therefore,

$$|Z^A(t)| \ge \sum_n |H^R(t - n\Delta t)|\, |u_n| \Delta t \le \overline{H}^R \Delta t \sum_n |u(n\Delta t)|.$$

The last series converges by the Hardy lemma, which holds for a function $u \in L^1$ of bounded variation **[8]**.

3) The first assertion again follows from the Hardy lemma. To prove the second assertion we apply the Poisson summation formula

$$\sum_k \varphi(k) = \sum_n \int \varphi(x) e^{-i2\pi nx}\, dx,$$

which holds for a function $\varphi(x) \in L^1$ of bounded variation **[8]**, to the function $\varphi(x) = u(x\Delta t)\exp\{i\omega x \Delta t\}\Delta t$.

4) To prove this statement one should substitute the expression for $H^R(t)$ into (0.9) and exchange the order of summation and integration; this exchange is justified since $\sum_n \int d\omega |\widehat{H}^R(\omega)|\, |u_n| < \infty$, see **[15]**. □

Formulas (0.2) and (0.7) yield the following expression for the regularization error $\Delta Z^R(t)$ defined by (0.33):

$$\Delta Z^R(t) = \frac{1}{2\pi} \int d\omega e^{-i\omega t} (R_\alpha(\omega) - 1)\widehat{L}(\omega)\widehat{u}(\omega). \tag{1.15}$$

The next proposition provides an expression for $Z^{R,T}(t)$ that differs from (0.9) and (0.10). It will be crucial in our analysis of the discretization error.

PROPOSITION 1.2. *Let the conditions of Proposition* 1.1 *be satisfied. Let, moreover, one of the following conditions be satisfied*:

1) $\widehat{u}(\omega) = O(|\omega|^{-1-\delta})$ *as* $|\omega| \to \infty$;

2) $\sum_n \max_{n \le t \le n+1} |u(t)| < \infty$ *and* $\omega \widehat{H}^R(\omega) \in L^1$.

Then

$$Z^{R,T}(t) = \frac{1}{2\pi} \sum_n e^{-i2n\Omega t} \int d\omega e^{-i\omega t} \widehat{H}^R(\omega + 2n\Omega)\widehat{u}(\omega). \tag{1.16}$$

PROOF. 1) If the first condition is satisfied, then the series converges absolutely and uniformly. Together with the condition $\widehat{H}^R \in L^1$ this implies that in (0.10) one can exchange summation and integration.

If the second condition is satisfied, (1.16) can be easily obtained by formal application of the Poisson summation formula to the function

$$\varphi(x) = H^R(t - x\Delta t)u(x\Delta t)\Delta t.$$

Therefore we must show only that the Poisson summation formula can be applied to $\varphi(x)$. It is clear that $\widehat{H}^R(\omega) \in L^1$ implies $|H^R(t)| \leq \overline{H}^R$ and $u(t) \in L^1$ implies $\varphi(x) \in L^1$. Let us prove that the function $\varphi(x)$ is bounded (by **[8]**, this would give the applicability of the Poisson formula.) By condition 2), $H^R(s)$ has a bounded derivative, $|(H^R)'(s)| \leq \overline{H}^{R\prime} < \infty$. Therefore (see **[16]**), we have $\operatorname{var}_{[a,b]} H(s) \leq \overline{H}^{R\prime}(b-a)$. Using properties of functions of bounded variation (see **[16]**), we get

$$\begin{aligned}\operatorname*{var}_{\mathbb{R}} \varphi(x) = \sum_n \operatorname*{var}_{[n,n+1]} \varphi(x) &\leq \sum_n \max_{x\in[n,n+1]} |H^R(t - x\Delta t)| \operatorname*{var}_{[n,n+1]} u(x\Delta t)\Delta t \\ &\quad + \sum_n \max_{x\in[n,n+1]} |u(x\Delta t)| \operatorname*{var}_{[t-n-1,t-n]} H(s)\Delta t \\ &\leq \overline{H}^R \Delta t \operatorname*{var}_{\mathbb{R}} u + \overline{H}^{R\prime}\Delta t \sum_n \max_{n\Delta t \leq s \leq (n+1)\Delta t} |u(s)| < \infty;\end{aligned}$$

the last inequality follows from the fact that

$$\sum_n \max_{n\leq t\leq n+1} |u(t)| < \infty$$

implies

$$\sum_n \max_{n\Delta t\leq t\leq (n+1)\Delta t} |u(t)| < \infty$$

for each Δt (see, for example, **[17]**). □

Using (0.7) and (1.16), we have the following expression for the discretization error (0.34):

$$\Delta Z^T(t) = (2\pi)^{-1} \sum_{n\neq 0} e^{-i2\pi\Omega t} \int d\omega e^{-i\omega t} \widehat{H}^R(\omega + 2\pi\Omega)\widehat{u}(\omega). \tag{1.17}$$

Let us formulate also the following useful corollary.

COROLLARY. *Let the conditions of Proposition* 1.1 *be satisfied and let the equality* (1.16) *hold. Let, in addition,* $\widehat{H}^R(\omega) = O(|\omega|^{-1-\delta})$ *as* $|\omega| \to \infty$ *and* $\widehat{u}(\omega) \in L^1$. *Then*

$$Z^A(t) = \frac{1}{2\pi} \int d\omega e^{-i\omega t} Q^R(\omega, t)\widehat{u}(\omega),$$

where

$$Q^R(\omega, t) = \sum_n e^{-i2\pi\Omega t} \widehat{H}^R(\omega + 2\pi\Omega).$$

PROOF. The condition $\widehat{H}^R(\omega) = O(|\omega|^{-1-\delta})$ guarantees that Q^R is well defined, and, together with the condition $\widehat{u}(\omega) \in L^1$, it enables us to exchange summation and integration in (1.16). □

For $R_\alpha \in \mathscr{R}(L)$, the condition on $\widehat{H}^R$ is automatically satisfied. The condition $\widehat{u}(\omega) \in L^1$ is satisfied, in particular, in the smooth case.

We have considered algorithms A_{RT} in the absence of noise, proved that they are well defined, and obtained convenient expressions for their regularization and discretization errors. It remains to obtain an expression for the variance of the statistical error. Since all the algorithms we consider are linear, the statistical error is given by

$$\Delta Z^{\sigma}(t) = \sum_n H^R(t - n\Delta t) v_n \Delta t.$$

Using (0.32) to compute variances, we easily get

$$\sigma_Z^2(t) = \sigma_u^2 \sum_n |H^R(t - n\Delta t)|^2 \Delta t^2. \tag{1.18}$$

The next proposition gives a convenient expression for the variance of the statistical error.

PROPOSITION 1.3. *If $\widehat{H}^R(\omega)$ belongs to $L^1 \cap L^2$ and has bounded variation, then*

$$\sigma_Z^2(t) = \frac{1}{2\pi} \sigma_u^2 \Delta t \sum_n e^{-i2\pi\Omega t} \int d\omega \widehat{H}^R(\omega) \widehat{H}^{R^*}(\omega - 2\pi\Omega). \tag{1.19}$$

PROOF. First of all, we remark that if $\widehat{H}^R(\omega) \in L^1$ is a function of bounded variation, then $H^R(s) = O(|s|^{-1})$ as $|s| \to \infty$. Therefore, the series (1.18) converges absolutely and uniformly and $\sigma_Z^2(t)$ is well defined by this series.

Since $\sum_n$ means $\lim_{N\to\infty} \sum_{n=-N}^{N}$, we can rewrite (1.18) in the form

$$\sigma_Z^2(t) = \frac{\sigma_u^2 \Delta t^2}{(2\pi)^2} \lim_{N\to\infty} \int d\omega e^{-i\omega t} \widehat{H}^R(\omega)$$
$$\times \int d\omega' e^{i\omega' t} \widehat{H}^{R^*}(\omega') \frac{\sin((\omega - \omega')\Delta t(N + 1/2))}{\sin(\frac{1}{2}(\omega - \omega')\Delta t)}.$$

Since $\widehat{H}^R(\omega)$ belongs to L^1 and has bounded variation, the same holds for $\widehat{H}^{R^*}(\omega')e^{i\omega' t}$, and, by the Hardy lemma **[8]**, the series

$$\sum_n \widehat{H}^{R^*}(\omega' + 2n\Omega) e^{i(\omega' + 2n\Omega)t}$$

converges absolutely and uniformly with respect to ω' (and, of course, with respect to t as well), and defines a function $h_t^*(\omega')$ of bounded variation with period 2Ω. Let us transform the last integral in the expression for $\sigma_Z^2(t)$ to the form

$$\sum_n \int_{-\Omega}^{\Omega} d\omega' \widehat{H}^{R^*}(\omega' + 2\pi\Omega) e^{i(\omega' + 2n\Omega)} \frac{\sin((\omega - \omega')\Delta t(N + 1/2))}{\sin(\frac{1}{2}(\omega - \omega')\Delta t)}.$$

By the Hardy lemma and the well-known theorem **[15]** we can exchange summation and integration in the last expression. We obtain

$$\sigma_Z^2(t) = \lim_{n\to\infty} \frac{\sigma_u^2 \Delta t}{2\pi} \int_{-\Omega}^{\Omega} d\omega h_t(\omega) S_N(h_t^*)(\omega),$$

where $h_t(\omega)$ is a 2Ω-periodic function,

$$h_t(\omega) = \sum_n \widehat{H}^R(\omega + 2n\Omega) e^{-i(\omega + 2\pi\Omega)t},$$

and $S_N(h_t^*)(\omega)$ is the Nth partial Fourier sum for the function h_t^*. Any Fourier series can be multiplied term by term by any function of bounded variation, and integrated term by term over any finite interval **[15]**. Since the variation of the function $h_t(\omega)$ over the period is bounded, we get

$$\sigma_Z^2(t) = \frac{\sigma_u^2 \Delta t}{2\pi} \int_{-\Omega}^{\Omega} d\omega h_t(\omega) h_t^*(\omega).$$

Using here the last formula for h_t and exchanging summation and integration, we obtain the desired formula (1.19). □

To obtain (1.19) we had to impose on $\widehat{H}^R(\omega)$ somewhat more restrictive conditions than in previous propositions. The fact that a regularizer belongs to a class of admissible regularizers ($R_\alpha \in \mathscr{R}(L)$) does not guarantee that the regularized kernel has bounded variation. The boundedness can be guaranteed by assuming that a regularizer is piecewise smooth and its first derivative is absolutely integrable. If $\widehat{L}(\omega)$ has a piecewise smooth derivative, the boundedness of the variation of the regularized kernel $\widehat{H}^R(\omega)$ can be guaranteed by certain conditions on the rate of decrease of the regularizer itself and of its first derivative. If all cases that are interesting from the practical point of view these conditions are satisfied and (1.19) holds.

Everywhere below we will assume that the right-hand side u belongs to a class of admissible right-hand sides $\mathscr{U}$ and the regularizer belongs to a class of admissible regularizers, so that Proposition 1.1 and its corollaries hold. In discussing the discretization error we will assume that Proposition 1.2 holds (usually the applicability of Proposition 1.2 is ensured by the smoothness of the right-hand side). Similarly, in analyzing the statistical error we will assume that Proposition 1.3 holds.

§1.3. Regularization error and statistical error

This section is devoted to the analysis of the asymptotic behavior of the discretization error and of the statistical error. In one way or other, this analysis was performed in a series of papers **[2–4]**. The results below are presented not for their novelty, but mostly for completeness; another reason is that we wish to formulate them in a convenient form.

Regularization error depends on a single parameter, namely the regularization parameter α, and, as we will see later, tends to 0 as $\alpha \to 0$. Below we obtain asymptotic expressions for homogeneous, Tikhonov, and Wiener regularizers. All answers are obtained for smooth right-hand sides (so that $\widehat{Z}(\omega)$ decreases sufficiently fast as $|\omega| \to \infty$). The asymptotic behavior of the regularization error for a Tikhonov regularizer easily yields an asymptotic bound that coincides with the corresponding bound from **[3]**. In **[3]**, the bound was obtained for a much wider class of problems, so that to compare it with our answer we must adapt the bound in **[3]** to our case. Let us note that in **[3]** the answer is for a smooth class of right-hand sides, which, however, is somewhat wider than our class.

The behavior of the statistical error depends on three parameters: α, Δt (or $\Omega = \pi/\Delta t$), and σ_u^2; the dependence on σ_u^2 is trivial (see (1.19). The behavior of the statistical error as $\Delta t \to 0$, $\alpha \to 0$, $\sigma_u^2 \to 0$ depends to a large extent on the way the limit is taken. If the noise is small (so that σ_u^2 is, in some sense, much smaller than α and Δt), the statistical error tends to 0. Otherwise the statistical error can tend to infinity. Below this is illustrated with the example of the kernel $\widehat{L}(\omega) = b|\omega|^p$, $p > 0$, and a homogeneous regularizer. In this case the complete analysis of the asymptotic behavior of the statistical error for all possible ways of passing to the limit is presented. All results can be immediately generalized to kernels of the form $\widehat{L}(\omega) = \sum_{i=0}^{I} b_i |\omega|^{p_i}$, and the leading terms in all asymptotic expansions remain the same (ρ should be replaced by $\rho_0 = \max\{\rho_i\}$).

We begin our analysis of the regularization error with the following result.

PROPOSITION 1.4. *Let a kernel L be given, and let $u \in \mathscr{U}(L)$, $R_\alpha \in \mathscr{R}(L)$. If $\widehat{Z}(\omega) \equiv \widehat{L}(\omega)\widehat{u}(\omega) \in L^1$, then as $\alpha \to 0$ the regularization error converges uniformly with respect to t, i.e.,*

$$\Delta Z^R \stackrel{\text{def}}{=} \sup_t |\Delta Z^R(t)| \to 0 \quad \text{as } \alpha \to 0.$$

PROOF. Rewrite (1.15) in the form

$$\Delta Z^R(t) = \frac{1}{2\pi} \int d\omega e^{-i\omega t}(R_\alpha(\omega) - 1)\widehat{Z}(\omega). \tag{1.20}$$

Then

$$\Delta Z^R \leq \frac{1}{2\pi} \int d\omega |R_\alpha(\omega) - 1| \cdot |\widehat{Z}(\omega)|,$$

and the proposition follows from the properties (1.10d), (1.10e). □

Proposition 1.4 guarantees the convergence of the regularization error for a smooth admissible right-hand side $u \in \mathscr{U}_M$. Therefore, the convergence of the algorithm A_{RT} on a smooth class $\{u\} \subset \mathscr{U}_M$ (inside the set $\mathscr{D} \equiv \mathscr{D}_{\overline{\beta}}$) is equivalent to the convergence of the discretization error on the same class (and inside the same set). Let us note that discontinuous functions $Z(t)$ (of the type $\chi_{[a,b]}(t)$) do not satisfy the condition of Proposition 1.4; in this proposition $Z(t)$ should be a continuous function with pointwise continuous first derivative.

Now let us consider the asymptotic behavior of the regularization error for homogeneous regularizes.

PROPOSITION 1.5. *Let $R_\alpha \in \mathscr{R}$ be a homogeneous regularizer, $R_\alpha(\omega) = S(\alpha\omega)$, with $S(\xi)$ satisfying the condition $S(\xi) \in C^{N+1}([-a, a])$, $a > 0$. Let $u \in U_M$, so that, in particular, (1.8) is satisfied:*

$$|\widehat{Z}(\omega)| \leq \widetilde{Z}|\omega|^{-M_Z}, \qquad M_Z \geq 1 + \delta.$$

Then the conditions

$$S^{(i)}(0) = 0, \qquad i = 1, 2, \ldots, k-1, \quad k \leq N$$

$$S^{(k)}(0) \neq 0, \qquad M_Z \geq k + 2 + \delta,$$

imply

$$\Delta Z^R(t) = \frac{i}{k!} S^{(k)}(0) Z^{(k)}(t)\alpha^k + O(\alpha^{k+1}), \qquad \alpha \to 0, \tag{1.21}$$

which implies

$$\Delta Z^R = \frac{1}{k!}|S^{(k)}(0)| \sup_t |Z^{(k)}(t)|\alpha^k + O(\alpha^{k+1}).$$

PROOF. The condition $M_Z \geq k + 2 + \delta$ is a smoothness condition for $Z(t)$: it guarantees the existence of continuous derivatives up to order $k + 1$, which tend to 0 at infinity. This, in turn, guarantees that $\sup_t |Z^{(k)}(t)| < \infty$. Rewrite (1.20) expressing $\Delta Z^R(t)$ as the sum of four terms

$$\Delta Z^R(t) = \sum_{j=1}^{4} \Delta_R^j(t),$$

where

$$\Delta_R^1(t) = \frac{1}{2\pi} \int d\omega e^{-i\omega t} \widehat{Z}(\omega) \frac{(\alpha\omega)^k}{k!} S^{(k)}(0);$$

$$\Delta_R^2(t) = \frac{1}{2\pi} \int_{-a}^{a} d\xi \, (1/\alpha) e^{-i\xi t/\alpha} \widehat{Z}(\xi/\alpha) \left(S(\xi) - 1 - \frac{S^{(k)}(0)}{k!} \xi^k \right);$$

$$\Delta_R^3(t) = \frac{1}{2\pi} \int_{|\xi|>a} d\xi \, (1/\alpha) e^{-i\xi t/\alpha} \widehat{Z}(\xi/\alpha)(S(\xi) - 1);$$

$$\Delta_R^4(t) = \frac{1}{2\pi} \int_{|\xi|>a} d\xi \, (1/\alpha) e^{-i\xi t/\alpha} \widehat{Z}(\xi/\alpha) S^{(k)}(0) \frac{\xi^k}{k!}.$$

The summand $\Delta_R^1(t)$ gives the principal contribution to (1.21), and the absolute values of other summands should be estimated from above. To estimate $\Delta_R^2(t)$, we use the integral form of the remainder in the Taylor formula **[18]**

$$S(\xi) - 1 - \frac{S^{(k)}(0)}{k!} \xi^k = \frac{1}{k!} \int_0^{\xi} (\xi - \eta)^k S^{(k+1)}(\eta) d\eta.$$

Substituting the expression for $\Delta_R^2(t)$ and estimating the absolute value, we obtain

$$|\Delta_R^2(t)| \leq \frac{1}{2\pi} \cdot \frac{1}{k!} \sup_{[-a,a]} |S^{(k+1)}(\eta)| \, \|\widehat{Z}(\omega)\omega^{k+1}\|_{L^1} \, \alpha^{k+1},$$

where $\|\widehat{Z}(\omega)\omega^{k+1}\|_{L^1} \stackrel{\text{def}}{=} \int d\omega |\widehat{Z}(\omega)\omega^{k+1}| < \infty$. To estimate $\Delta_R^3(t)$, we use (1.8):

$$|\Delta_R^3(t)| \leq \frac{1}{2\pi} \frac{1}{\alpha} \int_{|\xi|>a} d\xi \widetilde{Z}(|\xi|/\alpha)^{-M_Z} (\widetilde{S} + 1) \leq \frac{\widetilde{S} + 1}{2\pi} \widetilde{Z} \frac{2}{M_Z - 1} a^{-M_Z+1} \alpha^{M_Z-1}$$

(recall that $|S(\xi)| \leq \widetilde{S}$). Since $M_Z \geq k + 2 + \delta$, we have $|\Delta_R^3(t)| \leq C\widetilde{Z}\alpha^{k+1}$. The term $\Delta_R^4(t)$ is estimated similarly to $\Delta_R^3(t)$. □

REMARK 1. If all derivatives of S vanish at $\xi = 0$ and $M_Z \geq N + 2 + \delta$, then instead of (1.21) we evidently have

$$|\Delta^R(t)| \leq O(\alpha^{N+1}).$$

REMARK 2. Let $S(\xi) \in C^{\infty}([-a, a])$ and all derivatives vanish at $\xi = 0$; then the asymptotic behavior of the regularization error is determined by the smoothness of the right-hand sides (i.e., essentially by the parameter M_Z). If we assume that S

is regular near the origin (i.e., $S(\xi) \equiv 1$ in a neighborhood of the origin), simple estimates (similar to those used in the proof of Proposition 1.5) give

$$|\Delta Z^R(t)| \leq \Delta Z^R \leq O(\alpha^{M_Z-1}). \tag{1.22}$$

The last estimate holds, in particular, for a rectangular window, i.e., for a regularizer of the form

$$R_\alpha(\omega) = \begin{cases} 1 & \text{for } |\omega| \leq \Omega, \\ 0 & \text{for } |\omega| > \Omega. \end{cases}$$

Since under the assumptions $\widehat{Z}(\omega) \geq 0$ and $\widehat{Z}(\omega) = \widetilde{Z}|\omega|^{-M_Z}$ for $|\omega| \geq 1$, we have (for sufficiently small α)

$$\Delta^R(0) = \frac{\widetilde{Z}}{2\pi} \int_{|\xi|>a} d\xi |\xi|^{-M_Z}(S(\xi) - 1)\alpha^{M_Z-1};$$

in the general case the estimate (1.22) is sharp on the entire class of right-hand sides we are considering.

Proposition 1.5 together with the above two remarks solves the problem about the behavior, as $\alpha \to 0$, of the regularization error for a homogeneous regularizer.

Let us consider now generalized Tikhonov regularizers (1.13).

PROPOSITION 1.6. *Let our regularizer be a generalized Tikhonov regularizer. Let $u \in \mathscr{U}_M$ and M_Z in* (1.8) *satisfy the condition $M_Z \geq 2q_0 + 1 + \delta$, where q_0 is the degree of the quasipolynomial Q in the regularizer. Then*

$$\Delta Z^R(t) = -\frac{1}{2\pi} \int d\omega e^{-i\omega t} \widehat{Z}(\omega) Q(\omega/\omega_R)\alpha_T + O(\alpha_T^2), \qquad \alpha_T \to 0,$$

so that

$$\Delta Z^R = C(Z)\alpha_T + O(\alpha_T^2) \qquad \alpha_T \to 0; \tag{1.23}$$

the constant $C(Z)$ in (1.23) *depends on $Z(t)$ and satisfies*

$$0 \leq C(Z) \leq \frac{1}{2\pi} \int d\omega |\widehat{Z}(\omega)| \cdot |Q(\omega/\omega_R)| < \infty,$$

and $C(Z) > 0$ for some Z.

PROOF. By the conditions $C_0 = 1$, $q_0 > \cdots > q_I \geq 0$ imposed on the quasipolynomial Q, we have $\alpha_T Q(\omega/\omega_R) > -1/2$ for a sufficiently small α_T. Hence

$$\Delta Z^R(t) = -\frac{1}{2\pi} \int d\omega\, e^{-i\omega t} \widehat{Z}(\omega) Q(\omega/\omega_k)\alpha_T + \frac{1}{2\pi} \int d\omega\, e^{-i\omega t} \widehat{Z}(\omega) \frac{\alpha_T^2 Q^2(\omega/\omega_k)}{1 + \alpha_T Q(\omega/\omega_k)},$$

and the second term can be easily estimated using the condition $M_Z \geq 2q_0 + 1 + \delta$ and taking into account that $1 + \alpha_T Q(\omega/\omega_R) \geq 1/2$ for a sufficiently small α_T. □

Let us note that in the case $Q(\xi) = |\xi|^{q_0}$ (i.e., when $C_1 = \cdots = C_I = 0$) a Tikhonov regularizer becomes homogeneous after the substitution $\alpha_T \longrightarrow (\alpha\omega_0)^{q_0}$. If $q_0 = 2m$, $m = 1, 2, \ldots$, the corresponding homogeneous regularizer is smooth and the order of the nonvanishing (at the origin) derivative is $q_0 = 2m$. In this case the conditions of Proposition 1.5 are satisfied (provided that $M_Z \geq q_0 + 2 + \delta$), and instead of (1.23) we have

$$\Delta Z^R = C\alpha_T + O(\alpha_T^{1+1/q_0}).$$

The leading term in the asymptotic expansion coincides, of course, with that in (1.23). The case $q_0 = 2(\overline{p} + r)$, where $\overline{p}$ is the kernel growth indicator, admits a comparison with **[3]**. In both cases the estimate is $\Delta Z^R = O(\alpha_T)$. In our case it holds for $M_Z \geq 4(\overline{p} + r) + 1 + \delta$, and in **[3]** for $M_Z \geq 2\overline{p} + 1 + \delta$, i.e., in a somewhat wider class.

In conclusion, let us consider the Wiener regularizer (0.13).

PROPOSITION 1.7. *Let our regularizer be a Wiener regularizer. Let $u \in \mathscr{U}_M$, and let* (1.8) *be satisfied with some $M_Z \geq 1 + \delta$. Then*

$$|\Delta Z^R(t)| \leq \Delta Z^R \leq O[((\log(1/\alpha))^{1/q})^{-M_Z+1}]. \tag{1.24}$$

The estimate (1.24) *is sharp on the entire class of right-hand sides.*

PROOF. One can easily see that

$$\Delta Z^R \leq \frac{1}{2\pi} \int d\omega\, |\widehat{Z}(\omega)| \frac{\alpha|\omega/\omega_k|^h \exp(|\omega/\omega_k|^q)}{1 + \alpha|\omega/\omega_R|^h \exp(|\omega\omega_R|^q)}.$$

To estimate the last expression we divide the integration region into two parts

$$|\omega| \leq a\omega_R(\log(1/\alpha))^{1/q} \quad \text{and} \quad |\omega| \geq a\omega_R(\log(1/\alpha))^{1/q},$$

where a is an arbitrary number in $(0, 1)$. Denote the resulting integrals by Δ_R^1 and Δ_R^2, and estimate each of them separately. We have

$$\begin{aligned}
\Delta_R^1 &\leq \frac{1}{2\pi} a^h (\log(1/\alpha))^{h/q} \alpha^{1-a^q} \int_{|\omega| \leq a\omega_R(\log(1/\alpha))^{1/q}} d\omega\, |\widehat{Z}(\omega)| \\
&\leq C \parallel \widehat{Z} \parallel_{L^1} (\log(1/\alpha))^{h/q} \alpha^{(1-a^q)}, \\
\Delta_R^2 &\leq \frac{1}{2\pi} \int_{|\omega| \geq a\omega_R(\log(1/\alpha))^{1/q}} d\omega\, |\widehat{Z}(\omega)| \leq \frac{\widetilde{Z}}{2\pi} \int_{a\omega_R(\log(1/\alpha))^{1/q}}^{\infty} d\omega\, |\omega|^{-M_Z} \\
&= \frac{\widetilde{Z}}{2\pi} \frac{2}{M_Z - 1} (a\omega_R)^{-M_Z+1} ((\log(1/\alpha))^{1/q})^{-M_Z+1}.
\end{aligned}$$

It is clear that for small α we have

$$\Delta Z^R = \Delta_R^1 + \Delta_R^2 \leq C\widetilde{Z}((\log(1/\alpha))^{1/q})^{-M_Z+1}.$$

The estimate (1.24) is proved. Let us prove now that this estimate is sharp when considered on the entire class. If $\widehat{Z}(\omega) \geq 0$ and $\widehat{Z}(\omega) = \widetilde{Z}|\omega|^{-M_Z}$ ($\widetilde{Z} > 0$) for $|\omega| \geq 1$, then for sufficiently small α we have

$$\Delta Z^R \geq |\Delta Z^R(0)| \geq \frac{1}{2\pi} \int_{|\omega|>\omega_R(\log(1/\alpha))^{1/q}} d\omega\, \widehat{Z}(\omega) \frac{\alpha|\omega/\omega_R|^h \exp(|\omega/\omega_R|)^q}{1+\alpha|\omega/\omega_R|^h \exp(|\omega/\omega_R|)^q}$$

$$\geq \frac{1}{2\pi}\widetilde{Z}\left[1+\frac{1}{(\log(1/\alpha))^{h/q}}\right]^{-1} \cdot 2\int_{\omega_R(\log(1/2\pi))^{1/q}}^{\infty} d\omega\, \omega^{-M_Z}.$$

Therefore,

$$\Delta Z^R \geq C\widetilde{Z}((\log(1/\alpha))^{1/q})^{-M_Z+1} \qquad (C > 0),$$

and the sharpness is proved. □

REMARK. A similar result holds for a regularizer (1.14) of Wiener type with q replaced by the degree q_0 of the quasipolynomial Q.

Now let us consider the statistical error, which we assume to be defined by (1.19). Note that if we use a compactly supported regularization (i.e., the Nyquist condition is satisfied), then (1.19) can be simplified to

$$\sigma_Z^2(t) = \frac{1}{2\pi}\sigma_u^2 \Delta t \int_{-\sigma}^{\sigma} d\omega\, \widehat{H}^R(\omega)\widehat{H}^{R*}(\omega).$$

Now let $\widehat{L}(\omega) = b|\omega|^p$, $p \geq 0$, and assume that the regularizer is homogeneous. Formula (1.19) implies

(1.25)
$$\sigma_Z^2(t) = \frac{1}{2}|b|^2\sigma_u^2\Omega^{-1}\alpha^{-2p-1}\sum_k e^{-i2k\Omega t}\int d\xi\, |\xi|^p|2k\varepsilon_S - \xi|^p S(\xi)S(2k\varepsilon_S - \xi),$$

where $\varepsilon_S = \alpha\Omega$. Sometimes it will be more convenient to use another expression for $\sigma_Z^2(t)$, which is given by the following proposition. In it, we must strengthen our assumptions about the regularizer.

PROPOSITION 1.8. *Let* $\widehat{L}(\omega) = b|\omega|^p$, $p \geq 0$. *Let a regularizer* $R_\alpha \in \mathscr{R}$ *be homogeneous,* $R_\alpha(\omega) = S(\alpha\omega)$, *and* $\operatorname{Var}_{\mathbb{R}} |\omega|^p S(\omega) < \infty$. *Then*

$$(1.26) \qquad \sigma_Z^2(t) = \frac{1}{2}|b|^2\sigma_u^2\Omega^{-1}\alpha^{-2p-1} \cdot \frac{1}{2\varepsilon_S}\sum_k \left[\int d\xi\, |\xi|^p S(\xi) e^{i\pi(k-\tau)/\varepsilon_S}\right]^2,$$

$\varepsilon_S = \alpha\Omega$, $\tau = \{t/\Delta t\}$, $\{\cdot\}$ *being the symbol of the fractional part.*

PROOF. According to (1.25), let us consider the expression

$$A(t, \varepsilon_S) = \sum_k e^{-i2\pi k\tau}\int d\xi\, |\xi|^p|2k\varepsilon_S - \xi|^p S(\xi)S(2k\varepsilon_S - \xi).$$

and perform the following transformations (this is possible due to the assumptions of the proposition):

1) on the right-hand side, exchange the order of summation and integration;
2) apply the Poisson summation formula to the resulting expresssion;
3) once again exchange the order of summation and integration.

We obtain (1.26). □

Formulas (1.25) and (1.26) complement each other and together answer the question about the behavior of the statistical error in the case under consideration. Formula (1.25) can be used when $\alpha\Omega = \varepsilon_S \geq \underline{\varepsilon_S}$, and (1.26) when $\alpha\Omega = \varepsilon_S \leq \overline{\varepsilon_S}$.

PROPOSITION 1.9. *Let the condition of Proposition* 1.6 *be satisfied. Denote* $\beta = \frac{1}{2}|b|^2\sigma_u^2\Omega^{-1}\alpha^{-2p-1}$. *Then*:

1) *As* $\varepsilon_S \to \infty$,

$$\sigma_Z^2(t) = \beta\left(\int d\xi\, |\xi|^{2p} S(\xi)S(-\xi) + O(\varepsilon_S^{-\delta})\right).$$

2) *If* $\underline{\varepsilon_S} \leq \varepsilon_S \leq \overline{\varepsilon_S}$, $\underline{\varepsilon_S}, \overline{\varepsilon_S} = \text{const}$, *then*

$$\sigma_Z^2(t) = \beta A(t, \varepsilon_S), \quad \text{where } |A(t,\varepsilon_S)| \leq C_1\varepsilon_S^{-1} + C_2\varepsilon_S.$$

If $\varepsilon_S = \text{const}$, *we have* $\sigma_Z^2 = \beta C_3$, *and* $C_3 \neq 0$ *in the general case.*

3) *If* $\varepsilon_S \to 0$, *then*

$$\sigma_Z^2(t) = \beta\left((1/\tau)^2 + (1-\tau)^{-2} + O(1)\right) O(\varepsilon_S)$$

for $\tau = \{t/\Delta t\} \neq 0$, *i.e., for* $t \neq t_n$, *and*

$$\sigma_Z^2(t) = \beta\left(\frac{1}{\varepsilon_S}\frac{1}{2}\left[\int d\xi\, |\xi|^p S(\xi)\right]^2 + O(\varepsilon_S)\right)$$

for $\tau = 0$.

In the general case

$$\sigma_Z^2(t) = \beta\left(\frac{1}{\varepsilon_S}\frac{1}{2}\left[\int d\xi\, |\xi|^p S(\xi)\right]^2 + O(\varepsilon_S)\right).$$

All O-*estimates are uniform with respect to the parameters* σ_u, Ω, α *and with respect to* t. *Moreover, these estimates, as well as the constants* C_1, C_2, C_3, *can be explicitly computed*

PROOF. 1) The term with $k = 0$ in (1.25) gives the leading term in the asymptotic expansion. Next, we must estimate the expression

$$\sum_{k\neq 0}\int d\xi\, |\xi|^p|S(\xi)|\; |2k\varepsilon_S - \xi|^p|S(2k\varepsilon_S - \xi)|.$$

An accurate estimate using the properties

$$|\xi|^p|S(\xi)| \leq C_H, \qquad |\xi|^p|S(\xi)| \leq C_H'|\xi|^{-1-\delta}$$

yields the desired bound (with δ equal to δ in the last inequality).

2) Using (1.26), one easily obtains the following bound for A:

$$|A(t,\varepsilon_S)| = \left| \frac{1}{2\varepsilon_S} \left(\sum_{k=0,1} + \sum_{k\neq 0,1} \right) \left(\int d\xi\, |\xi|^p S(\xi) e^{i\pi(k-\tau)/\varepsilon_S} \right)^2 \right|$$

$$\leq \frac{1}{\varepsilon_S} \left(\int d\xi\, |\xi|^p |S(\xi)| \right)^2 + \left| \frac{1}{2\varepsilon_S} \sum_{k\neq 0,1} \left(\int d\xi\, |\xi|^p S(\xi) e^{i\pi(k-\tau)/\varepsilon_S} \right)^2 \right|.$$

Integration by parts yields

$$\left| \int d\xi\, |\xi|^p S(\xi) e^{i\pi(k-\tau)/\varepsilon_S} \right| \leq \frac{1}{\pi} \frac{\varepsilon_S}{|k-\tau|} \operatorname*{var}_{\mathbb{R}}(|\xi|^p S(\xi)), \tag{1.27}$$

and the second summand can be bounded from above as follows $(0 \leq \tau < 1)$:

$$\leq \frac{1}{\pi} \zeta(2) \operatorname*{var}_{\mathbb{R}}(|\xi|^p S(\xi)) \varepsilon_S,$$

where ζ is the Riemann zeta-function. This estimate for $|A(t,\varepsilon_S)|$ also implies the second assertion in 2).

3) Using (1.26) again, integrating by parts (see (1.27)), and separating terms with $k = 0, 1$, we obtain the first assertion for $\tau \neq 0$. If $\tau = 0$, we must first separate the term with $k = 0$:

$$\beta \frac{1}{2\xi_S} \left(\int d\xi\, |\xi|^p S(\xi) \right)^2,$$

and integrate by parts in all other terms. As a result, we obtain the second assertion. The last assertion in 3) follows from the first and the second. □

Chapter 2. Discretization Error

In this chapter we analyze the discretization error, thus concluding the complete study of the algorithm A_{RT} begun in the previous chapter. In our interpretation, the analysis of the discretization error can be reduced to the error analysis of a quadrature formula in the case when the integrand depends on the quadrature step (and is singular as $\Delta t \to 0$). Therefore, this chapter may be of independent interest.

In this chapter we assume that a regularizer belong to an admissible class, $R_\alpha \in \mathscr{R}$, and a right-hand side belongs to a class of admissible smooth right-hand sides, $u \in \mathscr{U}_M$. These assumptions guarantee that we can use Propositions 1.1 and 1.2, and the discretization error satisfies (1.17). The discretization error depends on parameters Δt (or Ω) and α. The behavior of the error as $\Delta t \to 0$, $\alpha \to 0$, depends not only on the kernel, the regularizer, and the right-hand side, but also on the path used in passing to the limit (a path in $\mathscr{D}_{(\Delta t,\alpha)}$). Choosing a class of kernels, a class of regularizers, and the region $\mathscr{D}_{(\Delta t,\alpha)}$ of admissible values of parameters, we can analyze the behavior of the error. The general structure of this chapter is such that by imposing stronger restrictions on classes of kernels and of regularizers we obtain more precise results for wider regions.

In §2.1 we consider kernels $L \in \mathscr{L}(\Lambda)$ of arbitrary growth, and admissible regularizers $R_\alpha \in \mathscr{R}(\Lambda)$. We obtain some estimates for compactly supported (i.e. satisfying the Nyquist condition) and almost compactly supported regularizations $\operatorname{Reg}(R_\alpha, \mathscr{D})$. These estimates prove the convergence of the error (in a smooth class of right-hand sides in $\mathscr{D}$). It is proved also that for a fast-growing kernel the essential violation of the Nyquist condition leads to the divergence of the regularization error.

In §2.2 we consider slow-growing kernels $L \in \mathscr{L}(\overline{p})$ and prove sufficient conditions (on regularizers) that ensure the convergence of the discretization error. We also present estimates for the so-called quasifinite regularizations and homogeneous regularizers.

In §2.3 we consider kernels of polynomial growth $L \in \mathscr{L}(\rho^{\pm})$ and monotone quasifinite regularizations. Necessary and sufficient conditions for convergence are obtained. As an example, we consider the Tikhonov regularizer and the Wiener regularizer.

The case of polynomial kernels $L \in \mathscr{L}_0(\rho_0^{\pm})$ and smooth regularizers is considered in §2.4. Most interesting here are smooth homogeneous regularizers. This problem admits a complete solution, i.e., the description of the error behavior for an arbitrary limiting path as $\Delta t \to 0$, $\alpha \to 0$. For the high-resolution case a convergence criterion for the discretization error is given.

Finally, in §2.5 we use the results of §2.4 to construct a convergent (in $\mathscr{D}_{\overline{\beta}} = [0, \Delta t_0] \times [0, \alpha_0]$) quadrature formula. This formula defines a new algorithm that converges for any passage to the limit as $\Delta t \to 0$, $\alpha \to 0$. The construction of this new quadrature formula is equivalent to the renormalization procedure in quantum field theory.

§2.1. Discretization error for kernels of arbitrary growth

We consider $L \in \mathscr{L}(\Lambda)$, $R_\alpha \in \mathscr{R}(\Lambda)$, $u \in \mathscr{U}_M(\Lambda)$. According to (1.17), the discretization error is of the form

$$\Delta Z^T(t) = \Delta D^a(t) + \Delta D^\infty(t),$$

$$\Delta D^a(t) = \frac{1}{2\pi}\sum_{n\neq 0} e^{-i2\pi\Omega t}\int_{-a\Omega}^{a\Omega} d\omega\, e^{-i\omega t}\widehat{H}^R(\omega + 2n\Omega)\widehat{u}(\omega), \tag{2.1}$$

$$\Delta D^\infty(t) = \frac{1}{2\pi}\sum_{n\neq 0} e^{-i2n\Omega t}\int_{|\omega|\geq a\Omega} d\omega\, e^{-i\omega t}\widehat{H}^R(\omega + 2n\Omega)\widehat{u}(\omega),$$

where $0 < a \leq 1$.

PROPOSITION 2.1. *Let $L \in \mathscr{L}(\Lambda)$, $R_\alpha \in \mathscr{R}(\Lambda)$, $u \in \mathscr{U}_M(\Lambda)$, and $M_Z \geq 2 + \delta$. Then for any $\widetilde{H}(\alpha)$ satisfying the condition*

$$|\widehat{H}^R(\omega)| \leq \widetilde{H}(\alpha)|\omega|^{-1-\sigma}, \qquad \sigma > 0, \tag{2.2}$$

we have

$$|\Delta D^\infty(t)| \leq C_1\widetilde{Z}\frac{\widetilde{H}(\alpha)}{\Lambda(a\Omega)}\Omega^{-M_Z-\sigma} + C_2\widetilde{Z}\Omega^{M_Z+1}, \tag{2.3}$$

where $\widetilde{Z}$ is the constant from (1.8) for $\widehat{Z}(\omega)$, and the constants C_1, C_2 do not depend on α, Ω, t and can be explicitly computed.

PROOF. First of all, let us remark that the existence of $\widetilde{H}(\alpha)$ follows from (1.10c). It suffice to prove (2.3) for

$$\Delta D_{\pm}^{\infty}(t) = \frac{1}{2\pi}\sum_{n=1}^{\infty} e^{\mp i2n\Omega t}\int_{|\omega|\geq a\Omega} d\omega\, e^{-i\omega t}\widehat{H}^R(\omega \pm 2n\Omega)\widehat{u}(\omega).$$

Let us consider ΔD_+^{∞}. It is clear that

$$|\Delta D_+^{\infty}(t)| \leq \frac{1}{2\pi}\sum_{n=1}^{\infty} I_n, \qquad I_n = \int_{|\omega|\geq a\Omega} d\omega\, |\widehat{H}^R(\omega + 2n\Omega)|\cdot|\widehat{u}(\omega)|.$$

To estimate I_n, we divide the integration region into four intervals: $(-\infty, -3n\Omega]$, $[-3n\Omega, -n\Omega]$, $[-n\Omega, -a\Omega]$, $[a\Omega, +\infty)$. Denote the corresponding integrals by I_n^p, $p = 1, \ldots, 4$. Using the properties of the function $\Lambda(\omega)$, formula (1.8), and condition (2.2), we have

$$I_n^1 \leq C\widetilde{Z}\frac{\widetilde{H}(\alpha)}{\Lambda(a\Omega)} n^{-M_Z-\sigma}\Omega^{-M_Z-\sigma}, \qquad I_n^2 \leq C\widetilde{Z}n^{-M_Z+1}\Omega^{-M_Z+1},$$

$$I_n^3 \leq C\widetilde{Z}\frac{\widetilde{H}(\alpha)}{\Lambda(a\Omega)} n^{-1-\sigma}\Omega^{-M_Z-\sigma}, \qquad I_n^4 \leq C\widetilde{Z}\frac{\widetilde{H}(\alpha)}{\Lambda(a\Omega)} n^{-M_Z-\sigma}\Omega^{-M_Z-\sigma}.$$

In each inequality, C is an explicitly computable constant independent of α, Ω, and t, different in different inequalities. Adding these estimates together and summing over n (using the condition $M_Z \geq 2+\delta$), we obtain the desired assertion. □

Next we prove a result about kernels that decrease at infinity.

PROPOSITION 2.2. *Under the assumption of Proposition* 2.1, *if* $\widehat{L}(\omega) = O(|\omega|^{-1-\delta})$, $|\omega| \to \infty$, *then*

$$|\Delta Z^T(t)| \leq \Delta Z^T \leq C_1\widetilde{Z}\Omega^{-M_Z+1} + C_2\|\widehat{u}\|_{L^1}\Omega^{-1-\delta}. \tag{2.4}$$

Therefore, the discretization error converges rapidly and uniformly inside any region $\mathcal{D}_{\overline{\beta}}$.

PROOF. Since $|R_\alpha(\omega)| \leq \widetilde{R}$, the condition (2.2) is satisfied with $\widetilde{H}(\alpha) \equiv \widetilde{H} =$ const. Therefore, to prove (2.4) it suffices to estimate ΔD^a (2.1). If $\widehat{L}(\omega) \leq \widetilde{L}|\omega|^{-1-\delta}$ for sufficiently large ω, then

$$\begin{aligned}|\Delta D^a(t)| &\leq \frac{1}{2\pi}\sum_{n\neq 0}\widetilde{L}\widetilde{R}(|2n-1|\Omega)^{-1-\delta}\int d\omega\,|\widehat{u}(\omega)| \\ &\leq \frac{1}{2\pi}\widetilde{L}\widetilde{R}\cdot\zeta(1+\delta)\|\widehat{u}\|_{L^1}\Omega^{-1-\delta}\end{aligned}$$

for sufficiently large Ω. □

Proposition 2.2 shows that in the analysis of the discretization error, terms of order $|\omega|^{-1-\sigma}$ in the kernel can be ignored, because they do not influence the convergence.

Proposition 2.1 implies the following result.

THEOREM 2.1. *Let* $L \in \mathcal{L}(\Lambda)$, $R_\alpha \in \mathcal{R}(\Lambda)$, $u \in \mathcal{U}_M(\Lambda)$, *and* $M_Z \geq 2+\delta$. *Let a regularization* $\operatorname{Reg}(R_\alpha, \mathcal{D})$ *be compactly supported, i.e., for any* $(\Delta t, \alpha) \in \mathcal{D}$

the Nyquist condition $R_\alpha(\omega) = 0$, $|\omega| \geq \Omega$, is satisfied. Then the discretization error satisfies

$$|\Delta Z^T(t)| \leq C\widetilde{Z}\Omega^{-M_Z+1}.$$

Therefore, the discretization error converges rapidly and uniformly on the class $\mathscr{U}_M$ inside the set $\mathscr{D}$.

PROOF. Take $a = 1$ in (2.3). The Nyquist condition gives the estimate $|\widehat{H}^R(\omega)| \leq \widetilde{R}\Lambda(\Omega)\Omega^{1+\sigma}|\omega|^{-1-\sigma}$. Hence

$$\widetilde{H}(\alpha) \leq \widetilde{R}\Lambda(\Omega)\Omega^{1+\sigma}, \qquad \frac{\widetilde{H}(\alpha)}{\Lambda(\Omega)}\Omega^{-M_Z-\sigma} \leq C\Omega^{-M_Z+1}.$$

Therefore in this case (2.3) implies $|\Delta D^\infty(t)| \leq C\widetilde{Z}\Omega^{-M_Z+1}$. Turning to $\Delta D^a(t)$, we have that for $a = 1$ the Nyquist condition implies $\Delta D^a(t) \equiv 0$. □

So, Theorem 2.1 says that the Nyquist condition is sufficient for the rapid uniform convergence of the discretization error. By the results of the previous chapter, this implies the convergence of the corresponding algorithm (including high-resolution RT-algorithms). A generalization of previous results is given by the following proposition.

PROPOSITION 2.3. *Let $L \in \mathscr{L}(\Lambda)$, $R_\alpha \in \mathscr{R}(\Lambda)$, $u \in \mathscr{U}_M(\Lambda)$, and $M_Z \geq 2+\delta$. Let a regularization satisfy the condition*

$$|\widehat{H}^R(\omega)| \leq C_H|\omega|^{-1-\sigma}, \qquad |\omega| \geq \Omega, \tag{2.5}$$

for each $(\Delta t, \alpha) \in \mathscr{D}$, where C_H does not depend on α and Ω, and $\sigma > 0$. Then for the discretization error the following estimate holds:

$$|\Delta Z^T(t)| \leq C_1\widetilde{Z}\Omega^{-M_Z+1} + C_2\|\widehat{u}\|_{L^1}\Omega^{-1-\sigma}. \tag{2.6}$$

The discretization error converges rapidly and uniformly on the class $\mathscr{U}_M$ inside $\mathscr{D}$.

PROOF. Again, let $a = 1$. The term ΔD^∞ is estimated in the same way as in the proof of Theorem 2.1. However, now $\Delta D^a(t) \not\equiv 0$ and needs to be estimated. We have

$$\begin{aligned} |\Delta D^{a=1}(t)| &\leq \frac{1}{2\pi}\sum_{n\neq 0} C_H(n\Omega)^{-1-\sigma}\int d\omega\, |\widehat{u}(\omega)| \\ &\leq \frac{1}{2\pi}C_H \cdot 2\zeta(1+\sigma)\|\widehat{u}\|_{L^1}\Omega^{-1-\sigma} = C_2\|\widehat{u}\|_{L^1}\Omega^{-1-\sigma}. \end{aligned}$$ □

Let us remark that (2.5) is a generalization of the Nyquist condition. Proposition 2.3 has the following corollary.

COROLLARY. *If $|\overline{\beta}| \to 0$ along the line $\Delta t = 0$, then the discretization error converges.*

PROOF. We must prove that $\Delta Z^T \to 0$ when first $\Delta t \to 0$ and then $\alpha \to 0$. For a fixed α, the condition (1.10c) shows that (2.5) is satisfied starting from some Ω. Then (2.6) implies that for the inner limit we have

$$\lim_{\substack{\Omega\to 0\\ \alpha=\text{const}}} \Delta Z^T = 0.$$ □

The last result is trivial, since the only thing it tells us is that the trapezoid quadrature formula converges (recall that the discretization error is the error of the trapezoid quadrature formula). If $\Delta t \to 0$ and $\alpha \to 0$ simultaneously (along some path), this argument does not apply, since, as we have already remarked, the integrand depends on Δt and becomes singular as $\Delta t \to 0$. Condition (2.5) is a restriction on the set of admissible regions $\mathscr{D} \equiv \mathscr{D}_{(\Delta t,\alpha)}$. It can be interpreted as follows. If $\Delta t \to 0$ $(\Omega \to \infty)$ and $\alpha \to 0$ simultaneously, then the discretization error converges if $\alpha \to 0$ not too rapidly compared to Δt. Indeed, according to (1.10c), for any α there exists ω_α such that $|\widehat{H}^R(\omega)| \le C_H |\omega|^{-1-\sigma}$ for $|\omega| \ge \omega_\alpha$. By (1.10e), $\omega_\alpha \to \infty$ as $\alpha \to 0$. For (2.5) to be satisfied as $\Delta t \to 0$, $\alpha \to 0$, the parameters should satisfy the condition $\Omega \equiv 2\pi/\Delta t \ge \omega_\alpha$. For example, in the case of a rectangular window (more generally, for any homogeneous regularizer with $\operatorname{supp} S \subset [-1,1]$) the Nyquist condition is satisfied for $\alpha \ge 1/\Omega$.

Proposition 2.3 shows that if the regularizer extends beyond the Nyquist interval (i.e., $R_\alpha(\omega) \not\equiv 0$ for $|\omega| > \Omega$), the discretization error can still converge. However, the extension beyond the Nyquist interval that is allowed by (2.5) is rather small. The next example shows that for kernels with fast growth the Nyquist condition cannot be weakened significantly. Let

$$\widehat{L} = e^{\omega^2}, \qquad \widehat{u}(\omega) = e^{-\omega^2}\frac{1}{1+\omega^{2n}}, \quad n = 1, 2, \dots,$$

$$R_\alpha(\omega) = \begin{cases} 1, & |\omega| \le C\Omega, \\ 0, & |\omega| > C\Omega, \end{cases} \qquad 1 < C < 2.$$

One can easily show that in this example the discretization error tends to infinity:

$$\begin{aligned}
\Delta Z^T \ge |\Delta Z^T(0)| &= \frac{1}{2\pi}\sum_{n\neq 0}\int_{-C\Omega}^{C\Omega} d\omega\, \widehat{u}(\omega - 2n\Omega)\widehat{L}(\omega) \\
&\ge \frac{1}{2\pi}\int_{-C\Omega}^{C\Omega} d\omega\, \widehat{u}(\omega - 2\Omega)\widehat{L}(\omega) = \frac{1}{2\pi}\int_{-C\Omega}^{C\Omega} d\omega\, \frac{e^{-(\omega-2\Omega)^2}e^{\omega^2}}{1+(\omega-2\Omega)^{2n}} \\
&\ge \frac{1}{2\pi}[1+((2+C)\Omega)^{2n}]^{-1}\int_{(1+C)\Omega/2}^{C\Omega} d\omega\, e^{\omega^2[1-(1-2\Omega/\omega)^2]} \\
&\ge \frac{1}{2\pi}[1+((2+C)\Omega)^{2n}]^{-1}\cdot\left(\frac{C-1}{2}\right)\cdot\Omega\cdot\exp\left(\frac{1+C}{2}\Omega^2\frac{C-1}{C+1}\frac{4}{C}\right) \to +\infty
\end{aligned}$$

as $\Omega \to +\infty$. Let us remark that since $M_Z = 2n$ in this example, the discretization error diverges for any a priori smoothness.

Therefore, the natural condition that guarantees the convergence of the discretization error in the class of fast-growing kernels is the Nyquist condition (that is, it is natural to consider compactly supported regularizations only).

§2.2. Slow-growing kernels

For slow-growing kernels $L \in \mathscr{L}(\overline{p})$ one can give certain sufficient convergence conditions that are weaker than the Nyquist condition.

Definition 2.1. A regularization $\operatorname{Reg}(R_\alpha, \mathscr{D} \equiv \mathscr{D}_{(\Delta t,\alpha)})$ is called *quasi compactly supported* if $R_\alpha \in \mathscr{R}(\overline{p})$ and there exist positive constants κ, C_R, and σ such that for any $(\Delta t, \alpha) \in \mathscr{D}$ the following condition is satisfied (at least for sufficiently large Ω):

$$(2.7) \qquad |R_\alpha(\omega)| \leq C_R |\omega|^{-\overline{p}-1-\sigma}, \qquad |\omega| \geq \kappa\Omega.$$

Let us remark that for $C_R = 0$ and $\kappa \leq 1$ we have a compactly supported regularization (condition (2.7) becomes the Nyquist condition). For $C_R \neq 0$ and $\kappa \leq 1$ we have a regularization of the type discussed in Proposition 2.3 (condition (2.7) becomes (2.5)).

PROPOSITION 2.4. *Let $L \in \mathscr{L}(\overline{p})$, $u \in \mathscr{U}_M(\overline{p})$, and $M_Z \geq 2+\delta$. Let $R_\alpha \in \mathscr{R}(\overline{p})$, and let $\operatorname{Reg}(R_\alpha, \mathscr{D})$ be a quasi compactly supported regularization. Then for sufficiently large Ω and $(\Delta t, \alpha) \in \mathscr{D}$ we have*

$$(2.8) \qquad |\Delta Z^T(t) - \Delta D^{a,n_0}(t)| \leq C_1 \widetilde{Z} \Omega^{-M_Z+1} + C_2 \|\widehat{u}\|_{L_1} \Omega^{-1-\sigma},$$

where $0 < a \leq 1$, $n_0 \geq \frac{1}{2}(\kappa + a)$, κ and σ are the constants from Definition 2.1, and

$$(2.9) \qquad \Delta D^{a,n_0}(t) = \frac{1}{2\pi} \sum_{\substack{n \neq 0 \\ |n| < n_0}} e^{-i2n\Omega t} \int_{-a\Omega}^{a\Omega} d\omega\, e^{-i\omega t} \widehat{H}^R(\omega + 2n\Omega) \widehat{u}(\omega).$$

Here C_1, C_2 do not depend on α, Ω, t and can be explicitly computed.

PROOF. We assume that $\Omega \geq \omega_L$ (see (1.1)) and that (2.7) holds. Then

$$|\widehat{H}^R(\omega)| \leq \frac{C_R \widetilde{L}}{\omega_L^{\overline{p}}} |\omega|^{-1-\sigma}, \qquad |\omega| \geq \kappa\Omega.$$

$$|\widehat{H}^R(\omega)| \leq \frac{\widetilde{R}\widetilde{L}}{\omega_L^{\overline{p}}} \kappa^{\overline{p}+1+\sigma} |\omega|^{-1-\sigma} \Omega^{\overline{p}+1+\sigma}, \qquad |\omega| < \kappa\Omega.$$

Therefore, for $\widetilde{H}(\alpha)$ in (2.2) we have $\widetilde{H}(\alpha) \leq C\Omega^{\overline{p}+1+\sigma}$, and, according to Proposition 2.1,

$$|\Delta D^\infty(t)| \leq C' \widetilde{Z} \Omega^{\overline{p}+1+\sigma} (a\Omega)^{-\overline{p}} \Omega^{-M_Z-\sigma} + C'' \widetilde{Z} \Omega^{-M_Z+1} = C_1 \widetilde{Z} \Omega^{-M_Z+1}.$$

Now (for the same Ω)

$$\left| \frac{1}{\pi} \sum_{|n| \geq n_0} e^{-i2n\Omega t} \int_{-a\Omega}^{a\Omega} d\omega\, e^{-i\omega t} \widehat{H}^R(\omega + 2n\Omega) \widehat{u}(\omega) \right|$$

$$\geq \frac{1}{2\pi} \cdot \zeta(1+\sigma) \frac{\widetilde{L} C_R}{\omega_L^{\overline{p}}} \|\widehat{u}\|_{L^1} \Omega^{-1-\sigma} = C_2 \|\widehat{u}\|_{L^1} \Omega^{-1-\sigma}. \qquad \square$$

Proposition 2.4 implies the following result.

THEOREM 2.2. *Let the conditions of Proposition 2.4 be satisfied. Then each of the conditions*

1) *there exists a', $0 < a' \leq 1$, such that for any $(\Delta t, \alpha) \in \mathscr{D}$ we have $R_\alpha(\omega) = 0$ for $\omega \in \bigcup_{n \neq 0, |n| \leq [\kappa/2]} [(2n - a')\Omega, (2n + a')\Omega]$ ($[x]$ is the integral part of x);*
2) *$\kappa < 2$*

is sufficient for the rapid uniform convergence of the discretization error on the class $\mathscr{U}_M$ inside the set $\mathscr{D}$.

For $(\Delta t, \alpha) \in \mathscr{D}$ *we have the estimate*

$$|\Delta Z^T(t)| \leq C_1 \widetilde{Z} \Omega^{-M_Z+1} + C_2 \|\widehat{u}\|_{L^1} \Omega^{-1-\sigma}, \tag{2.10}$$

where the constants C_1, C_2 *do not depend on* α, Ω, t *and can be explicitly computed.*

PROOF. When 1) is satisfied, we must take $a = \min(a', 2(1 - \{\kappa/2\})$ in Proposition 2.4 (here $\{x\}$ is the fractional part of x), and $n_0 = [\kappa/2] + 1$. It is evident that in this case $n_0 = \frac{1}{2}(\kappa + a)$, and by condition 1) $\widehat{H}^R(\omega + 2n\Omega) = 0$ for $\omega \in [-a\Omega, a\Omega]$, $n = \pm 1, \dots, \pm(n_0 - 1)$. Now (2.8) implies (2.10) since $\Delta D^{a,n_0}(t) \equiv 0$.

When 2) is satisfied, we take $a = \min(1, 2 - \kappa)$ in Proposition 2.4 and obtain $1 \geq \frac{1}{2}(\kappa + a)$. Therefore we can take $n_0 = 1$, and (2.8) becomes (2.10). □

Let us note that each of the conditions is considerably weaker than the Nyquist condition (and than the condition (2.5)).

Let us mention also the following result.

PROPOSTION 2.5. *Let the condition of Proposition* 2.4 *be satisfied and, in addition, let the kernel satisfy the condition* $\widehat{L}(\omega) = O(|\omega|^{-\delta})$, $|\omega| \to \infty$. *Then*

$$|\Delta Z^T(t)| \leq O(\Omega^{-M_Z+1}) + O(\Omega^{-1-\sigma}) + O(\Omega^{-\delta}), \qquad (\Delta t, \alpha) \in \mathscr{D},$$

with O-estimates that are uniform with respect to α *and* t. *The discretization error converges rapidly and uniformly on the class* $\mathscr{U}_M$ *inside the set* $\mathscr{D}$.

We omit the proof, which follows easily from (2.8). It is useful to compare this result with Proposition 2.2.

Now we consider homogeneous regularizers. It is convenient to rewrite the condition (1.11b) in the form

$$|S(\xi)| \leq \overline{S} |\xi|^{-\overline{p}-1-\sigma}, \qquad \sigma > 0.$$

One can easily see that in this case

$$|R_\alpha(\omega)| \leq \overline{S} \alpha^{-\overline{p}-1-\sigma} |\omega|^{-\overline{p}-1-\sigma},$$

$$|\widehat{H}^R(\omega)| \leq |\widetilde{L} + (\widetilde{L}/\omega_L^{\overline{p}})\omega^{\overline{p}}| \, \overline{S} \, |\omega|^{-\overline{p}-1-\sigma} \alpha^{-\overline{p}-1-\sigma},$$

i.e.,

$$|\widehat{H}^R(\omega)| \leq C \alpha^{-\overline{p}-1-\sigma} |\omega|^{-1-\sigma}. \tag{2.11}$$

It is clear that for a homogeneous regularization to be quasi compactly supported, the condition

$$\alpha^{-\overline{p}-1-\sigma} \Omega^{-(\sigma-\delta)} \leq C, \qquad 0 < \delta < \sigma,$$

must be satisfied for any $(\Delta t, \alpha) \in \mathscr{D}$. Here we can assume $\kappa < 2$ (this is guaranteed by the choice of C_R; see Definition 2.1). By Theorem 2.2, the discretization error converges rapidly and uniformly. However, the requirement for the regularization to be quasi compactly supported is too restrictive in this case. In particular, it excludes high-resolution regularizations (for these regularizations $\alpha\Omega = \varepsilon_S = \text{const}$). To improve the situation we prove the following result.

THEOREM 2.3. *Let* $L \in \mathscr{L}(\overline{p})$, $u \in \mathscr{U}_M(\overline{p})$, *and* $M_Z \geq 2+\delta$. *Let* $R_\alpha \in \mathscr{R}(\overline{p})$ *be a homogeneous regularizer. Let* $\mathscr{D}$ *be a set such that for any* $(\Delta t, \alpha) \in \mathscr{D}$ *the condition*

$$\alpha^{-\overline{p}-1-\sigma}\Omega^{-M_Z-\sigma-\overline{p}} \to 0, \qquad |\overline{\beta}| \to 0, \quad \overline{\beta} = (\Delta t, \alpha), \tag{2.12}$$

is satisfied. In order that the discretization error converge uniformly (*on* $\mathscr{U}_M$ *inside* $\mathscr{D}$) *it suffices that for each* $(\Delta t, \alpha) \in \mathscr{D}$ *the condition*

$$R_\alpha(\omega) = 0 \quad \text{for } \omega \in \bigcup_{n\neq 0}[(2n-a)\Omega, (2n+a)\Omega] \tag{2.13}$$

be satisfied with some a, $0 < a \leq 1$. *If, moreover,*

$$\alpha^{-\overline{p}-1-\sigma}\Omega^{-M_Z-\sigma-\overline{p}} \leq C\Omega^{-\delta_1}, \tag{2.14}$$

then

$$|\Delta Z^T(t)| \leq C_1\widetilde{Z}\Omega^{-M_Z+1} + C_2\widetilde{Z}\Omega^{-\delta_1},$$

and the convergence is rapid.

PROOF. The condition (2.11) easily implies that $\widetilde{H}(\alpha)$ in (2.2) can be estimated as follows:

$$\widetilde{H}(\alpha) \leq C\alpha^{-\overline{p}-1-\sigma}.$$

Now Theorem 2.3 follows from Proposition 2.1. □

Condition (2.12) allows us to consider high-resolution regularizations. In this case Theorem 2.3 implies the following result.

THEOREM 2.4. *Let* $L \in \mathscr{L}(\overline{p})$, $u \in \mathscr{U}_M(\overline{p})$, *and* $M_Z \geq 2+\delta$. *Let* $R_\alpha \in \mathscr{R}(\overline{p})$, *and let our regularization be a high-resolution regularization* ($\alpha\Omega = \varepsilon_S = \text{const}$). *Then the condition*

$$S(\xi) = 0 \quad \text{for } \xi \in \bigcup_{n\neq 0}[(2n-a)\varepsilon_S, (2n+a)\varepsilon_S] \tag{2.15}$$

for some a, $0 < a \leq 1$, *implies*

$$|\Delta Z^T(t)| \leq C\widetilde{Z}\Omega^{-M_Z+1},$$

and the discretization error converges fast and uniformly (C *is an explicitly computable constant that does not depend on* α, Ω, t).

PROOF. Since for a high-resolution regularization we have

$$\alpha^{-\overline{p}-1-\sigma}\Omega^{-M_Z-\sigma-\overline{p}} = (1/\varepsilon_S)^{\overline{p}+1+\sigma}\Omega^{-M_Z+1},$$

(2.14) holds with $\delta_1 = M_Z - 1$. Condition (2.15) follows from (2.13). □

Let us remark in conclusion that in most cases the sufficient conditions obtained in this section mean that the regularizer $R_\alpha(\omega)$ vanishes near points $2n\Omega$.

§2.3. Polynomial growth kernels and homogeneous regularizers

In these cases we can obtain not only sufficient but also necessary conditions for convergence.

We begin by defining the class of so-called monotone regularizers and giving a general theorem about necessary and sufficient conditions for convergence. Then these results will be applied to the analysis of some special classes of regularizers, namely to generalized Tikhonov regularizers and Wiener regularizers. We do not consider here monotone homogeneous regularizers, since the complete analysis of homogeneous regularizers using different ideas will be performed in the next section. Actually, generalized Tikhonov regularizers can also be analyzed in more detail using results of the next section. However, the basic properties of generalized Tikhonov regularizers can be easily derived from their monotonicity. As for Wiener regularizers, we do not know any other approach to their analysis, and the results derived from the monotonicity assumptions are essentially complete.

DEFINITION 2.2. A one-parameter regularizer $R_\alpha(\omega)$ is said to be *monotone* if it is real and there exists $\omega_m \geq 0$ independent of α such that for all (sufficiently small) α the function $R_\alpha(\omega)$ does not increase for $\omega \geq \omega_m$ and does not decrease for $\omega \leq -\omega_m$.

Let us give examples of monotone regularizers. If $S(\xi)$ is an even function that does not increase for $\xi \geq 0$, then the corresponding homogeneous regularizer is monotone. The Wiener regularizer is also monotone. Generalized Tikhonov regularizers and Wiener type regularizers are monotone, although for these regularizers $\omega_m \neq 0$ and α is bounded from above. Let us note that a monotone regularizer satisfies the condition $R_\alpha(\omega) \geq 0$ for $|\omega| \geq \omega_m$.

For monotone regularizers and kernels of polynomial growth (1.2), (1.3) the following result holds.

THEOREM 2.5. *Consider a kernel of polynomial growth $L \in \mathscr{L}(\rho^\pm)$ and a monotone regularizer $R_\alpha \in \mathscr{R}(\overline{\rho})$, where $\overline{\rho} = \max(\rho^+, \rho^-, 0)$. If the regularization* $\operatorname{Reg}(R_\alpha, \mathscr{D})$ *is quasi compactly supported, then the condition*

$$\Omega^{\rho^\pm} R_\alpha(\pm(2-a')) \to 0 \qquad \textit{for some } a',\ 0 < a' < 2, \tag{2.16}$$

is sufficient and the condition

$$\Omega^{\rho^\pm} R_\alpha(\pm 2\Omega) \to 0 \tag{2.17}$$

is necessary for the uniform convergence of the discretization error on the class $\mathscr{U}_M(\overline{\rho})$, $M_Z \geq 2+\delta$, inside the set $\mathscr{D}$ as $\alpha \to 0$, $\Omega \to \infty$, $(\Delta t, \alpha) \in \mathscr{D}$.

If the condition (2.16) *is satisfied, the rate of convergence of the discretization error is determined by the rate of convergence in this condition and by the terms $O(\Omega^{-M_Z+1})$ and $O(\Omega^{-1-\delta})$ in Proposition* 2.4.

PROOF. 1) We begin with the proof of sufficiency. By Proposition 2.4, we must estimate $\Delta D^{a,n_0}(t)$ (see (2.9)). We choose $n_0 = [\kappa/2]+1$, $a = \min(1, a', 2(1-\{\kappa/2\}))$ ($[x]$ and $\{x\}$ are the integral and the fractional part of x). This choice guarantees the condition $n_0 \geq \frac{1}{2}(\kappa + a)$. For a sufficiently large Ω (namely, for $\Omega \geq \omega_L$), $n \neq 0$, and $|\omega| < \Omega$ we have the following estimate for the kernel:

$$\begin{aligned}|\widehat{L}(\omega + 2n\Omega)| &\leq \frac{|\widetilde{L}^{\pm}|}{\omega_L^{\rho^\pm}} |\omega + 2n\Omega|^{\rho^\pm} \left(1 + \frac{C^{\pm}\omega_L^{\rho^\pm}}{|\widetilde{L}^{\pm}|} |\omega + 2n\Omega|^{-\delta^\pm}\right) \\ &\leq \frac{|\widetilde{L}^{\pm}|}{\omega_L^{\rho^\pm}} |\omega + 2n\Omega|^{\rho^\pm} (1 + C\Omega^{-\delta^\pm}),\end{aligned}$$

where the upper sign corresponds to $n \geq 1$ and the lower to $n \leq -1$. Therefore, for $\Omega \geq \omega_L$ we have

$$\begin{aligned}|\Delta D^{a,n_0}(t)| \leq &\frac{1}{2\pi} \sum_{n=1}^{[\kappa/2]} \int_{-a\Omega}^{a\Omega} d\omega \, |\widehat{u}(\omega)| \\ &\times \left(\frac{|\widetilde{L}^{+}|}{\omega_L^{\rho^+}} |\omega + 2n\Omega|^{\rho^+} (1 + C\Omega^{-\delta^+}) |R_\alpha(\omega + 2n\Omega)| \right. \\ &\left. + \frac{|\widetilde{L}^{-}|}{\omega_L^{\rho^-}} |\omega - 2n\Omega|^{\rho^-} (1 + C\Omega^{-\delta^-}) |R_\alpha(\omega - 2n\Omega)| \right).\end{aligned}$$

Using the monotonicity, we see that (since $a \leq a'$)

$$|\Delta D^{a,n_0}(t)| \leq C_1 \Omega^{\rho^+} R_\alpha((2 - a')\Omega) + C_2 \Omega^{\rho^-} R_\alpha(-(2 - a')\Omega)$$

for sufficiently large Ω (namely, for $\Omega \geq \max(\omega_L, \omega_m)$). This yields the sufficiency of (2.16). Let us note that if $\rho^+, \rho^- < 0$, then the condition (2.16) is satisfied automatically, so that in this case the discretization error converges (in accordance with Proposition 2.5).

2) *Necessity.* According to Theorem 2.2, for $\kappa < 2$ the discretization error converges and conditions (2.17) are satisfied automatically. The same is true if $\rho^+, \rho^- < 0$. Therefore, the only nontrivial case is the case when $\kappa \geq 2$ and one of the numbers (for example, ρ^+) is nonnegative. So, we assume $\kappa \geq 2$, $\rho^+ \geq 0$, $\widetilde{L}^+ \neq 0$ and prove that uniform convergence implies $\Omega^{\rho^+} R_\alpha(2\Omega) \to 0$ (the necessity of the second condition can be proved similarly). Let $\Delta Z^T(t) \to 0$ uniformly with respect to t. By Proposition 2.4, this means that $\Delta D^{a,n_0}(t) \to 0$ uniformly with respect to t for any right-hand side $u \in \mathcal{U}_M$. Since $\kappa \geq 2$, formula (2.9) for $\Delta D^{a,n_0}(t)$ contains at least two summands. Denote

$$I_{\pm}(\Omega, \widehat{u}) \equiv I_{\pm} \stackrel{\text{def}}{=} \int_{-\pi}^{\pi} \Delta D^{a,n_0}(t) e^{\pm i2\Omega t} \, dt.$$

The uniform convergence assumptions imply that for any $u \in \mathcal{U}_M$ we have $I_t \to 0$ as $\Omega \to \infty$. Integrating explicitly with respect to t, we obtain

$$\begin{aligned}I_{\pm} = &\int_{-a\Omega}^{a\Omega} d\omega \, \frac{\sin \omega\pi}{\omega\pi} \widehat{u}(\omega) \widehat{L}(\omega \pm 2\Omega) R_\alpha(\omega \pm 2\Omega) \\ &+ \sum_{\substack{|n| < n_0 \\ n \neq 0, \pm 1}} \int_{-a\Omega}^{a\Omega} d\omega \frac{\sin(2(n \pm 1)\Omega + \omega)\pi}{(2(n \pm 1) + \omega/\Omega)\pi} \frac{1}{\Omega} \widehat{u}(\omega) \widehat{L}(\omega + 2n\Omega) R_\alpha(\omega + 2n\Omega).\end{aligned}$$

Let us choose the functions $u_\pm \in \mathscr{U}_M$ satisfying the following conditions:

$$\widehat{u}_\pm(\omega) \text{ is real and nonnegative;}$$

$$\int d\omega \widehat{u}_\pm(\omega) = 1; \quad \operatorname{supp} \widehat{u}_+(\omega) \subset [-1/2, 0]; \quad \operatorname{supp} \widehat{u}_-(\omega) \subset [0, 1/2].$$

Taking into account the form of the kernel and the monotonicity of the regularizer, we obtain

$$\begin{aligned} I_\pm(\Omega, \widehat{u}_\pm) = &\widetilde{L}^\pm \Omega^{\rho^\pm} C_1^\pm \int_{\operatorname{supp} \widehat{u}_\pm} d\omega \frac{\sin \omega\pi}{\omega\pi} \widehat{u}_\pm(\omega) R_\alpha(\omega \pm 2\Omega) \\ &+ (O(\Omega^{\rho^\pm - \delta^\pm}) + O(\Omega^{\rho^\pm - 1}) + O(\Omega^{\rho^\pm - 1 - \delta})^\pm) R_\alpha(\pm 2\Omega) \\ &+ (O(\Omega^{\rho^\mp - 1}) + O(\Omega^{\rho^\mp - 1 - \delta^\mp})) R_\alpha(\mp 2\Omega), \qquad \Omega \to \infty, \end{aligned}$$

where $C_1^\pm$ are positive constants and the O-estimates are uniform with respect to α. We assume, of course, that $\omega \geq \omega_m$. Using the properties of $\widehat{u}_\pm$ and the monotonicity of the regularizer, we can rewrite the last formula as follows:

(2.18)
$$I_\pm(\Omega, \widehat{u}_\pm) = \widetilde{L}^\pm C_2^\pm \Omega^{\rho^\pm} J^\pm(\alpha) + O(\Omega^{\rho^\pm - \delta}) R_\alpha(\pm 2\Omega) + O(\Omega^{\rho^\mp - \delta}) R_\alpha(\mp 2\Omega),$$

where $C_2^\pm$ are positive constants, $J^\pm(\alpha)$ are real, and $J^\pm(\alpha) \geq R_\alpha(\pm 2\Omega) \geq 0$. We want to prove that if $\widetilde{L}^+ \neq 0$, then $\Omega^{\rho^+} R_\alpha(+2\Omega) \to 0$. We must consider the following 8 cases:

$$\begin{array}{llll} 1)\ \operatorname{Re} \widetilde{L}^+ > 0, & \operatorname{Re} \widetilde{L}^- \geq 0; & 2)\ \operatorname{Re} \widetilde{L}^+ < 0, & \operatorname{Re} \widetilde{L}^- \leq 0; \\ 3)\ \operatorname{Re} \widetilde{L}^+ > 0, & \operatorname{Re} \widetilde{L}^- \leq 0; & 4)\ \operatorname{Re} \widetilde{L}^+ < 0, & \operatorname{Re} \widetilde{L}^- \geq 0; \\ 5)\ \operatorname{Im} \widetilde{L}^+ > 0, & \operatorname{Im} \widetilde{L}^- \geq 0; & 6)\ \operatorname{Im} \widetilde{L}^+ < 0, & \operatorname{Im} \widetilde{L}^- \leq 0; \\ 7)\ \operatorname{Im} \widetilde{L}^+ > 0, & \operatorname{Im} \widetilde{L}^- \leq 0; & 8)\ \operatorname{Im} \widetilde{L}^+ < 0, & \operatorname{Im} \widetilde{L}^- \geq 0. \end{array}$$

Consider, as an example, case 1). Summing up the real parts of (2.18) corresponding to different signs, we obtain

$$\begin{aligned} &\operatorname{Re} I_+(\Omega, \widehat{u}_+) + \operatorname{Re} I_-(\Omega, \widehat{u}_-) \\ &\quad = \operatorname{Re} \widetilde{L}^+ C_2^+ \Omega^{\rho^+} R_\alpha(2\Omega) \left(\frac{J^+(\alpha)}{R_\alpha(2\Omega)} + \operatorname{Re} O(\Omega^{-\delta}) \right) \\ &\quad + \operatorname{Re} \widetilde{L}^- C_2^- \Omega^{\rho^-} R_\alpha(-2\Omega) \left(\frac{J^-(\alpha)}{R_\alpha(-2\Omega)} + \operatorname{Re} O(\Omega^{-\delta}) \right). \end{aligned}$$

By our assumptions for case 1), the expressions before the parenthesis are nonnegative. Moreover, $J^\pm(\alpha)/R_\alpha(\pm 2\Omega) \geq 1$. Therefore,

$$\begin{aligned} \operatorname{Re} I_+ + \operatorname{Re} I_- &\geq \tfrac{1}{2} \operatorname{Re} \widetilde{L}^+ C_2^+ \Omega^{\rho^+} R_\alpha(2\Omega) + \tfrac{1}{2} \operatorname{Re} \widetilde{L}^- C_2^- \Omega^{\rho^-} R_\alpha(-2\omega) \\ &\geq \tfrac{1}{2} \operatorname{Re} \widetilde{L}^+ C_2^+ \Omega^{\rho^+} R_\alpha(2\Omega) \geq 0, \end{aligned}$$

for sufficiently large Ω. Since $I_\pm(\Omega, \widehat{u}_\pm) \to 0$ as $\Omega \to \infty$, we have also $\operatorname{Re} I_+(\Omega, \widehat{u}_+) + \operatorname{Re} I_-(\Omega, \widehat{u}_-) \to 0$ as $\Omega \to \infty$. By the last inequality, this is possible only when $\Omega^{\rho^+} R_\alpha(2\Omega) \to 0$.

The seven other cases are treated similarly. □

REMARK 1. For a slow-growing kernel $L \in \mathscr{L}(\rho^-)$ only the sufficiency part of Theorem 2.5 remains, with (2.16) replaced by the condition

$$\Omega^{\rho^-} R_\alpha(\pm(2-a')\Omega) \to 0.$$

The proof repeats the corresponding part of the proof of Theorem 2.5.

REMARK 2. If the kernel is real and nonnegative, $L \in \mathscr{L}(\rho^\pm)$, $\widehat{L}(\omega) \geq 0$, the necessity of conditions (2.17) for *pointwise* convergence can be proved much more easily and without the assumption that the regularization is quasi compactly supported. Indeed, taking $\widehat{u}(\omega) = \widehat{u}_\pm(\omega)$ (see the proof of Theorem 2.5), we obtain, for $\Omega \geq \omega_m$,

$$\begin{aligned}\Delta Z^T(0) &= \sum_{n\neq 0} \int d\omega\, \widehat{u}_\pm(\omega)\widehat{L}(\omega + 2n\Omega)R_\alpha(\omega+2n\Omega)\\ &\geq \int d\omega\, \widehat{u}_\pm(\omega)\widehat{L}(\omega \pm 2n\Omega)R_\alpha(\omega \pm 2\Omega)\\ &\geq \widetilde{L}^\pm \frac{1}{\omega_L^{\rho^\pm}}(2\Omega - 1/2)^{\rho^\pm}(1 + O(\Omega^{-\delta^\pm}))R_\alpha(\pm 2\Omega).\end{aligned}$$

Now $\Delta Z^T(0) \to 0$ implies (2.27).

As a first example, let us confider a generalized Tikhonov regularizer.

PROPOSITION 2.6. *Let $L \in \mathscr{L}(\overline{\rho})$, $u \in \mathscr{U}_M(\overline{\rho})$, and $M_Z \geq 2+\delta$. Let $R_{\alpha_T} \in \mathscr{R}(\overline{\rho})$ be a homogeneous Tikhonov regularizer* (1.13) (*the degree q_0 of the quasipolynomial Q in the exponent satisfies $q_0 \geq \overline{\rho}+1+\delta$*). *Let $\mathscr{D} \equiv \mathscr{D}_{(\Delta t, \alpha_T)}$ be the set of admissible* (*by the regularization*) *values of parameters. Then*:

1) *The regularization is quasi compactly supported if*

$$\frac{1}{\alpha_T}\Omega^{-q_0+\overline{\rho}+1+\sigma} \leq C \tag{2.19}$$

for any $(\Delta t, \alpha) \in \mathscr{D}$; here C does not depend on α_T and Ω, and we can assume that $\kappa < 2$ (*changing C_R, if necessary*).

2) *If the condition* (2.19) *is satisfied, then the discretization error converges rapidly and uniformly on the class $\mathscr{U}_M$ inside the set $\mathscr{D}$.*

3) *if $L \in \mathscr{L}^\pm$, then a necessary condition for the convergence of the discretization error on the class $\mathscr{U}_M$ inside an arbitrary set $\mathscr{D}' \equiv \mathscr{D}'_{(\Delta t, \alpha_T)}$ is*

$$\frac{1}{\alpha_T}\Omega^{\rho - q_0} \to 0 \quad \text{as } \Delta t \to 0,\ \alpha_T \to 0,\ (\Delta t, \alpha_T) \in \mathscr{D}', \tag{2.20}$$

where $\rho = \max(\rho^+, \rho^-)$.

PROOF. This all follows easily from Definition 2.1 (of a quasi compactly supported regularization), Theorem 2.2, Remark 2 to Theorem 2.5, and the explicit form of the regularizer. □

Let us consider high-resolution regularization for a Tikhonov regularizer. It is convenient to rewrite the equation (0.58) in the form

$$k_T\Omega = \int_0^\infty R_{\alpha_T}(\omega)d\omega, \qquad k_T > 0.$$

For large Ω the solution $\alpha_T(\Omega)$ of this equation has the form

$$\alpha_T^{1/q_0} = C_T(q_0)[1 + O((\Omega/\omega_R)^{-\varepsilon})](\Omega/\omega_R)^{-1},$$

where

$$\varepsilon = \max_{1\le i\le I}(q_0 - q_i) > 0, \qquad C_T(q_0) = \frac{1}{k_T}\int_0^\infty \frac{d\xi}{1+\xi^{q_0}}.$$

One can easily see that for a high-resolution regularization the condition (2.19) is violated and the regularization is not quasi compactly supported. Furthermore, we have the following result.

COROLLARY. *Under the conditions of part* 3) *of Proposition* 2.6, *the discretization error for a high-resolution algorithm diverges.*

PROOF. Condition (2.20) for a high-resolution algorithm is clearly violated. □

Now let us consider the Wiener regularizer (0.13).

PROPOSITION 2.7. *Let* $L \in \mathscr{L}(\overline{p})$, $u \in \mathscr{U}_M(\overline{p})$, $M_Z \ge 2+\delta$, *and let* $R_{\alpha_T} \in \mathscr{R}(\overline{p})$ *be the Wiener regularizer. Let the set* $\mathscr{D}^v \equiv \mathscr{D}^v_{(\Delta t,\alpha)}$ *of admissible values of parameters satisfy the following condition*:

$$(2.21) \qquad (\log(1/\alpha))^{1/q} \le \overline{r}_v(\Omega/\omega_R) \quad \textit{for some } \overline{r}_v > 0$$

for any $(\Delta t, \alpha) \in \mathscr{D}^v$. *Then*:

1) *The regularization* $\operatorname{Reg}(R_\alpha, \mathscr{D}^v)$ *is quasi compactly supported*; $\kappa \ge \overline{r_v} + \delta > \overline{r_v}$.

2) *If* $\overline{r_v} < 2$, *then the discretization error (on* $\mathscr{U}_M$ *inside* $\mathscr{D}^v$*) converges uniformly; the convergence rate is determined by the smoothness of* M_Z, *i.e.*, $\Delta Z^T(t) = O(\Omega^{-M_Z+1})$, *uniformly with respect to* α *and* t.

3 *If* $L \in \mathscr{L}(p^\pm)$, $p = \max(p^+, p^-) \ge 0$, *and there is an* r_v, $2 < r_v \le \overline{r_v}$, *such that in an arbitrary small neighborhood of* $\overline{\beta} = 0$ *there exists* $(\Delta t, \alpha) \in \mathscr{D}^v$ *with*

$$(\log(1/\alpha))^{1/q} \ge r_v(\Omega/\omega_R),$$

then the discretization error does not converge uniformly in $\mathscr{D}^v$.

PROOF. 1) By the definition (0.13) of $R_\alpha(\omega)$, for $|\omega| \ge \kappa\Omega$ and $\kappa \ge \overline{r_v} + \delta > \overline{r_v}$ we have

$$0 < R_\alpha(\omega) \le |\omega/\omega_R|^{-h} \exp[-|\omega/\omega_R|^q(1 - (\overline{r}_v/\kappa)^q)],$$

so that $R_\alpha(\omega)$ decreases exponentially. The same is true for $\widehat{H}^R(\omega) = \widehat{L}(\omega)R_\alpha(\omega)$ for $L \in \mathscr{L}(\overline{p})$. Note that σ in the definition of a quasi compactly supported regularizer can be taken arbitrary large ($\sigma = \pm\infty$).

2) For $\overline{r_v} < 2$ we can take $\kappa < 2$. Convergence follows from Theorem 2.2, and the desired estimate follows from (2.10) (taking into account that $\sigma = +\infty$).

3) Consider $R_\alpha(2\Omega)$. For a sufficiently large Ω we have

$$R_\alpha(2\Omega) \geq \{1 + (2\Omega/\omega_R)^h \exp[(-r_v\Omega/\omega_R)^q(1 - (2/r_v)^q)]\}^{-1} \geq \delta > 0,$$

since

$$(2\Omega/\omega_R)^h \exp[-(r_v\Omega/\omega_R)^q(1 - (2/r_v)^q)] \to 0, \qquad \Omega \to \infty,$$

for $r_v > 2$, and so for $\rho = \max(\rho^+, \rho^-) \geq 0$ the necessary convergence condition from Theorem 2.5 is violated. □

REMARK 1. According to Remark 2 to Theorem 2.5, in the case $\widehat{L}(\omega)$ (for example, when $\widehat{L}(\omega) = |\omega|^\rho$, $\rho \geq 0$) the inequality

$$(\log(1/\alpha))^{1/q} \geq r_v(\Omega/\omega_R), \qquad r_v > 2,$$

implies the divergence of the discretization error even without the assumption (2.21). Furthermore, in this case the error at the point $t = 0$ grows as Ω^ρ.

REMARK 2. Let us consider here the class of fast-growing kernels $\mathscr{L}(\Lambda)$, $\Lambda(\omega) = \exp|\omega/\omega_L|^\rho$. The Wiener regularizer R_α belongs to $\mathscr{R}(\Lambda)$ for $q > \rho$. Parts 1) and 2) in the proof of Proposition 2.7 show that for $\overline{r_v} < 1$ the set $\mathscr{D}^v$ satisfies the condition (2.5) from Proposition 2.3 with $\sigma = +\infty$. Therefore, for these classes $\mathscr{L}(\Lambda)$ and appropriate $\mathscr{U}_M$ the discretization error converges rapidly and uniformly inside $\mathscr{D}^v$. Similarly to part 3) of the proof, one can show that for $r_v > 1$ there is a $c > 0$ such that $R_\alpha(\omega) \geq \delta > 0$ for $|\omega| \leq (1 + c)\Omega$. Similarly to the corresponding example in §1.1, one can prove that for kernels of the form $\widehat{L}(\omega)\exp|\omega/\omega_L|^\rho$, $\rho > 0$, the discretization error diverges. Therefore we obtain a practically precise description of the convergence region.

Let us remark that for any fixed ω the Wiener regularizer $R_\alpha(\omega)$ increases when α decreases, and that $R_{+\infty} = 0$, $R_0 = 1$. This means that the function $h_R(\alpha)$ (see (0.56)) is continuous and monotone decreasing to 0 as α decreases to 0. Therefore, the Wiener regularizer admits high resolution. Let us consider high-resolution regularizations for $R_\alpha(\omega)$. By definition, the parameters α and Δt are related by the condition (0.58), which can be conveniently written in the form

$$k_v\Omega = I(\alpha) = \int_0^\infty R_\alpha(\omega)\, d\omega.$$

For large Ω the function $\alpha_{k_v}(\Omega)$ has the following asymptotic behavior:

$$\begin{aligned}(k_v\Omega/\omega_R)^q[1 - A_1\Omega^{-q}] &\leq \log\left(1/\alpha_{k_v}(\Omega)\right) \\ &\leq (k_v\Omega/\omega_R)^q\left[1 + A_2\Omega^{-q/2} + A_3\Omega^{-q} + A_2A_3\Omega^{-3q/2}\right],\end{aligned} \tag{2.22}$$

where

$$A_1 = 8\Gamma(1+q)\frac{q+1}{q^2}\left(\frac{2\omega_R}{k_v}\right)^q, \qquad A_2 = \left(1 + \frac{h}{q}\right)\left(\frac{2\omega_R}{k_v}\right)^{q/2},$$
$$A_3 = 4\Gamma(1+q)\left(\frac{2\omega_R}{k_v}\right)^q,$$

$\Gamma(x)$ being the Euler function gamma. Using Proposition 2.7, we obtain from (2.22) that the high-resolution regularization for the Wiener regularizer is quasi compactly supported for any $k_v > 0$. The discretization error converges for $k_v < 2$ and diverges for $k_v > 2$ (we assume that $L \in \mathscr{L}(\rho^{\pm})$, $\rho = \max(\rho^+, \rho^-) \geq 0$). The case $k_v = 2$ must be analyzed separately. Skipping the details, we formulate the final result.

PROPOSITION 2.8. *Let $L \in \mathscr{L}(\rho^{\pm})$, $\rho = \max(\rho^+, \rho^-) \geq 0$, and let $u \in \mathscr{U}_M$ and $M_Z \geq 2 + \delta$. Then for the Wiener regularizer and the high-resolution regularization $(\alpha = \alpha_{k_v})$ we have*

1) *if $k_v < 2$, then the discretization error converges and $\Delta Z^T \leq O(\Omega^{-M_Z+1})$ uniformly with respect to t and α;*
2) *if $k_v \geq 2$, then the discretization error diverges.*

It is interesting to mention the behavior of the Wiener regularizer $R_\alpha(r\Omega)$ at high resolution, i.e., the behavior of $R_{\alpha_{k_v}(\Omega)}(r\Omega)$ as $\Omega \to \infty$:

1) $R_\alpha(r\Omega)$ exponentially decreases to zero for $r > k_v$;
2) $R_\alpha(r\Omega) \geq C > 0$ for $r = k_v$;
3) $R_\alpha(r\Omega)$ exponentially tends to 1 for $r < k_v$.

Therefore, up to exponentially small terms, the Wiener regularizer at high resolution is similar to the rectangular window with the cutoff frequency $k_v\Omega$. Let us remark in conclusion that all the results hold for Wiener type regularizers (1.14), with q replaced by q_0. We omit the proof, since it is very cumbersome and follows similar lines.

§2.4. Polynomial kernels and smooth regularizers

In this section we study the asymptotic behavior of the discretization error for polynomial kernels and smooth regularizers with an arbitrary convergence path $\Delta t \to 0$, $\alpha \to 0$. In particular, we completely describe the convergence set $\mathscr{D}_{(\Delta t, \alpha)}$ for smooth homogeneous regularizers. This section contains complete proofs of results from **[10]**, as well as the formulation of Lemma 2 and the correction of an error in Theorem 2 from **[10]**.

Let us note that Proposition 2.2 describes the behavior of the part of the discretization error corresponding to the summand $\Delta\widehat{L}_0(\omega)$ of the kernel $\widehat{L}(\omega) \in \mathscr{L}_0(\rho_0^{\pm})$ (see (1.4), (1.5)). Below we will use the linearity of the problem and assume that $\Delta\widehat{L}_0 \equiv 0$. All the results of this section remain true in the general case if we add the term corresponding to $\Delta\widehat{L}_0(\omega)$. Therefore, in this and the next section $L \in \mathscr{L}_0$ means that

$$\widehat{L}(\omega) = \sum_{i=0}^{I^{\pm}} l_i^{\pm} |\omega/\omega_L|^{\rho_i^{\pm}}, \qquad |\omega| > \omega_L,$$

with + sign for $\omega \geq \omega_L$ and − sign for $\omega \leq -\omega_L$; furthermore, $|\widehat{L}(\omega)| \leq \widehat{L}$ for $|\omega| \leq |\omega_L|$. The numbers $\rho_i^{\pm}$ are ordered in the standard way: $\rho_0^+ > \rho_1^+ > \cdots > \rho_{I^+}^+$, $\rho_0^- > \rho_1^- > \cdots > \rho_{I^-}^-$. We introduce the following additional notation:

$$\rho = \max(\rho_0^+, \rho_0^-), \qquad \overline{\rho} = \max(\rho, 0), \qquad \overline{\rho}_{\max} = \max_i(|\rho_i^+|, |\rho_i^-|),$$

$$b_i^{\pm} = l_i^{\pm}\omega_L^{-\rho_i^{\pm}}, \qquad \overline{b}_{\max} = \max_i(|b_i^+|, |b_i^-|), \qquad \overline{I} = \max(I^+, I^-).$$

Also, it will be convenient to use the notation $\widehat{H}_\alpha(\omega) \equiv \widehat{H}^R(\omega)$. Denote

$$B_k^\rho = \begin{cases} \rho(\rho-1)\cdots(\rho-k+1), & k = 1, 2, \dots, \\ 1, & k = 0. \end{cases}$$

By linearity, it is often sufficient to consider the simplest polynomial kernel of the form

$$(2.23)\qquad \widehat{L}_0(\omega) = \begin{cases} b^+|\omega|^{\rho^+} \equiv l^+|\omega/\omega_L|^{\rho^+}, & \omega \geq \omega_L, \\ b^-|\omega|^{\rho^-} \equiv l^-|\omega/\omega_L|^{\rho^-}, & \omega \leq -\omega_L, \end{cases}$$

with $|\widehat{L}(\omega)| \leq \widehat{L}$ for $|\omega| \leq |\omega_L|$. Everywhere below we assume that L_0 is such a kernel, with at least one of the numbers $b^{\pm}$ nonzero. In this case we set $\rho = \max(\rho^+, \rho^-)$.

Now let us introduce the notion of a smooth regularizer.

DEFINITION 2.3. A regularizer $R_\alpha \in \mathscr{R}(\overline{p})$ is said to be $(N+1)$-*smooth* if the following conditions are satisfied:

$$(2.24)\qquad \begin{cases} \text{a) } R_\alpha(\omega) \in C^{N+1}(\mathbb{R}\setminus 0) \text{ for any } \alpha; \\ \text{b) } |R_\alpha^{(m)}(\omega)| = O(|\omega|^{-\overline{p}-1-\delta}), \quad |\omega| \to \infty, \\ \qquad \text{for } m = 0, 1, \dots, N+1 \text{ and for any } \alpha; \\ \text{c) } |R_\alpha^{(m)}(\omega)| \leq \widetilde{R}_m |\omega|^{-m} \text{ for any } \alpha; \\ \text{d) } |R_\alpha^{(m)}(\omega)| \leq \overline{R}_m \text{ for any } \alpha; \\ \qquad \text{the constants } \widetilde{R}_m, \overline{R}_m \text{ do not depend on } \alpha. \end{cases}$$

We remark that condition d) is not uniform in α.

Let us give examples of homogeneous regularizers. Suppose we have a homogeneous regularizer and the function $S(\xi)$ satisfies, in addition to (1.11), the following conditions:

$$(2.25)\qquad \begin{cases} \text{a) } S(\xi) \in C^{N+1}(\mathbb{R}\setminus 0); \\ \text{b) } |S^{(m)}(\xi)| = O(|\xi|^{-\overline{p}-1-\delta}), \quad |\xi| \to \infty, m = 0, 1, \dots, N+1; \\ \text{c) } |S^{(m)}(\xi)| \leq \widetilde{S}_m |\xi|^{-m}. \end{cases}$$

Then $R_\alpha(\omega) = S(\alpha\omega)$ is an $(N+1)$-smooth regularizer with $\widetilde{R}_m = \widetilde{S}_m$. Conditions (2.25) are satisfied for a wide class of functions $S(\xi)$, for example for $S(\xi) = e^{-|\xi|^q}$, $q > 0$, and for $S(\xi) = [1 + Q(\xi)]^{-1}$, $Q(\xi)$ is a quasipolynomial. Generalized Tikhonov regularizers are also smooth.

Now let us consider a regularizer of the form

$$R_{\overline{\alpha}}(\omega) \equiv R_{(\alpha_1,\alpha_2)}(\omega) = R_{\alpha_1}(\omega) R_{\alpha_2}(\omega).$$

If $R_{\alpha_1}, R_{\alpha_2} \in \mathscr{R}(\overline{p}_{1,2})$, $\overline{p}_1 + \overline{p}_2 \geq \overline{p}$, are $(N+1)$-smooth, then $R_{\overline{\alpha}} \in \mathscr{R}(\overline{p})$ is $(N+1)$-smooth.

The following result forms a basis for further analysis.

THEOREM 2.6. *Let* $L \in \mathscr{L}_0(\rho_0^{\pm})$, $\rho = \max(\rho_0^+, \rho_0^-)$, *and let* $R_\alpha \in \mathscr{R}(\overline{p})$, $\overline{p} = \max(\rho, 0)$, *be an* $(N+1)$-*smooth regularizer with* $N \geq \rho + \delta$. *Let* $u \in \mathscr{U}_M(\overline{p})$ *with* $M_u \geq N + 2 + \delta$ (*so that* $M_u \geq \overline{p} + 2 + \delta$). *Then*

$$(2.26)\qquad \Delta Z^T(t) = \sum_{k=0}^{N} u^{(K)}(t) T_K(t) + Q_{N+1}(t)$$

and

$$(2.27)\qquad |Q_{N+1}(t)| \leq O(\Omega^{-(M_u - \overline{p} - 1)}) + O(\Omega^{-(N+1-\rho)}),$$

uniformly with respect to τ and α. The functions $T_k(t) = T_k^+(t) + T_k^-(t)$ are given by

$$T_k^{\pm}(t) = \frac{i^k}{k!} \sum_{n=1}^{\infty} e^{\mp i 2n\Omega t} \widehat{H}_\alpha^{(k)}(\pm 2n\Omega), \qquad \widehat{H}_\alpha \equiv \widehat{H}^R. \tag{2.28}$$

PROOF. We begin with some elementary estimates. Since $|\widehat{L}(\omega)| \leq \widetilde{L}$ for $|\omega| \leq \omega_L$, we have

$$|\widehat{H}_\alpha(\omega)| \leq \widetilde{L}\widetilde{R}_0, \qquad |\omega| \leq \omega_L. \tag{2.29}$$

By (2.23),

$$\widehat{L}^{(j)}(\omega) = \sum_{i=0}^{I^{\pm}} (\pm 1)^j b_i^{\pm} B_j^{p_i^{\pm}} |\omega|^{p_i^{\pm} - j},$$

with the upper sign for $\omega \geq \omega_L$ and the lower sign for $\omega \leq -\omega_L$. Since

$$\widehat{H}_\alpha^{(m)}(\omega) = \sum_{j=0}^{m} \binom{m}{j} \widehat{L}^{(j)}(\omega) R_\alpha^{(m-j)}(\omega),$$

using (2.24c) and the previous formula we obtain

$$|\widehat{H}_\alpha^{(m)}(\omega)| \leq C_H |\omega|^{p-m}, \qquad |\omega| \geq \omega_L. \tag{2.30}$$

For $m = 0, \dots, N+1$ the constant C_H can be taken to be

$$C_H = (N+1)2^{N+1}(\overline{I}+1)\overline{b}_{\max}(\overline{p}_{\max} + N + 1)^{N+1} \max_{0 \leq m \leq N+1} \widetilde{R}_m.$$

2) By (2.24b), the $T_k^{\pm}(t)$ are well defined and the corresponding series converge absolutely and uniformly. The sum on the right-hand side of (2.26) corresponds to the Taylor series expansions of the function $\widehat{H}_\alpha(\omega) = \widehat{H}^R(\omega)$ (see (1.17)) near points $2n\Omega$. Hence

$$|Q_{N+1}(t)| \leq \sum_{n=1}^{\infty} (I_n^+ + I_n^-),$$

where

$$I_n^{\pm} = \frac{1}{2\pi} \int d\omega |\widehat{u}(\omega)| \left| \widehat{H}_\alpha(\omega \pm 2n\Omega) - \sum_{k=0}^{N} \frac{\widehat{H}_\alpha^{(k)}(\pm 2n\Omega)}{k!} \omega^k \right|.$$

3) The next step of the proof is to estimate $I_n^{\pm}$. Considering, for example, I_n^+ (I_n^- can be treated similarly), we have

$$I_n^+ \leq I_n^{+1} + I_n^{+2} + I_n^{+3},$$

where

$$I_n^{+1} = \frac{1}{2\pi} \int_{|\omega| > n\Omega} d\omega \, |\widehat{u}(\omega)| \cdot |\widehat{H}_\alpha(\omega + 2n\Omega)|,$$

$$I_n^{+2} = \frac{1}{2\pi} \int_{|\omega| > n\Omega} d\omega \, |\widehat{u}(\omega)| \sum_{k=0}^{N} \frac{|\widehat{H}_\alpha^{(k)}(2n\Omega)|}{k!} |\omega|^k,$$

$$I_n^{+3} = \frac{1}{2\pi} \int_{-n\Omega}^{n\Omega} d\omega \, |\widehat{u}(\omega)| \left| \widehat{H}_\alpha(\omega + 2n\Omega) - \sum_{k=0}^{N} \frac{\widehat{H}_\alpha^{(k)}(2n\Omega)}{k!} \omega^k \right|.$$

To estimate $I_n^{+1,2}$ we must use (1.9) ($|\widehat{u}(\omega)| \leq \widetilde{u}|\omega|^{-M_u}$), (2.30), and, for the interval $\omega \in [-2n\Omega - \omega_L, -2n\Omega + \omega_L]$ in I_n^{+1}, also (2.29), as well as the conditions $M_u \geq N + 2 + \delta$, $N \geq \rho + \delta$, $M_u \geq \overline{\rho} + 2 + \delta$. To estimate I_n^{+1} it is convenient to divide the integration interval into six parts: $(-\infty, -4n\Omega]$, $[-4n\Omega, -2n\Omega - \omega_L]$, $[-2n\Omega - \omega_L, -2n\Omega + \omega_L]$, $[-2n\Omega + \omega_L, -n\Omega]$, $[n\Omega, 2n\Omega]$, $[2n\Omega, \infty)$. To estimate I_n^{+2} it suffices to consider two intervals: $(-\infty, -n\Omega]$, $[n\Omega, +\infty)$. As a result, we obtain

$$I_n^{+1,2} \leq C\widetilde{u}(n, \Omega)^{-M_u + \overline{\rho} + 1} \tag{2.31}$$

with an explicitly computable constant C that does not depend on n, α, Ω.

Now consider I_n^{+3}. For $\omega \in [-n\Omega, n\Omega]$ the condition on the smoothness of the regularizer and on the form of the kernel imply that the function $\widehat{H}_\alpha(\omega + 2n\Omega)$ has $N + 1$ continuous derivatives. Using the integral form of the remainder in the Taylor formula, we obtain

$$\widehat{H}_\alpha(\omega + 2n\Omega) - \sum_{k=0}^{N} \frac{1}{k!} \widehat{H}_\alpha^{(k)}(2n\Omega)\omega^k$$
$$= \frac{1}{N!} \int_{2n\Omega}^{2n\Omega+\omega} d\omega' \, (2n\Omega + \omega - \omega')^N \widehat{H}_\alpha^{(N+1)}(\omega').$$

Substituting this in the formula for I_n^{+3}, we get

$$I_n^{+3} \leq \frac{1}{2\pi} \int_{-n\Omega}^{n\Omega} d\omega \, |\widehat{u}(\omega)| \frac{1}{N!} |\omega|^{N+1} C_H (n\Omega)^{-N-1+\rho}$$

(we have used (2.30) and the fact that $\omega' \in [n\Omega, 3n\Omega]$). Since $M_u \geq N + 2 + \delta$, the last inequality implies

$$I_n^{+3} \leq C \|\widehat{u}(\omega)\omega^{N+1}\|_{L^1} (n\Omega)^{-N-1+\rho}, \tag{2.32}$$

with a constant C that can be easily computed and does not depend on n, α, Ω.

4) It remains to add together the estimates (2.31), (2.32) for I_n^{+1}, I_n^{+2}, I_n^{+3} and to sum over n taking into account that $N \geq \rho + \delta$, $M_u \geq \overline{\rho} + 2 + \delta$. □

Theorem 2.6 reduces the analysis of the behavior of the discretization error to the analysis of $T_k(t)$. Let us note that it was more convenient to formulate the smoothness condition in terms of smoothness of u: the condition $M_u \geq \overline{\rho} + 2 + \delta$ corresponds to the condition $M_Z \geq 2 + \delta$ that was used earlier.

Now let us consider $(N + 1)$-smooth homogeneous regularizers. For such regularizers we have

$$T_k^{\pm}(t) = \frac{i^k}{k!} \sum_{n=0}^{I^{\pm}} b_n^{\pm} \Omega^{\rho_n^{\pm} - k} \sum_{j=0}^{k} (\pm 1)^{k-j} \varepsilon_S^k \binom{k}{j} B_{k-j}^{\rho_n^{\pm}} Q_{k,j;n}^{\pm}(t), \tag{2.33}$$

$$Q_{k,j;n}^{\pm}(t) = \sum_{p=1}^{\infty} e^{\mp i 2p\Omega t} (2p)^{\rho_n^{\pm} - k + j} S^{(j)}(\pm 2p\varepsilon_S), \qquad \varepsilon_S = \alpha\Omega. \tag{2.34}$$

We note that $T_k^{\pm}$ is a linear combination of the corresponding expressions for kernels of the form $\widehat{L}_0(\omega) = b^{\pm}|\omega|^{\rho^{\pm}}$. Formulas for $T_k^{\pm}$ for these simplest kernels differ from (2.33) and (2.34) in that they do not contain the summation over n and the index n is absent.

Formulas (2.33) and (2.34), together with Theorem 2.6, answer the question about the asymptotic behavior of the regularization error for polynomial kernels and smooth homogeneous regularizers in the case $\alpha\Omega = \varepsilon_S \geq \underline{\varepsilon_S} = \text{const}$. Indeed, we have the following result.

PROPOSITION 2.9. *For an $(N+1)$-smooth homogeneous regularizer let the conditions of Theorem 2.6 be satisfied. Let the parameters α and Ω satisfy the condition $\alpha\Omega = \varepsilon_S \geq \underline{\varepsilon_S} = \text{const}$. Then, for $k \leq N$:*

1) *The equality*

$$T_k^{\pm} = \sum_{n=0}^{I^{\pm}} b_n^{\pm} \Omega^{\rho_n^{\pm} - k} \psi_{n,k}^{\pm}(2t\Omega, \varepsilon_S) \tag{2.35}$$

holds, where $\psi_{n,k}^{\pm}(\tau, \varepsilon_S)$ are continuous 2π-periodic functions defined by

$$\begin{aligned} \psi_{n,k}^{\pm}(\tau, \varepsilon_S) &= \frac{i^k}{k!} \sum_{j=0}^{k} (\pm 1)^{k-j} \varepsilon_S^k \binom{k}{j} B_{k-j}^{\rho_n^{\pm}} Q'^{\pm}_{k,j;n}(\tau), \\ Q'^{\pm}_{k,j;n}(\tau) = Q^{\pm}_{k,j;n}(\tau/2\Omega) &= \sum_{p=1}^{\infty} e^{\mp ip\tau} (2p)^{\rho_n^{\pm} - k + j} S^{(j)}(\pm 2p\varepsilon_S). \end{aligned} \tag{2.36}$$

Moreover,

$$\psi_{n,k}^{\pm}(\tau, \varepsilon_S) \leq C(\underline{\varepsilon_S}), \tag{2.37}$$

where $C(\underline{\varepsilon_S})$ is a constant that depends on $\underline{\varepsilon_S}$ but not on ε_S, n, k.

2) *If $\alpha \to 0$, $\Delta t \to 0$ in such a way that $\alpha\Omega \geq \underline{\varepsilon_S}$, then the divergence part of the discretization error is completely determined by T_k with $k = 0, 1, \ldots, [\rho]$, where $[x]$ is the integral part of x.*

PROOF. 1) Formulas (2.35), (2.36) follow directly from (2.33), (2.34). To obtain the bound (2.37) we need the upper estimate

$$|Q'^{\pm}_{k,j;n}(\tau)| \leq \sum_{p=1}^{\infty} (2p)^{\rho_n^{\pm} - k + j} |S^{(j)}(\pm 2p\varepsilon_S)|.$$

Here we have used the following arguments. Condition (2.25b) means that there exist ξ_m and c_m such that $|S^{(m)}(\xi)| \leq c_m |\xi|^{-\overline{\rho} - 1 - \delta}$. Let $\overline{\xi} = \max_{0 \leq m \leq N+1} \xi_m$ and $\overline{c} = \max_{0 \leq m \leq N+1} c_m$. Then for $p \geq [\overline{\xi}/2\underline{\varepsilon_S}]$ we have

$$|S^{(j)}(\pm 2p\varepsilon_S)| \leq \overline{c}(2p\varepsilon_S)^{-\overline{\rho} - 1 - \delta} \leq \overline{c} p^{-\overline{\rho} - 1 - \delta} (2\underline{\varepsilon_S})^{-\overline{\rho} - 1 - \delta}.$$

For terms with $1 \leq p \leq [\overline{\xi}/2\underline{\varepsilon_S}]$ we must use the boundedness of $S^{(j)}$.

2) The second statement follows immediately from the first one. □

Proposition 2.9 shows that the bound (2.27) in Theorem 2.6 is sharp (for $\overline{\rho} = \rho = \max(\rho_0^+, \rho_0^-) \geq 0$). Indeed, the main contribution to (2.27) is from the second term, since the first one is related to the smoothness of the right-hand side and M_u can be arbitrary large. Proposition 2.9 shows that $T_N \sim \Omega^{\rho - N}$, and the second term in (2.27) is $O(\Omega^{\rho - N - 1})$.

Now let us consider the *high-resolution* case $\alpha\Omega = \varepsilon_S = \text{const}$. In this case Theorem 2.6 and Proposition 2.9 together yield a criterion for the convergence of the discretization error.

THEOREM 2.7. *Let the condition of Theorem 2.6 be satisfied, and let the regularizer be homogeneous. The discretization error for the high-resolution regularization* $\alpha\Omega = \varepsilon_S = \text{const}$ *converges (on the entire class* $\mathcal{U}_M$*) if and only if*

$$S^{(m)}(\pm 2p\varepsilon_S) = 0, \qquad m = 0, 1, \dots, [\rho_0^{\pm}], \quad p = 1, 2, \dots, \tag{2.38}$$

i.e., if $R_\alpha^{(m)}(\pm 2p\Omega) = 0$. *If these conditions are satisfied, then the convergence is rapid and uniform. Otherwise the discretization error diverges at any point* t.

PROOF. *Sufficiency.* According to Theorem 2.6, we must prove that $T_k^{\pm}(t) \to 0$ as $\Omega \to \infty$ ($\varepsilon_S = \text{const}$) uniformly with respect to t (for $k = 0, \dots, N$). For $k > [\rho_0^{\pm}]$ this follows immediately from Proposition 2.9, and we have the estimate

$$T_t^{\pm}(t) = O(\Omega^{\rho_0^{\pm} - k}) = O(\Omega^{-\delta}),$$

which is uniform with respect to t. Now let $k \le [\rho_0^{\pm}]$. In this case conditions (2.38) imply $Q'^{\pm}_{k,j;n}(t) \equiv 0$, hence for these k we have $T_k^{\pm}(t) \equiv 0$.

Necessity. 1) According to Theorem 2.6, we need $\sum_{k=0}^{N} T_k(t) u^{(k)}(t) \to 0$. Since this must be satisfied on the entire class $\mathcal{U}_M$, we need $T_k(t) \to 0$ for $k = 0, 1, \dots, N$. By the above, these conditions holds automatically for $k = [\rho_0^{\pm}], \dots, N$. Let us examine the conditions $T_k(t) \to 0$ as $\Omega \to \infty$ for $k = 0, 1, \dots, [\rho_0^{\pm}]$.

2) Let us consider first the case $\rho_0^+ \ne \rho_0^-$; without loss of generality we can assume $\rho_0^+ > \rho_0^-$, $b_0^+ \ne 0$. Using (2.37) and this assumption, we obtain from (2.35)

$$T_k(t) = b_0^+ \Omega^{\rho_0^{\pm} - k} [\psi_{0,k}^+(2t\Omega, \varepsilon_S) + O(\Omega^{-\delta})], \qquad \Omega \to \infty,$$

with an O-bound that is uniform with respect to t and k.

Since $\psi_{0,k}^+(\tau, \varepsilon_S)$ is a 2π-periodic function, the condition $T_k(x) \to 0$ for $k = 0, 1, \dots, [\rho_0^{\pm}]$ and each t implies $\psi_{0,k}^+(\tau, \varepsilon_S) \equiv 0$. Indeed, if $\psi_{0,k}^+(\tau_0, \varepsilon_S) \ne 0$, then, taking for an arbitrary $t = t_0$ the increasing sequence $\Omega_i = \tau_0 / 2t_0 + 2\pi i$, we get the increasing to infinity (at the rate $\Omega_i^{\rho_0^+ - k}$ as $i \to \infty$) sequence $T_k(t_0)$. Now, by (2.36)

$$\psi_{0,0}^+(\tau, \varepsilon_S) = Q'^{+}_{0,0;0}(\tau) = \sum_{p=1}^{\infty} e^{-ip\tau} (2p)^{\rho_0^+} S(2p\varepsilon_S);$$

also, $\psi_{0,0}^+ \equiv 0$ if and only if $S(2p\varepsilon_S) = 0$, $p = 1, 2, \dots$. We have thus obtained one of the required conditions. Now we use induction. Let $S^{(m)}(2p\varepsilon_S) = 0$, $p = 1, 2, \dots$, $m = 0, 1, \dots, k_0$, and $k_0 \le [\rho_0^+] - 1$. We show that all conditions are satisfied for $m = k_0 + 1$. We know that $\psi_{0,k_0+1}^+ \equiv 0$. Using the induction assumptions for ψ_{0,k_0+1}^+, we obtain from (2.36) the formula

$$\psi_{0,k_0+1}^+(\tau, \varepsilon_S) = \frac{i^{k_0+1}}{(k_0+1)!} \varepsilon_S^{k_0+1} \sum_{p=1}^{\infty} e^{-ip\tau} (2p)^{\rho_0^+} S^{(k_0+1)}(2p\varepsilon_S).$$

Therefore $S^{(k_0+1)}(2p\varepsilon_S) = 0$, $p = 1, 2, \dots$. Conditions (2.38) corresponding to the

$+$ sign are proved. Let us note that if these conditions are satisfied, then $\psi^+_{n,k} \equiv 0$ for $n = 1, 2, \dots, I^+$. Using (2.37), we obtain from (2.35) that

$$T_k(t) = b_0^- \Omega^{\rho_0^- - k}[\psi^-_{0,k}(2t\Omega, \varepsilon_s) + O(\Omega^\delta)].$$

Similarly to the above, we prove the remaining conditions in (2.38).

3) Let us briefly outline the proof in the case $\rho_0^+ = \rho_0^- = \rho_0$, $b_0^\pm \neq 0$. Formulas (2.35), (2.37) imply

$$T_k(t) = \Omega^{\rho_0 - k}[b_0^+ \psi^+_{0,k}(2t\Omega, \varepsilon_S) + b_0^- \psi^-_{0,k}(2t\Omega, \varepsilon_S) + O(\Omega^{-\delta})].$$

The function

$$\varphi_{0,k}(\tau, \varepsilon_S) = b_0^+ \psi^+_{0,k}(\tau, \varepsilon_S) + b_0^- \psi^-_{0,k}(\tau, \varepsilon_S)$$

is 2π-periodic; hence $T_k \to 0$ for $k = 0, \dots, [\rho_0]$ implies $\varphi_{0,k}(\tau, \varepsilon_S) \equiv 0$. This is satisfied if and only if $S^{(m)}(\pm 2p\varepsilon_S) = 0$ for $m = 0, 1, \dots, [\rho_0]$, $p = 1, 2, \dots$. □

Now let us consider the "low" resolution case, i.e., the passage to the limit as $\Delta t \to 0$ and $\alpha \to 0$ so that $\varepsilon_S = \alpha\Omega \to \infty$. According to (2.25), we have

$$|S^{(j)}(\xi)| \leq \overline{S}_j |\xi|^{-\sigma_j}, \qquad j = 0, 1, \dots, N+1, \tag{2.39}$$

where $\overline{S}_j$, σ_j are positive constants with

$$\sigma_j \geq \max(\overline{\rho} + 1 + \delta, j). \tag{2.40}$$

Denote

$$\overline{\sigma}_k = \min_{j \leq k}(\sigma_j - j), \qquad k = 0, 1, \dots, N+1.$$

By (2.40), $\overline{\sigma}_k \geq 0$ for all k and $\overline{\sigma}_k > 0$ for $k \leq [\rho] + 1$. We recall that $\rho = \max(\rho_0^+, \rho_0^-)$, and $[x]$ is the integral part of x.

Proposition 2.10. *Let the conditions of Theorem 2.6 be satisfied for a homogeneous regularizer. Assume that the set $\mathcal{D}$ of admissible values of parameters is such that if $\Delta t \to 0$, $\alpha \to 0$ inside $\mathcal{D}$, then $\varepsilon_S = \alpha\Omega \to \infty$. Then a sufficient condition for the convergence the discretization error on $\mathcal{U}_M$ inside $\mathcal{D}$ is*

$$\alpha\Omega^{1-(\rho-k)/\overline{\sigma}_k} \to +\infty, \qquad k = 0, 1, \dots, [\rho], \tag{2.41}$$

for $\Delta t \to 0$, $\alpha \to 0$, $(\Delta t, \alpha) \in \mathcal{D}$.

Proof. Without loss of generality, we prove the proposition for the simplest kernel $\widehat{L}_0(\omega)$. By Theorem 2.6, we must prove that $T_k^\pm \to 0$ uniformly with respect to t. Taking (2.39) and (2.40) into account, we obtain from (2.34)

$$|Q^\pm_{k,j}(t)| \leq C_{k,j} \varepsilon_S^{-\sigma_j}, \qquad k = 0, 1, \dots, N+1, \quad j = 0, 1, \dots, k,$$

where the positive constants $C_{j,k}$ do not depend on t. The index n is omitted since we consider the simplest kernel. Now (2.33) yields

$$|T_k^\pm(t)| \leq \Omega^{\rho^\pm - k} \sum_{j=0}^{k} \binom{k}{j} B^{\rho^\pm}_{k-j} C_{k,j} \varepsilon_S^{-(\sigma_j - j)}.$$

For $\varepsilon_S \to \infty$ the last inequality can be rewritten as

$$|T_k^\pm(t)| \leq C_k \Omega^{\rho^\pm - k} \varepsilon_S^{-\overline{\sigma}_k}.$$

For $k \geq [\rho]+1$, $T_k^{\pm}(t) \to 0$ uniformly with respect to t, because $\sigma_k \geq 0$ and $\sigma_k > 0$ for $k = [\rho]+1$. Taking $k = 0, 1, \dots, [\rho]$, we obtain (2.41). □

Let us note also that for $[\rho] \geq 0$ formula (2.41) implies $\varepsilon_S \to \infty$.

When the bounds (2.39) are sharp, (2.41) become necessary conditions for low-resolution regularizations.

As an example, let us consider the simplest Tikhonov regularizer (reducible to a homogeneous one), $S(\xi) = 1/(1+|\xi|^q)$, $q \geq \overline{p}+1+\delta$. In this case $\sigma_j = q+j$ and $\overline{\sigma}_k = q$. The conditions (2.41) imply the following sufficient condition:

$$\alpha\Omega^{1-p/q} \to +\infty. \tag{2.42}$$

Let us compare the sufficient condition (2.42) with the necessary condition (2.20), where we must replace α_T by α^q and q_0 by q. Then (2.20) becomes $\alpha^{-q}\Omega^{p-q} \to 0$, i.e., we again obtain (2.42), in agreement with what was said above.

Hence, we must consider the case of "superresolution" , i.e., the asymptotic behavior of the discretization error as $\Delta t \to 0$, $\alpha \to 0$, $\varepsilon_S = \alpha\Omega \to 0$. This problem reduces to the analysis of the asymptotic behavior of $Q^{\pm}_{k,j;n}(t)$ (see (2.34)). In turn, this reduces to the analysis of the asymptotic behavior of expressions of the form

$$G(g(\varepsilon) \mid \tau, \beta, \varepsilon) = \sum_{p=1}^{\infty} e^{i2\pi p\tau} p^{\beta} g(\varepsilon p) \tag{2.43}$$

as $\varepsilon \to 0$, where $0 \leq \tau < 1$ and $g(\xi)$ is a smooth decreasing function. Therefore, we need a discrete version of the Erdélyi lemma. This problem, which may be of independent interest, admits a complete solution. The exposition of this solution goes beyond the scope of this paper. Here we only present some results generalizing those from **[10]**.

Denote

$$h(s,\tau) = (2\pi)^{-s}\Gamma(s)\big(e^{i\pi s/2}\zeta(s,\tau) + e^{-i\pi s/2}\zeta(s,1-\pi)\big), \tag{2.44}$$

where $\Gamma(s)$ is the Euler gamma function and $\zeta(s,\tau)$ is the generalized Riemann zeta function **[19]**. Using the properties of $\zeta(s,\tau)$, we can establish the following properties of the function $h(s,\tau)$. For any τ from the interval $0 < \tau < 1$, $h(s,\tau)$ is an entire function of s. For real s and $\tau \to 0$ the function $h(s,\tau)$ has the asymptotics

$$h(s,\tau) = \begin{cases} \dfrac{\Gamma(s)}{(2\pi)^s} e^{i\pi s/2} \dfrac{1}{\tau^s} + \varphi(s,\tau), & s > 0, \\ \log(1/\tau) + \varphi(s,\tau), & s = 0, \\ \varphi(s,\tau), & s < 0, \end{cases} \tag{2.45}$$

where $|\varphi(s,\tau)| \leq C_s$ and C_s is a constant that does not depend on τ.

The asymptotic behavior of the function $G(d|\tau, b, \varepsilon)$ as $\varepsilon \to +0$ is given by the following lemma.

LEMMA (The Discrete Erdélyi Lemma). *Let $g(x) \in C^L([0,+\infty))$, $L \geq 2$. Let $g(x)$ and its derivatives decrease sufficiently rapidly, i.e., $g^{(l)}(x) = O(|x|^{-\overline{p}-1-\delta})$ as $x \to \infty$, $\overline{p} \geq 0$. Then for $\beta \leq \overline{p}$ the function $G(g(\xi) \mid \tau, \beta, \varepsilon)$ defined by* (2.43) *has the following asymptotic behavior as $\varepsilon \to +0$:*

1) *Case* $0 < \tau < 1$:

$$G(g \mid \tau, \beta, \varepsilon) = \sum_{k=0}^{l-1} \varepsilon^k \frac{g^{(k)}(+0)}{k!} h(\beta + k + 1, \tau) + \Delta_l G(g \mid \tau, \beta, \varepsilon).$$

The function $h(\cdot, \cdot)$ *is defined by* (2.44).

For $\beta \geq 0$, l *can be taken to be an arbitrary number from the interval* $1 \leq l \leq L$. *In this case*

$$|\Delta_l G| \leq \varepsilon^{l-\beta-1} \left(\left(\frac{1}{\tau}\right)^{l-[-\beta]} + \left(\frac{1}{1-\tau}\right)^{l-[\beta]} + O(1) \right) O(1).$$

For $\beta < 0$, *we can take* $l = 1$. *In this case*

$$|\Delta_1 G| \leq \begin{cases} (\sin \pi\tau)^{-1} O(1) & \text{if } -1 \leq \beta < 0, \\ O(1) & \text{if } -2 \leq \beta < -1, \\ O(\varepsilon) & \text{if } \beta < -2. \end{cases}$$

2) *Case* $\tau = 0$:

$$G(g \mid 0, \beta, \varepsilon) = \varepsilon^{-\beta-1} C_{-1}(g \mid \beta, \varepsilon) + \sum_{k=0}^{l-1} \varepsilon^k \frac{g^{(k)}(+0)}{k!} C_k(\beta) + \Delta_l G(g \mid 0, \beta, \varepsilon).$$

For $\beta \geq 0$, l *can be an arbitrary number from the interval* $2 \leq l \leq L$. *For* $\beta < 0$, *we must take* $l = 1$. *Here*

$$C_{-1}(g|\beta, \varepsilon) = \begin{cases} \int_0^\infty x^\beta g(x)\, dx, & \beta \geq 0, \\ -\frac{1}{\beta+1} \int_0^\infty x^{\beta+1} g^{(1)}(x)\, dx, & -1 < \beta < 0 \text{ or } -2 < \beta < -1, \\ g(0) \log(1/\varepsilon), & \beta = -1, \\ 0, & \beta \leq -2, \end{cases}$$

$$C_0(\beta) = \begin{cases} \frac{2\Gamma(\beta+1)}{(2\pi)^{\beta+1}} \cos \frac{\pi}{2}(\beta+1)\zeta(\beta+1), & \beta > 0, \\ -\frac{1}{2}, & \beta = 0, \\ \frac{1}{2} - \frac{\beta}{12} + H_0(\beta), & \beta = -1, \\ \frac{1}{2} - \frac{\beta}{12} - \frac{1}{\beta+1} + H_0(\beta), & \beta < 0, \quad \beta \neq 1, \end{cases}$$

where

$$H_0(\beta) = -\frac{1}{2\pi^2} \beta(\beta - 1) \sum_{p=1}^{\infty} \frac{1}{p^2} \int_1^\infty t^{\beta-2} \cos 2\pi pt\, dt,$$

$\zeta(s)$ *is the Riemann zeta function,*

$$C_k(\beta) = 2\frac{\Gamma(k+\beta+1)}{(2\pi)^{k+\beta+1}} \cos \frac{2}{\pi}(k+\beta+1)\zeta(k+\beta+1) \qquad k = 1, 2, \ldots, \quad \beta \geq 0$$

(*for* $\beta < 0$ *we take* $l = 1$ *and there are no terms* C_k *with* $k \geq 1$).

Also,

$$|\Delta_l G| \leq \begin{cases} O(\varepsilon^{\rho-\beta-1}) & \text{if } \beta \geq 0 \ (l \geq 2), \\ O(\varepsilon \log(1/\varepsilon)) & \text{if } \beta < 0 \ (l = 2). \end{cases}$$

All O*-estimates are uniform with respect to* τ *and* β *and can be computed efficiently;* $O(1)$ *for* $\varepsilon \to +0$ *means that the term is bounded for small* ε.

This lemma enables us to answer the question about the asymptotic behavior of $T_k(t)$ (hence, about the asymptotic behavior of the discretization error) as $\varepsilon_S \to 0$. Below we will consider only the simplest kernels of the form $\widehat{L}_0(\omega) = b^{\pm}|\omega|^{\rho^{\pm}}$. For such a kernel formula (2.34) can be rewritten in the form

$$Q^{\pm}_{k,j}(t) = 2^{\rho^{\pm}-k+j} \sum_{p=1}^{\infty} e^{i2\pi p\{\mp t/\Delta t\}} p^{\rho^{\pm}-k+j} S^{(j)}(\pm p2\varepsilon_S).$$

We recall that $k = 0, 1, \ldots, N$, $j = 0, 1, \ldots, k$, and $\{x\}$ denotes the fractional part of x. We can easily see that

$$Q^{\pm}_{k,j}(t) = 2^{\rho^{\pm}-k+j} G(S^{(j)}(\pm\xi) \mid \{\mp t/\Delta t\}, \rho^{\pm} - k + j, 2\varepsilon_S).$$

Using this formula, from (2.33) we obtain

(2.46)
$$T^{\pm}_k(t) = \frac{i^k}{k!} b^{\pm}(2\Omega)^{\rho^{\pm}-k} \sum_{j=0}^{k} (\pm 1)^{k-j} \binom{k}{j} B^{\rho^{\pm}}_{k-j} \varepsilon^j G(S^{(j)}(\pm\xi) \mid \tau_{\pm}, \rho^{\pm} - k + j, \varepsilon),$$
$$\varepsilon = 2\varepsilon_S, \qquad \tau_{\pm} = \{\mp t/\Delta t\} \equiv \{\mp t\Omega/\pi\}.$$

The asymptotic behavior of $T_k(t)$ depends on whether $t \neq t_n = n\Delta t$ or $t = t_n$. Accordingly, we formulate two separate propositions. In these propositions and until the end of this section $[x]$ and $\{x\}$ denote the integral and the fractional part of x. All O-bounds for $\varepsilon \to +0$ are uniform with respect to parameters (like Ω, $\tau_{\pm}$, etc.) and can be efficiently computed. The parameters ε and $\tau_{\pm}$ are the same as in (2.46).

PROPOSITION 2.11. *Consider a kernel of the form* $\widehat{L}_0(\omega) = b^{\pm}|\omega|^{\rho^{\pm}}$, $\omega \geq$ *or* $\leq \pm\omega_L$, $\rho = \max(\rho^+, \rho^-)$, *and* $\overline{\rho} = \max(\rho, 0)$. *Let* $u \in \mathscr{U}_M$, $M_Z \geq \overline{\rho} + 2 + \delta$, *and let a regularizer* $R_\alpha \in \mathscr{R}(\overline{\rho})$ *be homogeneous and* $(N+2)$*-smooth* $(N \geq \rho + \delta)$. *Then for* $t \neq t_n$ *we have*:

1) *for* $0 \leq k \leq [\rho^{\pm}]$

$$T^{\pm}_k(t) = \frac{i^k}{k!} b^{\pm}(\pm 1)^k B^{\rho^{\pm}}_k (2\Omega)^{\rho^{\pm}-k} h(\rho^{\pm} - k + 1, \tau_{\pm})$$
$$+ \left(\left(\frac{1}{\tau_{\pm}}\right)^{-2[-\rho^{\pm}]+2-k} + \left(\frac{1}{1-\tau_{\pm}}\right)^{-2[-\rho^{\pm}]+2-k} + O(1) \right) O(\varepsilon)\Omega^{\rho^{\pm}-k};$$

2) *for* $k \geq [\rho^{\pm}] + 1$

$$T^{\pm}_k(t) = \left(\left(\frac{1}{\tau_{\pm}}\right)^{2-[-\rho^{\pm}]} + \left(\frac{1}{1-\tau_{\pm}}\right)^{2-[-\rho^{\pm}]} + O(1) \right) O(1)\Omega^{\rho^{\pm}-k}.$$

PROOF. 1) We note that this case does not occur if $\rho^{\pm} < 0$. Let $0 \leq k \leq [\rho^{\pm}]$. Then $\rho^{\pm} - k + j \geq 0$ for all $j = 0, 1, \ldots, k$. Consider the expression $\varepsilon^j G(S^{(j)}(\pm\xi)|\tau_{\pm}, \rho^{\pm} - k_j, \varepsilon)$ in (2.46). The function $S^{(j)}$ has $N + 2 - j \geq$

$\rho^{\pm} + \delta + 2 - j \geq -[-\rho^{\pm}] - k + 2 \geq 2$ derivatives. Using the first part of the previous lemma with $l = -[-\rho^{\pm}] - k + 2 \geq 2$, we obtain

$$\varepsilon^j G(S^{(j)}(\pm\xi) \mid \tau_{\pm}, \rho^{\pm} - k + j) = \varepsilon^j \sum_{m=0}^{l-1} \varepsilon^m \frac{S^{(j+m)}(\pm 0)}{m!} h(\rho^{\pm} - k + j + m + 1, \tau_{\pm})$$

$$+ \varepsilon^j \varepsilon^{l-\rho^{\pm}+k-j-1} \left(\left(\frac{1}{\tau_{\pm}}\right)^{l-[-\rho^{\pm}]-k+j} + \left(\frac{1}{1-\tau_{\pm}}\right)^{l-[-\rho^{\pm}]-k+j} + O(1) \right) O(1).$$

Using the properties of the function $h(\cdot,\cdot)$ (see (2.45)), the choice $l = -[-\rho^{\pm}] - k + 2$, and the property $S(0) = 1$, we have

$$\varepsilon^j G(S^{(j)}(\pm\xi) | \tau_{\pm}, \rho^{\pm} - k + j, \varepsilon) = \begin{cases} h(\rho^{\pm} - k + 1, \tau_{\pm}) + A, & \text{if } j = 0, \\ A, & \text{if } j \neq 0, \end{cases}$$

where

$$A = \left(\left(\frac{1}{\tau_{\pm}}\right)^{-2[-\rho^{\pm}]+2-k} + \left(\frac{1}{1-\tau_{\pm}}\right)^{-2[-\rho^{\pm}]+2-k} + O(1) \right) O(\varepsilon).$$

Substituting this in (2.46), we obtain the first equality of the proposition.

2) Let $k > [\rho^{\pm}]$. Then $\rho^{\pm} - k + j$ can be either positive or negative. Since $k \leq N$ and $S(\xi) \in C^{N+2}$, $S^{(j)}$ has at least two continuous derivatives for each $j = 0, 1, \ldots, k$. Let us take in the first part of the previous lemma $l = 2$ if $\rho^{\pm} - k + j \geq 0$ and $l = 1$ otherwise. We obtain

$$\varepsilon^j G(S^{(j)}(\pm\xi) | \tau_{\pm}, \rho^{\pm} - k + j, \varepsilon) = \varepsilon^j \sum_{m=0}^{l-1} \varepsilon^m \frac{S^{(j+m)}(\pm 0)}{m!} h(\rho^{\pm} - k + j + m + 1, \tau_{\pm})$$

$$+ \begin{cases} O(\varepsilon), & \text{if } \rho^{\pm} - k + j < -2, \\ O(1), & \text{if } -2 \leq \rho^{\pm} - k + j < -1, \\ \left(\frac{1}{\tau_{\pm}} + \frac{1}{1-\tau_{\pm}} + O(1)\right) O(\varepsilon), & \text{if } -1 \leq \rho^{\pm} - k + j < 0, \\ \left(\left(\frac{1}{\tau_{\pm}}\right)^{2-[-\rho^{\pm}]} + \left(\frac{1}{1-\tau_{\pm}}\right)^{2-[-\rho^{\pm}]} + O(1)\right) O(\varepsilon), & \text{if } \rho^{\pm} - k + j \geq 0. \end{cases}$$

Using the properties of the function $h(\cdot,\cdot)$ (see (2.45)), we have

$$\varepsilon^j G(S^{(j)}(\pm\xi) | \tau_{\pm}, \rho^{\pm} - k + j, \varepsilon)$$
$$= \left(\left(\frac{1}{\tau_{\pm}}\right)^{2-[-\rho^{\pm}]} + \left(\frac{1}{1-\tau_{\pm}}\right)^{2-[-\rho^{\pm}]} + O(1) \right) O(1).$$

Substituting this in (2.46), we obtain the second equality of the proposition. □

PROPOSITION 2.12. *Under the conditions of Proposition* 2.11, *let* $t = t_n$. *Then*

$$T_0^\pm(t_n) = b^\pm(2\Omega)^{\rho^\pm}\left(\varepsilon^{-\rho^\pm-1}E_{-1}^\pm(\rho^\pm) + E_0^\pm(\rho^\pm) + \log(1/\varepsilon)O(\varepsilon)\right),$$

$$T_k^\pm(t_n) = \frac{i^k}{k!}b^\pm(2\Omega)^{\rho^\pm-k}\left(E_0^\pm(\rho^\pm,k) + \log(1/\varepsilon)O(\varepsilon)\right), \qquad k = 1,2,\dots,N.$$

Here

$$E_{-1}^\pm(\rho^\pm) = \begin{cases} \int_0^\infty x^{\rho^\pm}S(\pm x)\,dx, & \rho^\pm \geq 0,\\ \dfrac{(\mp1)^{-[\rho^\pm]}}{(\rho^\pm+1)\cdots\{\rho^\pm\}}\int_0^\infty x^{\{\rho^\pm\}}S^{(-[\rho^\pm])}(x)\,dx, & -1 < \rho^\pm < 0, \textit{ or}\\ & -2 < \rho^\pm < -1,\\ \log(1/\varepsilon), & \rho^\pm = -1,\\ 0 & \rho^\pm \leq -2, \end{cases}$$

$$E_0^\pm(\rho^\pm) = C_0(\rho^\pm),$$

$$E_0^\pm(\rho^\pm,k) = \begin{cases} B_k^{\rho^\pm}C_0(\rho^\pm-k), & k \neq \rho^\pm+1,\ k = 1,2,\dots,N,\\ B_k^{\rho^\pm}C_0(\rho^\pm-k) - (\pm1)^k(k-1)!, & k = \rho^\pm+1, \end{cases}$$

and the function C_0 *is as in the above lemma.*

PROOF. 1) To get the asymptotic behavior of $\varepsilon^j G(S^{(j)}(\pm\xi) \mid 0, \rho^\pm - k + j, \varepsilon)$ we use the second part of the lemma. For $\rho^\pm - k + j \geq 0$ we take $l = -[-\rho^\pm] - k + 2$ in this lemma; otherwise $l = 1$ (this is possible since $k \leq N$ and $S(\xi) \in C^{N+2}$, so that $S^{(j)}$ has at least two continuous derivatives, and for $\rho^\pm - k + j \geq 0$, $S^{(j)}$ has at least $N + j - 2 \geq -[-\rho^\pm] - k + 2$ continuous derivatives). We have

$$\begin{aligned}\varepsilon^j G(S^{(j)}(\pm\xi) \mid 0, \rho^\pm - k + j, \varepsilon) &= \varepsilon^{-\rho^\pm+k-1}C_{-1}(S^{(j)}(\pm\xi)|\rho^\pm - k + j, \varepsilon)\\ &\quad + \varepsilon^j\sum_{m=0}^{l-1}\varepsilon^m\frac{S^{(j+m)}(\pm0)}{m!}C_m(\rho^\pm - k + j)\\ &\quad + \begin{cases} \varepsilon^{-[-\rho^\pm]-\rho^\pm+1}O(1), & \rho^\pm - k + j \geq 0,\\ \varepsilon^{j+1}\log(1/\varepsilon)O(1), & \rho^\pm - k + j < 0. \end{cases}\end{aligned}$$

Since $S(0) = 1$, the last formula yields

$$\begin{aligned}\varepsilon^j G(S^{(j)}(\pm\xi)|0, \rho^\pm - k + j, \varepsilon) =& \varepsilon^{-\rho^\pm+k-1}C_{-1}(S^{(j)}(\pm\xi)|\rho^\pm - k + j, \varepsilon)\\ &+ \log(1/\varepsilon)O(\varepsilon) + \begin{cases} C_0(\rho^\pm - k), & j = 0\\ 0, & j \neq 0. \end{cases}\end{aligned}$$

Now (2.46) gives

$$T_k^\pm(n) = \frac{i^k}{k!}b^\pm(2\Omega)^{\rho^\pm-k}(\varepsilon^{-\rho^\pm+k-1}\widetilde{E}_{-1,k}^\pm(\rho^\pm) + B_k^{\rho^\pm}C_0(\rho^\pm-k) + \log(1/\varepsilon)O(\varepsilon)),$$

where

$$\widetilde{E}_{-1,k}^\pm(\rho^\pm) = \sum_{j=0}^k(\pm1)^{k-j}\binom{k}{j}B_{k-j}^{\rho^\pm}C_{-1}(S^{(j)}(\pm\xi) \mid \rho^\pm - k + j, \varepsilon).$$

2) We must analyze the behavior of $\widetilde{E}^{\pm}_{-1,k}(\rho^{\pm})$. The simplest way to do this is to consider separately seven cases:

$$\rho^{\pm} \geq k; \qquad \rho^{\pm} = 0,\ k = 1, 2, \dots; \qquad \rho^{\pm} = -1;$$
$$\rho^{\pm} = -2, -3, \dots; \qquad \rho^{\pm} < 0,\ \{\rho^{\pm}\} > 0;$$
$$\rho^{\pm} = 1, 2, \dots,\ k > \rho^{\pm}; \qquad k > \rho^{\pm} > 0,\ \{\rho^{\pm}\} > 0.$$

Let us consider the first case $\rho^{\pm} \geq k$. In this case $\rho^{\pm} - k + j \geq 0$ and (see the lemma)

$$C_{-1}(S^{(j)}(\pm\xi) \mid \rho^{\pm} - k + j, \varepsilon) = \int_0^{\infty} x^{\rho^{\pm}-k+j} S^{(j)}(\pm x)\, dx.$$

Therefore,

$$\begin{aligned}
\widetilde{E}^{\pm}_{-1,k}(\rho^{\pm}) &= \sum_{j=0}^{k} (\pm 1)^{(k-j)} \binom{k}{j} B^{\rho^{\pm}}_{k-j} \int_0^{\infty} x^{\rho^{\pm}-k+j} S^{(j)}(\pm x)\, dx \\
&= (\pm 1)^k \int_0^{\infty} \frac{d}{dx^k}(x^{\rho^{\pm}} S(\pm x))\, dx = \begin{cases} \int_0^{\infty} x^{\rho^{\pm}} S(\pm x)\, dx, & k = 0, \\ 0, & k \neq 0. \end{cases}
\end{aligned}$$

So, for $\rho^{\pm} \geq k$ we have

$$\widetilde{E}^{\pm}_{-1,k}(\rho^{\pm}) = \begin{cases} \int_0^{\infty} x^{\rho^{\pm}} S(\pm x)\, dx, & k = 0, \\ 0, & k \neq 0. \end{cases}$$

The other cases can be considered similarly:
Case $\rho^{\pm} = 0$, $k = 1, 2, \dots$:

$$\widetilde{E}^{\pm}_{-1,k}(\rho^{\pm}) = \mp S^{(k-1)}(\pm 0).$$

Case $\rho^{\pm} = -1$:

$$\widetilde{E}^{\pm}_{-1,k}(\rho^{\pm}) = S^{(k)}(\pm 0) \log(1/\varepsilon).$$

Case $\rho^{\pm} = -2, -3, \dots$:

$$\widetilde{E}^{\pm}_{-1,k}(\rho^{\pm}) = 0.$$

Case $\rho^{\pm} < 0$, $\{\rho^{\pm}\} > 0$:

$$\widetilde{E}^{\pm}_{-1,k}(\rho^{\pm}) = \begin{cases} \frac{(\mp 1)^{[\rho^{\pm}]}}{(\rho^{\pm}+1)\cdots\{\rho^{\pm}\}} \int_0^{\infty} x^{\{\rho^{\pm}\}} (\pm 1)^{[\rho^{\pm}]} S^{(-[\rho^{\pm}])}(x)\, dx, & k = 0, \\ 0, & k = 1, 2, \dots. \end{cases}$$

Case $\rho^{\pm} = 1, 2, \dots$, $k > \rho^{\pm}$ (hence, $k \geq 2$):

$$\widetilde{E}^{\pm}_{-1,k}(\rho^{\pm}) = -(\pm 1)^{\rho^{\pm}+1} \rho^{\pm}! \binom{k-1}{\rho^{\pm}} S^{(k-1-\rho^{\pm})}(\pm 0).$$

Case $k > \rho^{\pm} > 0$, $\{\rho^{\pm}\} > 0$ (hence, $k \geq 1$):

$$\widetilde{E}^{\pm}_{-1,k}(\rho^{\pm}) = 0.$$

Combining 1) and 2), we complete the proof of Proposition 2.12. □

Propositions 2.11 and 2.12 completely describe the asymptotic behavior of $T_k(t)$ as $\Omega \to \infty$, $\alpha \to 0$ in such a way that $\varepsilon_S = \alpha\Omega \to 0$. Furthermore, we have the following result.

PROPOSITION 2.13. *Let $L \in \mathscr{L}_0(\rho_0^{\pm})$, $\rho = \max(\rho_0^+, \rho_0^-)$, $\overline{\rho} = \max(\rho, 0)$. Let $u \in \mathscr{U}_M$ for $M_Z \geq \overline{\rho} + 2 + \delta$, and let $R_\alpha \in \mathscr{R}(\overline{\rho})$ be a homogeneous $(N+2)$-smooth regularizer. Let $\Delta t \to 0$, $\alpha \to 0$ in such a way that $\varepsilon_S = \alpha\Omega \to 0$. Then the discretization error converges for $\rho < -1$ and diverges for $\rho \geq -1$. The divergence is caused by terms with $k = 0, 1, \dots, [\rho]$. The divergence part of the discretization error is given by the differential operator $\sum_{k=0}^{\max(0,[\rho])} u^{(k)}(t)T_k(t)$. For $t \neq t_n \equiv \pi N/\Omega$ and sufficiently small ε_S there exist constants D_k that do not depend on α, Ω, t and can be computed efficiently, such that*

$$|T_k^{\pm}(t_n)| \leq D_k d^{-4-2\overline{\rho}}\Omega^{\rho_0^{\pm}-k}.$$

Here d is the distance between t and the nearest node t_n divided by the lattice step Δt. For $t = t_n$, sufficiently small ε_S, and $k = 1, 2, \dots$ there exist constants $\widetilde{D_k}$ that do not depend on α and Ω and can be explicitly computed, such that

$$|T_k^{\pm}(t_n)| \leq \widetilde{D_k}\Omega^{\rho_0^{\pm}-k}.$$

Without loss of generality one can take $D_k = \widetilde{D_k}$.

PROOF. It suffices to consider a kernel $\widehat{L}_0(\omega)$ of the simplest form. For such a kernel the proof follows immediately from the asymptotic formulas in Propositions 2.11 and 2.12. □

Under the conditions of Theorem 2.7 and Propositions 2.11, 2.12 we have the following corollary.

COROLLARY. *For polynomial kernels and smooth homogeneous regularizers the discretization error convergence set $\mathscr{D}$ consists of the region described by* (2.41) *and, in the case when the conditions* (2.41) *are satisfied, of some straight lines $\alpha\Omega = \varepsilon_S = \mathrm{const}$.*

The general Theorem 2.6 allows a similar analysis for the case of a generalized Tikhonov regularizer (1.13). However, it is clear that in the quasipolynomial $Q(\xi)$ one can disregard all lower terms, therefore reducing the regularizer to a homogeneous one with convergence region described by (2.42). We formulate and prove the corresponding result.

PROPOSITON 2.14. *Let $L \in \mathscr{L}_0(\rho_0^{\pm})$ with $\rho = \max(\rho_0^+, \rho_0^-)$, $\overline{\rho} = \max(0, \rho)$. Let R_{α_T} be a generalized Tikhonov regularizer with $q_0 \geq +1+\delta$, and $u \in \mathscr{U}_M$ with $M_u \geq N+2+\delta$, $N \geq \rho + \delta$. Then:*

1) *Theorem* 2.6 *holds.*

2) *For all $k \leq N$, all sufficiently large Ω, and all sufficiently small α_T $(\alpha_T \leq 1)$,*

$$|T_k^{\pm}(t)| \leq C\alpha_T^{-1}\Omega^{\rho_0^{\pm}-q_0-k},$$

with a constant C that can be explicitly computed and does not depend on α_T, Ω, t.

3) *The discretization error converges uniformly (on $\mathscr{U}_M$) inside the region $\mathscr{D}$ defined by the condition*

$$\alpha_T^{-1}\Omega^{\rho-q_0} \to 0. \tag{2.47}$$

4) *For real nonnegative kernels of the form $\overline{L}(\omega) = |\omega|^\rho$ the region $\mathscr{D}$ defined by* (2.47) *is the largest convergence region.*

PROOF. Let us note that it suffices to prove the proposition for the kernel of the form $\widehat{L}_0(\omega) = b_0^{\pm}|\omega|^{\rho_0^{\pm}}$. The proof is based on the easily verified fact that the

Tikhonov regularizer of the form $R_{\alpha_T} = (1 + \alpha_T Q(\omega/\omega_R))$ satisfies, for a sufficiently large ω, the condition

$$(2.48) \qquad |R^{(j)}_{\alpha_T}(\omega)| \leq C^T_j \alpha^j_T \omega^{-j} |R_{\alpha_T}(\omega)|,$$

where the constants C^T_j do not depend on α_T and ω.

1) Since $R_{\alpha_T} \in C^\infty(\mathbb{R} \setminus \{0\})$ and (2.48) holds, the conditions of Theorem 2.6 are satisfied for any N.

2) Let us consider the upper sign. Using (2.28) and taking (2.48) into account, we obtain

$$\begin{aligned} |T^+_k(t)| &\leq \frac{|b^+_0|}{k!} \sum_{j=0}^{\infty} \sum_{j=0}^{k} \binom{k}{j} |R^{(j)}_{\alpha_T}(2n\Omega)| \cdot |B^{p^\pm}_{k-j}| \cdot |2n\Omega|^{\rho^+_0 - k + j} \\ &\leq C_1 \sum_{n=1}^{\infty} \frac{(2n\Omega)^{\rho^+_0 - k}}{1 + \alpha_T (2n\Omega)^{q_0}(1 + O(\Omega^{-\delta}))}. \end{aligned}$$

Here the O-term is uniform with respect to α_T and n, $\delta = q_0 - q_1 > 0$. Next, for a sufficiently large Ω we have

$$|T^+_k(t)| \leq C_1 \sum_{n=1}^{\infty} \frac{(2n\Omega)^{\rho^+_0 - k}}{\frac{1}{2}\alpha_T (2n\Omega)^{q_0}} \leq C_1 \cdot \tfrac{1}{2} \cdot 2^{\rho^\pm - k - q_0} \alpha_T^{-1} \Omega^{\rho^+_0 - k - q_0} \zeta(q_0 + k - \rho^+_0),$$

and part 2) is proved.

3) follows from Theorem 2.6 and part 2).

4) follows from Remark 2 to Theorem 2.5 and the condition (2.17). □

Replacing α_T by α^q in (2.47), we obtain (2.42).

In conclusion, we consider the case when a smooth regularizer is the product of two smooth regularizers, one being homogeneous.

PROPOSITION 2.15. *Let the conditions of Theorem 2.6 be satisfied with a regularizer of the form $R_{\overline{\alpha}}(\omega) = R^1_{\alpha_1}(\omega) R^2_{\alpha_2}(\omega)$, with R^1, R^2 being $(N+1)$-smooth and R^1 being also homogeneous. Let $\mathscr{D}^0_\beta = \mathscr{D}^1_{(\Delta t, \alpha_1)} \times [0, \overline{\alpha}_2]$, where $\overline{\alpha}_2 > 0$ and $\mathscr{D}^1_{(\Delta t, \alpha_1)}$ is the high-resolution region for R^1, i.e., $\alpha_1 \Omega = \varepsilon_S = \text{const}$. If the conditions (2.38) are satisfied, then the discretization error converges on $\mathscr{U}_M$ inside $\mathscr{D}^0_\beta$ fast and uniformly.*

PROOF. Conditions (2.38) guarantee that $T^\pm_k(t) \equiv 0$ for $k = 0, 1, \dots, [\rho^\pm_0]$. For $k > [\rho^\pm_0]$, we estimate $T^\pm_k(t)$ similarly to Proposition 2.9, using the Leibniz formula, the boundedness (uniform with respect to a_2) of derivatives of R^2, and (2.38). This yeilds an estimate of the form $O(\Omega^{\rho^\pm_0 - k})$ for $T^\pm_k(t)$ with $k > [\rho^\pm_0]$, which is uniform with respect to α_2, t. □

Proposition 2.15 shows that the conditions (2.38) are sufficient for convergence inside the entire region $\mathscr{D}^0_\beta$. The next proposition deals with the case when (2.38) is violated.

PROPOSITION 2.16. *Under the conditions of Proposition 2.15 let $R^2_{\alpha_2} = R_{\alpha_T}$ be a Tikhonov regularizer (with the quasipolynomial of degree q_0), and let (2.38) be replaced by*

$$S^{(j)}(2n\varepsilon_S) = 0, \qquad j = 0, \dots, k^{\pm}, \tag{2.49}$$

with at least one of the numbers $k^{\pm}$ being smaller than the corresponding $[\rho_0^{\pm}]$. Then a sufficient condition for the rapid and uniform convergence of the discretization error on $\mathcal{U}_M$ inside a region $\mathcal{D}_{\overline{\beta}} \subset \mathcal{D}^0_{\overline{\beta}}$ is

$$\alpha_T^{-1}\Omega^{\max_{+,-}(\rho_0^{\pm}-k^{\pm}-1)-q_0} \to 0 \tag{2.50}$$

as $|\overline{\beta}| \to 0$, $\overline{\beta} \in \mathcal{D}_{\overline{\beta}}$. For a sufficiently smooth right-hand side the convergence rate is determined by the convergence rate in (2.50).

PROOF. It suffices to consider the kernel $\widehat{L}_0(\omega) = b_0^{\pm}|\omega|^{\rho_0^{\pm}}$ of the simplest form. For this kernel Theorem 2.6 holds. Let us confider $T_k^{\pm}$. For $k = 0, 1, \dots, k^{\pm}$ the conditions (2.49) guarantee $T_k^{\pm} \equiv 0$. By the previous proposition, $T_k^{\pm}(t) = O(\Omega^{\rho_0^{\pm}-k})$ for $k > [\rho_0^{\pm}]$. Therefore, it remains to consider $T_k^{\pm}(t)$ for $k = k^{\pm}+1, \dots, [\rho_0^{\pm}]$. From (2.28) we have

$$|T_k^{+}(t)| \le \frac{|b_0^{+}|}{k!}\sum_{n=1}^{\infty}\sum_{j=0}^{k}\binom{k}{j}|R_{\overline{\alpha}}^{(j)}(2n\Omega)|\cdot|B_{k-j}^{\rho_0^{+}}|\cdot|2n\Omega|^{\rho_0^{\pm}-k+j}.$$

Using (2.48) and taking (2.49) into account, we obtain

$$|T_k^{+}(t)| \le \frac{|b_0^{+}|}{k!}\sum_{n=1}^{\infty}\sum_{j=k^{+}+1}^{k}\sum_{m=0}^{i-k^{+}-1}C_{k,j,m}\alpha_T^m\frac{(2n)^{\rho_0^{+}-k+j-m}S^{(j-m)}(2n\varepsilon_S)}{1+\alpha_T(2n\Omega)^{q_0}(1+O(\Omega^{-\delta}))}\Omega^{\rho_0^{+}-k},$$

where the explicitly computable constants $C_{k,j,m}$ do not depend on Ω, α_T, or t, and the O-bound is uniform with respect to α_T, t. The last inequality easily implies that

$$|T_k^{+}(t)| \le C_1\Omega^{\rho_0^{+}-k}\alpha_T^{-1}\Omega^{-q_0}\sum_{n=1}^{\infty}n^{\rho_0^{+}-q_0} \le C\alpha_T^{-1}\Omega^{\rho_0^{+}-k-q_0}$$

for a sufficiently large Ω and a sufficiently small α_T. The constant C does not depend on Ω, α_T, t. A similar estimate can be obtained for T_k^{-}. It is clear that (2.50) guarantees that $T_k^{\pm}(t) \to 0$ uniformly with respect to t for $k = k^{\pm}+1, \dots, [\rho_0^{\pm}]$.

Therefore, if (2.49), (2.50) are satisfied, $T_k(t) \to 0$ uniformly for all $k \ge N$, and the proposition follows from Theorem 2.6. □

For $\widehat{L}(\omega) \sim |\omega|^{\rho}$, the region described by (2.50) appears to be the largest convergence region inside $\mathcal{D}^0_{\overline{\beta}}$.

§2.5. Algorithm with renormalization

Using the results of the previous section, we construct here the so-called algorithm with renormalization A^{ren}, which, for smooth kernels and homogeneous regularizers, converges on a class of sufficiently smooth right-hand sides inside any set $\mathcal{D}_{(\Delta t,\alpha)}$ of parameter values. We remark that on the entire real line $\mathbb{R}$ the convergence is only pointwise: the uniformity fails near nodes $t = t_n$. On the other hand, on the set

$$\mathcal{J} = \left(\mathbb{R} \setminus \bigcup_n [t_n - d\Delta t, t_n + d\Delta t]\right) \cup \left(\bigcup_n \{t_n\}\right),$$

$d = \text{const}$, $0 < d < 1/2$, the convergence is uniform. This means that the algorithm converges uniformly on the lattice $l\widetilde{\Delta t} = \widetilde{t_l}$, $l = 0, \pm 1, \pm 2, \dots$, $\widetilde{\Delta t} = \Delta t/m$ or $\widetilde{\Delta t} = m\Delta t$, $m = 1, 2, \dots$, which is usually sufficient in practical applications.

The algorithm A^{ren} is obtained from the algorithm $Z^{A_{RT}(R)}$ by subtracting the divergent part of the discretization error (by analogy with quantum field theory **[20]** we call this procedure *renormalization*; hence the name of the algorithm). Therefore, the algorithm can be interpreted as an application of a special quadrature formula to the integral $Z^R(t)$ (0.8).

We prove the convergence of the algorithm for smooth homogeneous regularizers. The class of regularizers can by somewhat extended so as to include, for example, a rectangular window. Furthermore, our proof requires a strong smoothness condition on the right-hand side. Numerical experiments allow us to conjecture that the algorithm actually converges under very weak smoothness assumptions for $u(t)$.

Throughout this section we assume the conditions of Proposition 2.13 (and hence of Proposition 2.9) to be satisfied. According to Proposition 2.13, the divergent part of the discretization error is described by the differential operator

$$\sum_{k=0}^{\max(0,[p])} u^{(k)}(t)T_k(t).$$

For any N_1, $\overline{p} \le N_1 \le N$, define

$$Z_{N_1}^{R,T}(t) = Z^{R,T}(t) - \sum_{k=0}^{\infty} u^{(k)}(t)T_k(t).$$

PROPOSITION 2.17. *As $\Omega \to \infty$, and for $\overline{p} \le N_1 \le N$, the function $Z_{N_1}^{R,T}(t)$ converges pointwise to $Z^R(t)$. The following estimate holds*:

$$\begin{aligned} |Z_{N_1}^{R,T}(t) - Z^R(t)| \le & O(\Omega^{-M_u+\overline{p}+1}) + O(\Omega^{-N-1+p}) \\ & + \begin{cases} d^{-4-2\overline{p}} O(\Omega^{-N_1-1+p}), & t \ne t_n, \\ O(\Omega^{-N_1-1+p}), & t = t_n, \end{cases} \end{aligned} \tag{2.51}$$

with explicitly computable O-bounds that are uniform with respect to α and t. Here $d = \inf_n(|t - t_n|/\Delta t)$ is the distance from t to the nearest node t_n, measured in Δt units.

PROOF. By Theorem 2.6,

$$Z_{N_1}^{R,T}(t) - Z^R(t) = \sum_{k=N_1+1}^{N} u^{(k)}(t)T_k(t) + Q_{N+1}(t),$$

and $Q_{N+1}(t)$ can be estimated as in (2.27). By Proposition 2.13, for a sufficiently small $\alpha\Omega = \varepsilon_S$ ($\varepsilon_S \le \underline{\varepsilon}_S$) we have

$$|T_k(t)| \le D_k d^{-4-2\overline{p}} \Omega^{p-N_1-1} \quad \text{if } t \ne t_n,$$
$$|T_k(t)| \le \widetilde{D_k} \Omega^{p-N_1-1} \quad \text{if } t = t_n \text{ and } k \ge 1.$$

For $\varepsilon_S > \underline{\varepsilon}_S$ we use Proposition 2.9:

$$|T_k(t)| \leq C(\underline{\varepsilon_S})C\Omega^{\rho-N_1-1}.$$

Since $\sup_t |u^{(k)}(t)| < \infty$ for $k = 0, 1, \ldots, N$, we obtain (2.51). □

The process of passing from $Z^{R,T}$ to $Z^{R,T}_{N_1}$ by subtracting divergent (infinite) terms is called the renormalization of order N_1. Therefore, the construction of convergent quadrature formulas (i.e., of an algorithm that converges inside any $\mathscr{D}_{(\Delta t,\alpha)}$) reduces to a problem of numerical differentiation. Let us consider the simplest version of the solution **[10]**, which is based on an application of Lagrange polynomials. The possibility of constructing convergent quadratures is related to fact that the $T_k(t)$, $k \geq 1$, are independent of ε_S. Denote by $u(t,n)$ the Lagrange interpolation polynomial for the function $u(t)$ constructed from the values $u_{r+1}, \ldots, u_{r+n}$ ($t \in [t_{r+1}, t_{r+2}]$, $t_i = i\Delta t$), and by $u^{(k)}(t,n)$ its kth derivative. Denote also

$$Z^{R,T}_{N_1,n} \stackrel{\text{def}}{=} Z^{A^{\text{ren}}(R)}(t) = Z^{R,T} - \sum_{k=0}^{N_1} u^{(k)}(t,n)T_k(n). \tag{2.52}$$

Unlike $Z^{R,T}_{N_1}$, $Z^{R,T}_{N_1,n}$ is expressed explicitly in terms of samples of the function $u(t)$.

THEOREM 2.8. *Let the conditions of Proposition* 2.13 *be satisfied and let the function u be sufficiently smooth, so that n and N_1 can be chosen in such a way that*

1) $n \geq N_1 > \max(0, [\rho])$; $N_1 \leq N$,
2) $n + N_1 < [M_u] - 1$,

where $[\cdot]$ again denotes the integral part. Then $Z^{R,T}_{N_1,n}$ (defined by (2.52)) *yields a convergent quadrature formula for Z^R that converges uniformly with respect to α (i.e., $Z^{R,T}_{N_1,n} \to Z^R$ as $\Omega \to \infty$ uniformly with respect to α), so that the algorithm A^{ren} converges on $\mathscr{U}_M$ inside any region $\mathscr{D}_{[\Delta t,\alpha)}$. Furthermore,*

$$\begin{aligned}|Z^{R,T}_{N_1,n}(t) - Z^R(t)| \leq{}& O(\Omega^{-M_u+\overline{\rho}+1}) + O(\Omega^{-N-1+\rho}) \\ &+ \begin{cases} d^{-4-2\overline{\rho}}\left(O(\Omega^{-n+\rho}) + O(\Omega^{-N_1-1+\rho})\right), & t \neq t_n, \\ O(\Omega^{-n+\rho}) + O(\Omega^{-N_1-1+\rho}), & t = t_n, \end{cases}\end{aligned}$$

with O-bounds that are uniform with respect to α and t; here d is the distance to the nearest node measured in Δt units.

PROOF. By Proposition 2.9 and 2.13,

$$T_k(t) \leq \begin{cases} C_k d^{-4-2\overline{\rho}}\Omega^{\rho-k}, & t \neq t_r, \\ C_k\Omega^{\rho-k}, & t = t_r, \quad k \geq 1, \end{cases} \tag{2.53}$$

where the constants C_k do not depend on α, Ω, t and can be computed explicitly (see the proof of the previous proposition). We have

$$\begin{aligned}&|Z^{R,T}_{N_1,n}(t) - Z^R(t)| \\ &\quad \leq \sum_{k=0}^{N_1} |u^{(k)}(t,n) - u^{(k)}(t)| \cdot |T_k(t)| + \left|\sum_{k\geq N_1+1} u^{(k)}(t)T_k(t)\right| + |Q_{N+1}(t)|.\end{aligned}$$

For Q_{N+1} we have the estimate (2.27). Consider the first term in the previous formula.

Since $u(t,n)$ is the Lagrange polynomial for $u(t)$, we have, by **[21]**,

$$|u^{(k)}(t,n) - u^{(k)}(t)| \leq \sum_{j=0}^{k} \frac{k!}{(k-j)!(n+j)!} \widetilde{u}^{(n+j)} |\omega_n^{(k-j)}(t)|,$$

where

$$\widetilde{u}^{(n+j)} \stackrel{\text{def}}{=} \sup_{t\in[t_{r+1},t_{r+n}]} |u^{(n+j)}(t)|, \qquad \omega_n(t) = \prod_{i=1}^{n}(t - t_{r+i}).$$

Since $t \in [t_{r+1}, t_{r+n}]$, we have on this interval

$$|\omega_n^{(k-j)}(t)| \leq \widetilde{B}_{n,k-j}\Omega^{-n+k-j},$$

with certain constants $\widetilde{B}_{n,k-j}$. Therefore, if $u(t)$ has $n+k$ bounded derivatives, then

$$|u^{(k)}(t,n) - u^{(k)}(t)| \leq B_{kn}\Omega^{-n+k}, \tag{2.54}$$

where the constants B_{nk} are such that

$$\sum_{j=0}^{k} \frac{k!}{(k-j)!(n+j)!} \widetilde{u}^{(n+j)} \widetilde{B}_{n,k-j} \frac{1}{\Omega^j} \leq B_{nk}.$$

Condition 2) in the formulation of the theorem implies that the function $u(t)$ has $n+N_1$ continuous derivatives ($n \in L^1$, $|\widehat{u}(\omega)| \leq \widetilde{u}|\omega|^{-M_u}$). Now let $t \neq t_n$. The first inequality in (2.53), together in (2.54), yields the inequality

$$|u^{(k)}(t,n) - u^{(k)}(t)|\,|T_k(t)| \leq C_k B_{kn} d^{-4-2\overline{p}}\Omega^{p-n},$$

and the estimate $O(\Omega^{-n+p})d^{-4-2\overline{p}}$ for the first term. If $t = t_r$, then $u(t_r, n) = u(t_r)$ and the term with $k = 0$ in the sum corresponds to an appropriate term on the right-hand side. For $k \geq 1$, (2.53) and (2.54) give the estimate $O(\Omega^{-n+p})$. It remains to recall that condition 1) in the formulation of the theorem implies Proposition 2.17 and the estimate (2.51). □

Chapter 3. Algorithms for the Construction of Solutions on Lattices

In this chapter we consider algorithms for the construction of solutions on the lattice $t_n = \Delta t n$ with a finite number $(2N+1)$ of nodes ($n = -N, -N+1, \dots, N$), so that $\mathcal{J} = \bigcup_{n=-N}^{N}\{t_n\}$. Since in practice we are usually interested in the solutions inside a finite interval $|t| \leq T_Z$, and values of a function at the nodes allow us to construct its values at other points (using interpolation), the information about values at the nodes is usually sufficient (one must only satisfy the condition $N \geq T_Z/\Delta t$). In addition to the usual smoothness conditions for the right-hand side u, we assume that u has compact support; the case of non-compactly-supported u will be discussed only briefly. The compact support requirement is not very essential, but it simplifies and shortens the proofs; furthermore, it is often satisfied in practice.

We start in §3.1 with the realization of an algorithm for the construction of solutions on the lattice using the *finite discrete Fourier transform* (FDFT). Here we introduce the necessary notation.

In §3.2 we consider the algorithm $A_1(R)$. This algorithm is constructed using FDFT from a *seed regularizer* R_α and depends (in the case when R_α is one-dimensional) on the parameters $\overline{\beta} = (\Delta t, N^{-1}, \alpha)$. The analysis of this algorithm is based on the fact that if $|\overline{\beta}| \to 0$ in such a way that $N\Delta t \to \infty$, the solution $Z^{A_1}(t_n)$ differs only slightly from the solution $Z^{A_0(\widetilde{R})}(t_n)$, which is obtained using the RT-algorithm A_0 with the regularizer $\widetilde{R}(\omega) = R_\alpha(\omega)\chi_\Omega(\omega)$. This approach enables us to prove the convergence of algorithms $A_1(R)$ for smooth right-hand sides inside the regions $\mathscr{D}$ such that $|\overline{\beta}| \to 0$ implies $N\Delta t \to \infty$. Let us remark that in practice the number of nodes is chosen from the relation $N\Delta t = \text{const}$. The results below significantly clarify the situation, and conditions of the form $N\Delta t \to \infty$ are related only to the method of the proof. Algorithm A_1 provides a construction of an efficient regularizer R^{ef}; the explicit form of this regularizer is given below. For $|\overline{\beta}| \to 0$ and $N\Delta t \to \infty$ we have $R^{\text{eff}} \sim \widetilde{R}(\omega) = R_\alpha(\omega)\chi_\Omega(\omega)$.

In §3.3 we consider the algorithm A_T (see **[5]** and the Introduction). This algorithm can be used in the case when $K(t)$ (defined by $\widehat{K}(\omega) = \widehat{L}^{-1}(\omega)$) is a classical function. The algorithm A_T depends on the parameters $\overline{\beta} = (\Delta t, N^{-1}, \alpha)$. To study A_T we apply one of several possible approaches, namely the approach when we estimate the difference between the solution $Z_n^{A_T}$ and the solution obtained by using a certain RT-algorithm with the regularizer depending on the kernel $\widehat{K}(\omega)$ and the stabilizing factor $M(\omega)$. Using this approach, we prove the convergence in the region of the form $\mathscr{D}_{\widetilde{\beta}} = \mathscr{D}_{(\Delta t, N^{-1})} \times [0, \overline{\alpha}_T]$, where the region $\mathscr{D}_{(\Delta t, N^{-1})} \subset \mathbb{R}^2$ satisfies certain conditions to ensure that N grows faster than Ω. In the examples below these conditions take the form $N \geq C\Omega^{1+\delta}$ with δ depending on the kernel. We can enlarge the region for which the convergence of A_T is proved both by improving our approach and by using other approaches. However, these improvements do not seem to be too important.

§3.1. Realization of RT-algorithms on a finite lattice

We start this section with a simple but important remark about compactification. After that we define FDFT and construct a realization of the algorithm A_{RT} for a finite lattice. Usually, this realization has smaller complexity (i.e., we requires a smaller number of operations) than the one based on formula (0.9). The algorithm A_{RT} is given by the formulas

$$Z^{R,T}(t) = \sum_n H(t - n\Delta t)u_n\Delta t, \qquad \widehat{H}(\omega) = \widehat{L}(\omega)R_\alpha(\omega).$$

Here and later we omit the upper index R in the notation of regularized kernels. In practice we take only a finite sum over n, i.e., we consider

$$Z^{R,T,N_u}(t) = \sum_{n=-N_u}^{N_u} H(t - n\Delta t)u_n\Delta t \overset{\text{def}}{=} Z^{A_{RT}^{N_u}}(t).$$

This introduces an additional error, which will be called the *compactification error* ΔC ($\Delta C(t) = Z^{A_{RT}^{N_u}}(t) - Z^{A_{RT}}(t)$), and the solution $Z^{A_{RT}^{N_u}}$ depends now on the additional parameter N_u. It is clear that if $\alpha, \Omega = \text{const}$ and $N_u \to \infty$, then $\Delta C \to 0$. If we know the behavior of $u(t)$ as $t \to \infty$, the compactification error can be easily estimated.

As an example, let us consider the case when $L \in \mathscr{L}(\overline{p})$, $R_\alpha \in \mathscr{R}(\overline{p})$, the Nyquist condition is satisfied, and $u(t) = O(|t|^{-L})$, $L > 1$. In this case

$$|\Delta C(t)| \leq C\Omega^{\overline{p}+L} N_u^{-L+1}.$$

This estimate can be proved by elementary means and (partly because of this) is rather rough. If $u(t)$ is compactly supported ($u(t) = 0$ for $|t| > T_u$) and $N_u \geq T_u/\Delta t$, the algorithms A_{RT} and $A_{RT}^{N_u}$ coincide:

$$Z^{A_{RT}(R)}(t) \equiv Z^{A_{RT}^{N_u}(R)}(t), \qquad \Delta C \equiv 0.$$

This remark, although trivial, is nevertheless very important. Everywhere below (unless explicitly mentioned) we assume that $u(t)$ is compactly supported and $N_u \geq T_u/\Delta t$.

Now we construct solutions on a lattice. Let us assume that we are interested in the values of the solution at the points $t_n = n\Delta t$, $|n| \leq N_Z$, $N_Z \Delta t = T_Z$. Let the function $u(t)$ have compact support and $N_u \Delta t = T_u$. We write the solution in the form

$$\begin{gathered} Z_n^A = \sum_{j=-N_u}^{N_u} H_{n-j} u_j \Delta t, \\ Z_n^A \equiv Z^A(t_n), \qquad H_k \equiv H(k\Delta t), \qquad n \leq N_Z. \end{gathered} \tag{3.1}$$

Let us show how (3.1) can be realized using the FDFT. We start with the *definition of FDFT.* Let f_n^N be an $(2N+1)$-periodic sequence. The direct FDFT is defined by

$$\widetilde{f}_m^N = \sum_n{}^N e^{i2\pi nm/(2N+1)} f_n^N,$$

where $\sum^N$ means the summation over a period (i.e., the sum of any $2N+1$ consecutive elements of the sequence). It is clear that the resulting sequence is also $(2N+1)$-periodic. The inversion formula is of the form

$$f_n^N = \frac{1}{2N+1} \sum_m{}^N e^{-i2\pi nm/(2N+1)} \widetilde{f}_m^N.$$

Let us note that for FDFT there exists an analog of the convolution theorem (if $h_n^N = \sum_j{}^N g_{n-j}^N f_j^N$ then $\widetilde{h}_n^N = \widetilde{f}_n^N \widetilde{g}_n^N$) and an analog of the Plancherel formula ($\sum^N |f_n|^2 = \frac{1}{2N+1}\sum^N |\widetilde{f}_n|^2$). Of course, FDFT can be defined for functions with period of even length as well, but we will not need it.

Now let $f_n = f(n\Delta t)$ be samples of the function $f(t)$. Denote by f_n^N the $(2N+1)$-periodic sequence defined as follows:

$$f_n^N = \begin{cases} f_n & \text{for } |n| \leq N, \\ \text{determined by the periodicity condition for other } n. \end{cases} \tag{3.2}$$

If $f(t)$ is a compactly supported function, $\operatorname{supp} f \subset [-T_f, T_f]$, and $N\Delta t > T_f$, then for

$$\omega_j = j\Delta\omega, \qquad \Delta\omega = \frac{2\Omega}{2N+1} \qquad \left(\Delta\omega\Delta t = \frac{2\pi}{2N+1}\right),$$

we have

$$\widetilde{f}_n^N \Delta t = \widehat{f}^T(\omega_j).$$

Now let us describe the realization of the algorithm. Define u_n^N and H_n^N following (3.2) and assuming that $N \geq N_u + N_Z$. Since $|n-j| \leq N$ for $|j| \leq N_u$, $|n| \leq N_Z$, (3.1) can be rewritten in the form

$$Z_n^A = \sum_{j=-N_u}^{N_u} H_{n-j}^N u_j^N \Delta t$$

and, using the compactness of the support of $u(t)$, the summation can be extended to the entire period:

$$Z_n^A = \sum_j{}^N H_{n-j}^N u_j^N \Delta t, \qquad n \leq N_Z.$$

The last sum can be computed using the discrete convolution theorem:

$$Z_n^A = \frac{\Delta t}{2N+1} \sum_j{}^N e^{-i2\pi nj/(2N+1)} \widetilde{H}_j^N \widetilde{u}_j^N. \tag{3.3}$$

Therefore, the realization of the algorithm requires the computation of the direct and of the inverse FDFT. The existing fast algorithms allow us to compute FDFT for $\sim N \log N$ operations. In the most common case $T_Z \sim T_u$ we have $N \sim N_Z \sim N_u$, and the realization of the algorithm requires $\sim N \log N$ operations. Note that the straightforward realization of (0.9) requires $\sim N^2$ operations. Finally, we note that

$$\widetilde{H}_j^N = \sum_{k=-N}^{N} H_k \exp\left(i \frac{2\pi}{2N+1} kj\right), \qquad H_k = \frac{1}{2\pi} \int d\omega e^{-i\omega t_k} \widehat{H}(\omega),$$
$$\widehat{H}(\omega) = \widehat{L}(\omega) R(\omega), \qquad t_k = k\Delta t,$$

can be computed in advance.

§3.2. The algorithm A_1

In this section we consider the following algorithm A_1 for computing solutions of a finite lattice:

$$Z_n^{A_1} = \frac{1}{2N+1} \sum_{j=-N}^{N} e^{-i2\pi nj/(2N+1)} \widehat{H}_j \widetilde{u}_j^N, \qquad |n| \leq N_Z < N,$$
$$\widehat{H}_j \equiv \widehat{H}(\omega_j) \equiv \widehat{H}(j\Delta\omega), \qquad \Delta\omega = \frac{2\Omega}{2N+1}. \tag{3.4}$$

Here $\widetilde{u}_j^N$ is the FDFT of the function u_n^N, $\widehat{H}(\omega) = \widehat{L}(\omega)R(\omega)$, and $R(\omega)$ is called the *seed regularizer*. We prove that A_1 converges for large N, and construct an efficient regularizer $R^{\text{ef}}(A_1)$ for A_1.

Comparison of (3.4) with (3.3) reveals that the algorithm A_1 differs from the previous algorithm in that instead of $\widetilde{H}_j^N \Delta t$ in the main period we use $\widehat{H}(\omega_j)$. The algorithm A_1 itself is reduced to two FDFT's, and its complexity is $N \log N$. Note that we can assume the regularized kernel $\widehat{H}(\omega)$ and the regularizer $R(\omega)$ to be cut off at the Nyquist frequency, because the values of the kernel for $|\omega| > \Omega$ do not enter formula (3.4), which defines the algorithm. The algorithm depends on three parameters $\overline{\beta} = (\Delta t, N^{-1}, \alpha)$; for simplicity we assume that the seed regularizer is one-parametric. We are interested in the limit as $|\overline{\beta}| \to 0$, i.e., as $\Delta t \to 0$, $N \to \infty$, $\alpha \to 0$. To analyze the algorithm A_1, we reduce it to an appropriate RT-algorithm.

We start with the following simple formal remark. For $\widetilde{H}_j^N \Delta t$ with $|j| \le N$ we have

$$\begin{aligned}\widetilde{H}_j^N \Delta t &= \sum_{k=-N}^{N} H_k e^{-it_k\omega_j} \Delta t \simeq \sum_{k=-\infty}^{\infty} H_k e^{-it_k\omega_j} \\ &= \sum_k \widehat{H}(\omega_j + 2n\Omega) = \widehat{H}(\omega_j).\end{aligned} \tag{3.5}$$

The next to last equality in (3.5) is the Poisson formula, and the last one follows from the fact that the support of $\widehat{H}(\omega)$ lies inside the Nyquist interval. It is clear that the precision of the approximation in (3.5) increases when N increases. Therefore it is natural to assume that for large N (as $N \to \infty$) we have $Z^{A_1} \sim Z^{A_0}$ ($Z^{A_1} \to Z^{A_0}$), where Z^{A_0} is the solution obtained by the RT-algorithm A_0 with the regularized kernel $\widehat{H}(\omega)$. Let us note that while estimating the error introduced by extending the summation in (3.5) to all values of k, we can transform these formal arguments into rigorous ones. This can be done, for example, in the case $H_k = O(k^{-1-\delta})$.

Now let us try to estimate the difference $|Z_n^{A_1} - Z^{A_0}(t_n)|$ directly. We must mention that this difference cannot be considered as an additional error of the algorithm A_1 (similar to the discretization and regularization errors): it is an error of the approach (reduction of A_1 to A_0), and not of the algorithm itself.

Following Proposition 1.1, we rewrite the solution $Z^{A_0}(t_n)$ of the RT-algorithm A_0 in the form (0.10). Since the function $u(t)$ is compactly supported and $\operatorname{supp} u \subset [-N\Delta t, N\Delta t]$, we have

$$\widetilde{u}_j^N \equiv \frac{1}{\Delta t} \widehat{u}^T(\omega_j).$$

We assume, of course, that $u \in \mathscr{U}_M$, i.e., $\widehat{u}(\omega) = O(|\omega|^{-1-\delta})$. The last equality gives

$$Z_n^{A_1} = \frac{1}{2\pi} \sum_{j=-N}^{N} e^{-i\omega_j t_n} \widehat{H}(\omega_j) \widehat{u}^T(\omega_j) \Delta\omega \tag{3.6}$$

(here we take into account that the definition (3.4) of the step in ω gives $\Delta t \Delta\omega = 2\pi/(2N+1)$). Comparing (0.10) and (3.6), we see that as $\Delta\omega = 2\pi/(2N+1) \to 0$, we have $Z_n^{A_1} \to Z^{A_0}(t_n)$ (assuming the appropriate smoothness of $\widehat{H}(\omega)\widehat{u}^T(\omega)$).

PROPOSITION 3.1. *Let $L \in \mathscr{L}(\Lambda)$, $R_\alpha \in \mathscr{R}(\Lambda)$, and let $u \in \mathscr{U}_M(\Lambda)$ be a compactly supported function with* $\operatorname{supp} u \subset [-N\Delta t, N\Delta t]$. *Furthermore, let the following conditions be satisfied*:

$$\left| \frac{d}{d\omega} \widehat{L}(\omega) \right| \le O(|\omega|^{\rho'}) \Lambda(\omega), \qquad \rho' \ge 0, \quad |\omega| \to \infty, \tag{3.7}$$

$$\left| \Lambda(\omega) \frac{d}{d\omega} \widehat{u}(\omega) \right| \le \widetilde{Z}^1 |\omega|^{\rho' - M_Z} + \widetilde{Z}^2 |\omega|^{-1-\delta} \tag{3.8}$$

for some $\widetilde{Z}^1$, $\widetilde{Z}^2$, and

$$\left| \frac{d}{d\omega} R_\alpha(\omega) \right| \le \overline{R}_1 \quad \textit{uniformly with respect to } \alpha. \tag{3.9}$$

Then for $M_Z \ge \rho' + 1 + \delta$ and

$$N \ge T_u/\Delta t \ge 3 \tag{3.10}$$

we have the estimate

$$|Z_n^{A_1(R)} - Z^{A_0(\widetilde{R})}(t_n)| \leq C\Omega/N, \tag{3.11}$$

where $Z^{A_0(\widetilde{R}}(t_n)$ *is the solution that is obtained at nodes* t_n *using the* RT*-algorithm* A_0 *with the regularizer*

$$\widetilde{R}_\alpha(\omega) = R_\alpha(\omega)\chi_\Omega(\omega). \tag{3.12}$$

The constant C *depends on* $\widetilde{\widetilde{Z}}$ *(1.8),* $\widetilde{Z}^1$*,* $\widetilde{Z}^2$*,* $\|u(t)\|_{L^1}$*,* T_u*,* T_Z *and does not depend on* N*,* Ω*,* α*, and* t*.*

PROOF. The proof is based on formulas (0.10) and (3.6), which evidently hold under the conditions of the proposition, and on the error estimate for the trapezoid quadrature formula

$$\left|\int_a^b f(x)\,dx - (b-a)f((b-a)/2)\right| \leq \frac{(b-a)^2}{2}\sup_{[a,b]}|f'(x)|$$

According to this formula we have

$$|Z_n^{A_1} - Z^{A_0}(t_n)| \leq \frac{1}{2\pi}\frac{\Delta\omega^2}{2}\sum_{j=-N}^{N}\sup_{[\omega_j-\Delta\omega/2,\omega_j+\Delta\omega/2]}|f'(\omega)| \tag{3.13}$$

where

$$f(\omega) = e^{-i\omega t_n}\widehat{H}(\omega)\widehat{u}^T(\omega).$$

We must estimate the derivative of f for $|\omega| \leq \Omega$. We have

$$\begin{aligned}|f'(\omega)| \leq T_Z\widetilde{R}\left|\widehat{L}(\omega)\sum_n \widehat{u}(\omega+2n\Omega)\right| + \overline{R}_1\left|\widehat{L}(\omega)\sum_n \widehat{u}(\omega+2n\Omega)\right| \\ + \widetilde{R}\left|\widehat{L}^{(1)}\sum_n \widehat{u}(\omega+2n\Omega)\right| + \widetilde{R}\left|\widehat{L}(\omega)\left(\sum_n \widehat{u}(\omega+2n\Omega)\right)'\right|,\end{aligned}$$

where $T_Z = N_Z\Delta t$. Using the properties of $\Lambda(\omega)$, we have from (3.8)

$$\widehat{u}^{(1)}(\omega) = O(|\omega|^{-\rho'-M_Z}) + O(|\omega|^{-1-\delta}), \qquad |\omega| \to \infty.$$

Since $M_Z \geq \rho' + 1 + \delta$ and $\rho' \geq 0$, we have

$$\left(\sum_n \widehat{u}(\omega+2n\Omega)\right)' = \sum_n \widehat{u}^{(1)}(\omega+2n\Omega).$$

Taking into account the condition $|\widehat{L}(\omega)| \leq \Lambda(\omega)$ and formula (3.7), we get

$$\begin{aligned}|f'(\omega)| \leq \left[T_Z\widetilde{R} + \overline{R}_1 + \widetilde{R}O(|\omega|^{\rho'})\right]\left|\Lambda(\omega)\sum_n \widehat{u}(\omega+2\pi\Omega)\right| \\ + \widetilde{R}\left|\Lambda(\omega)\sum_n \widehat{u}^{(1)}(\omega+2\pi\Omega)\right|.\end{aligned} \tag{3.14}$$

Let us consider $|\Lambda(\omega)\sum_n \widehat{u}(\omega+2\pi\Omega)|$ for $|\omega|\leq\Omega$. Using the properties of $\Lambda(\omega)$ and (1.8), we have

$$\left|\Lambda(\omega)\sum_n \widehat{u}(\omega+2n\Omega)\right| \leq \widetilde{Z}|\omega|^{-M_Z}+2\widetilde{Z}\zeta(M_Z)\Omega^{-M_Z}, \qquad |\omega|\leq\Omega. \tag{3.15}$$

The last inequality is rather inconvenient for $|\omega|\leq 1$; for these values of ω we will replace it by the inequality

$$\left|\Lambda(\omega)\sum_n \widehat{u}(\omega+2n\Omega)\right| \leq \Lambda(1)\|u(t)\|_{L^1}+2\widetilde{Z}\zeta(M_Z)\Omega^{-M_Z}, \qquad |\omega|\leq 1. \tag{3.16}$$

Similarly, using (3.8) we obtain

$$\begin{aligned}\left|\Lambda(\omega)\sum_n \widehat{u}^{(1)}(\omega+2n\Omega)\right| \leq & 2\widetilde{Z}^1\zeta(M_t-p')\Omega^{p'-M_Z}+2\widetilde{Z}^2\zeta(1+\delta)\Omega^{-1-\delta} \\ & +\begin{cases}\widetilde{Z}^1|\omega|^{-M_Z+p'}+\widetilde{Z}^2|\omega|^{-1-\delta}, & |\omega|\leq\Omega,\\ \Lambda(1)\|u(t)\|_{L^1}T_u, & |\omega|\leq 1.\end{cases}\end{aligned}$$

Therefore, we have the following estimates for the derivative (separately for $|\omega|\leq\Omega$ and for $|\omega|\leq 1$):

$$\begin{aligned}|f'(\omega)| \leq & C_1\Omega^{-M_Z+p'}+C_2\Omega^{-1-\delta} \\ & +\begin{cases}C_3|\omega|^{-M_Z+p'}+C_4|\omega|^{-1-\delta}, & |\omega|\leq\Omega,\\ C_5+C_6\Omega^{-M_Z}, & |\omega|\leq 1.\end{cases}\end{aligned} \tag{3.17}$$

The constants $C_1,\ldots,C_6$ in (3.17) can be easily written down explicitly. They depend on various combinations of $\widetilde{Z}$ (1.8), $\widetilde{Z}^1$, $\widetilde{Z}^2$, $\|u(t)\|_{L^1}$, T_u, T_Z and do not depend on the parameters (the same applies to all constants below). Since under the conditions of the proposition we have $\Omega\geq\Omega_0=2\pi/T_u$, (3.17) implies the boundness of f':

$$|f'(\omega)|\leq C_7, \qquad |\omega|\leq\Omega. \tag{3.18}$$

To estimate $|Z_n^{A_1}-Z^{A_0}(t_n)|$ we break the right-hand side of (3.13) into three parts Σ_0, Σ_+, Σ_- as follows:

$$\Sigma_0=\frac{1}{2\pi}\frac{\Delta\omega^2}{2}\sum_{j=-J_0}^{J_0}\sup_{[\omega_j-\Delta\omega/2,\omega_j+\Delta\omega/2]}|f'(\omega)|,$$

and Σ_+, Σ_- differ from Σ_0 in that the summation in j goes from (J_0+1) to N and from $-N$ to $-(J_0+1)$ respectively. Here

$$J_0=\left[\frac{2\pi}{T_u\Delta\omega}\right]\equiv\left[\frac{2N+1}{T_u/\Delta\omega}\right],$$

By (3.10), J_0 satisfies the following conditions:

$$2\leq J_0\leq N, \qquad \pi/T_u\leq J_0\Delta\omega\leq 2\pi/T_u. \tag{3.19}$$

Taking (3.18) into account, we easily obtain the following estimate for Σ_0:

$$\Sigma_0\leq C_8\Delta\omega< C_8\Omega/N.$$

Now we estimate Σ_+ using (3.17):

$$\Sigma_+ \leq \frac{1}{2\pi}\frac{\Delta\omega^2}{2}\sum_{j=J_0+1}^{N}(C_1\Omega^{-M_Z+\rho'}+C_2\Omega^{-1-\delta})$$

$$+\frac{1}{2\pi}\frac{\Delta\omega^2}{2}\sum_{j=J+1}^{N}(C_3(\Delta\omega(j-1/2))^{-M_Z+\rho'}+C_4(\Delta\omega(j-1/2))^{-1-\delta}).$$

Since, by (3.19),

$$\sum_{j=J_0+1}^{N}((j-1/2)\Delta\omega)^{-M_Z+\rho'}\Delta\omega \leq \int_{(J_0-1/2)\Delta\omega}^{\infty}\omega^{-M_Z+\rho'}\,d\omega$$

$$= \frac{((J_0-1/2)\Delta\omega)^{-M_Z+\rho'+1}}{M_Z-\rho'-1} \leq \frac{1}{M_Z-\rho'-1}\left(\frac{\pi}{2T_u}\right)^{-M_Z+\rho'+1},$$

and similarly, for $\sum_{j=J_0+1}^{N}((j-1/2)\Delta\omega)^{-1-\delta}\Delta\omega$, we take into account the equality $\Delta\omega(2N+1) = 2\Omega$ and obtain

$$\Sigma_+ \leq C_9\Omega^{-M_Z+\rho'+1}\Delta\omega + C_{10}\Omega^{-\delta}\Delta\omega + C_{11}\Delta\omega;$$

Σ_- has a similar estimate. Since, by (3.10), $\Omega \geq 2\pi/T_u$ and $\Delta\omega = (2\Omega)/(2N+1) < \Omega/N$, we complete the proof of the proposition by summing up estimates for Σ_0, Σ_+, and Σ_-. □

Let us note that the conditions (3.7)–(3.9) are not too restrictive. For example, the condition (3.7) is satisfied for polynomial kernels like $|\omega|^\rho$ (and, more generally, for $L \in \mathcal{L}_0(\rho_0^\pm)$ with $\Delta L_0 \equiv 1$; see (1.4), (1.5)), and for exponentially growing kernels like $e^{|\omega|^\rho}$. Condition (3.9) follows from smoothness of the regularizer. Condition (3.8) is an a priori requirement for the smoothness of the solution. For example, it is satisfied if we require that the exact solution has piecewise differentiable derivative such that $tZ'(t) \in L^1$ (and assume (3.7)).

The proposition we have proved reduces the analysis of the algorithm $A_1(R)$ as $\Omega/N \to 0$ to the analysis of the RT-algorithm $A_0(\widetilde{R})$ with the regularizer $\widetilde{R}_{(\Delta t,\alpha)}(\omega) = R_\alpha(\omega)\chi_\Omega(\omega) \in \mathcal{N}$.

THEOREM 3.1. *Under the conditions of Proposition 3.1 the algorithm A_1 converges uniformly (on the set $t_n \leq n\Delta t$, $|n| \leq N_Z$) for the appropriate class of right-hand sides inside the set $\mathcal{D}_{\bar{\beta}} = \{(\Delta t, N^{-1}, \alpha)\}$ defined by the condition*

$$\Omega/N \to 0 \quad \text{as } |\bar{\beta}| \to 0, \hat{\beta} \in \mathcal{D}_{\bar{\beta}},$$

(that is, for large N).

PROOF. This immediately follows from (3.11) and the fact that the Nyquist condition is sufficient for the convergence of an RT-algorithm. □

Let us comment a little on the case when $u(t)$ is not compactly supported. In this case the equality $\tilde{u}_j^N = (1/\Delta t)\hat{u}^T(\omega_j)$ used to obtain (3.6) does not hold, so that the algorithm A_1 cannot be written in the form (3.6). Hence we must estimate the difference $\tilde{u}_j^N - (1/\Delta t)\hat{u}^T(\omega_j)$ and the corresponding error in (3.6). This can be easily done if we know the rate of decrease of $u(t)$.

Now we briefly discuss the approach to the study of A_1 related to the construction of an efficient regularizer. The samples $\widehat{H}_j = \widehat{H}(\omega_j)$ in formula (3.4) were obtained from the kernel $\widehat{H}(\omega)$. It is clear that any other kernel $\widehat{H}'(\omega)$ that coincides with the initial kernel at the lattice nodes (that is, such that $\widehat{H}'(\omega) = \widehat{H}(\omega)$) yields the same result. We write this symbolically in the form $A_1(H) = A_1(H')$. For example, this can be applied to the kernel

$$\widehat{H}'(\omega) = \sum_{k=-N}^{N} \frac{1}{2N+1} \frac{\sin(((N+1)/2)(\omega - \omega_k)\Delta t)}{\sin(\frac{1}{2}(\omega - \omega_k)\Delta t)} \widehat{H}(\omega_k)\chi_\Omega(\omega). \tag{3.20}$$

Inside the Nyquist interval $[-\Omega, \Omega]$ the kernel $\widehat{H}'(\omega)$ is a trigonometric polynomial of degree N that interpolates the function $\widehat{H}(\omega)$ at the lattice nodes. Let $A_0^{H'}$ denote the algorithm that consists in the computation of $Z^{A_0^{H'}}(t)$ using formula (0.9) with the kernel $H'(t)$. Then the following result holds.

PROPOSITION 3.2. *Let L be a kernel and $u \in \mathscr{U}(L)$ be a compactly supported function with* $\operatorname{supp} u \subset [-T_u, T_u]$. *Then for $N > N_u + N_Z$ $(N_u \geq T_u/\Delta t)$ we have*

$$Z_n^{A_1} = Z^{A_0^{H'}}(t_n) \quad \textit{for } |n| \leq N_Z.$$

PROOF. The direct computation of $H'(t)$ from (3.20) gives

$$H'(t) = \sum_{m=-N}^{N} \frac{1}{2N+1} \sum_{j=-N}^{N} e^{-i2\pi mj/(2N+1)} \widehat{H}(\omega_j) \frac{\sin((t - m\Delta t)\Omega)}{(t - m\Delta t)\Omega} \frac{1}{\Delta t}.$$

Since $u(t)$ is compactly supported and $N > N_u + N_Z$, we have

$$Z^{A_0^{H'}}(t_n) = \sum_{k=-N}^{N} \frac{1}{2N+1} \sum_{j=-N}^{N} e^{-i2\pi(n-k)j/(2N+1)} \widehat{H}(\omega_j) u_k^N.$$

Using the discrete convolution theorem, we can write $Z^{A_0^{H'}}(t_n)$ in the form (3.4). □

The above proposition shows that a natural candidate for the formal expression for an efficient regularizer is the expression obtained by dividing (3.20) by $\widehat{L}(\omega)$:

(3.21)

$$R^{\mathrm{ef}}(A_1)(\omega) = \widehat{L}^{-1}(\omega) \sum_{k=-N}^{N} \frac{1}{2N+1} \frac{\sin(((N+1)/2)(\omega - \omega_k)\Delta t)}{\sin(\frac{1}{2}(\omega - \omega_k)\Delta t)} \widehat{L}(\omega_k) R_\alpha(\omega_k) \chi_\Omega(\omega),$$

where $R_\alpha(\omega)$ is the seed regularizer. The efficient regularizer $R^{\mathrm{ef}}(A_1)$ depends on $\overline{\alpha} = (\Delta t, N^{-1}, \alpha)$. Using the fact that $\widehat{H}'(\omega)$ is a trigonometric interpolation polynomial, we can prove that $R^{\mathrm{ef}}(A_1)$ is indeed a regularizer (i.e., satisfies the necessary conditions) and $R^{\mathrm{ef}}(A_1) \simeq R_\alpha(\omega)\chi_\Omega(\omega)$ (for large N). This is also clear from Proposition 3.1. Therefore, for large N the role of an efficient regularizer can be played by the regularizer (3.12); in particular, this regularizer can be used in estimates for the resolution and the noise.

§3.3. The Tikhonov algorithm A_T

Let us consider a finite lattice algorithm for numerical solution of the convolution equation (0.3). We assume that

$$\widehat{K}(\omega) \equiv \widehat{L}^{-1}(\omega) \neq 0.$$

Moreover, following the general assumption for this chapter we assume that the right-hand side is compactly supported ($\operatorname{supp} u \subset [-T_u, T_u]$) and that we are looking for the solution at the nodes $t_n = n\Delta t$, $|n| \leq N_Z$. Instead of (0.3), consider its discrete analog

$$\sum_j K_{n-j}^N Z_j^N \Delta t = u_n^N. \tag{3.22}$$

We use the notation adopted in this chapter and assume that $N \geq N_u + N_Z$, $N_u \geq T_u/\Delta t$. As a periodic solution $Z_n^{A_T}$, we use the minimum of a certain discrete approximation of the regularizing function **[5]**

$$Z_n^{A_T} = \frac{1}{2N+1} \sum_j^N e^{-i2\pi j/n(2\nu+1)} \frac{\widetilde{K}_j^{N*} \widetilde{u}_j^N \Delta t}{|\widetilde{K}_j^N|^2 \Delta t^2 + \alpha_T M_j^N}. \tag{3.23}$$

Here $\widetilde{K}_j^N$, $\widetilde{u}_j^N$ are the FDFT of K_j^N, u_j^N and M_j^N is a certain $(2N+1)$-periodic sequence that depends not only on the form of the stabilizing factor but also on the method of the discrete approximation of the stabilizing functional. For simplicity, we consider the case

$$M_j^N = \begin{cases} M(\omega_j) \equiv M(j\Delta\omega) & \text{for } |j| \leq N, \\ \text{periodic with period } (2N+1), \end{cases}$$

where $\Delta\omega\Delta t = \frac{2\pi}{2N+1}$, and $M(\omega)$ is defined by (0.26). This corresponds to the choice of the stabilizing factor in the form (0.25) with the following approximation for it:

$$\widetilde{\Omega}[Z_n] = \frac{1}{2\pi} \sum_n^N M_n^N |\widetilde{Z}_n{}^N|^2 \Delta t^2 \Delta\omega.$$

Let us note that for $\alpha_T = 0$ formula (3.23) corresponds to the solution (3.22) obtained from it by the FDFT.

The algorithm A_T depends on the parameters $\overline{\beta} = (\Delta t, N^{-1}, \alpha_T)$. Since $u(t)$ is compactly supported and the condition $N_u < N$ holds, (3.23) can be rewritten in the form

$$Z_n^{A_T} = \frac{1}{2\pi} \sum_{j=-N}^{N} e^{-i\omega_j t_n} \frac{1}{\widehat{K}^{T,N}(\omega_j)} \left(1 + \alpha_T \frac{M(\omega_j)}{|\widehat{K}^{T,N}(\omega_j)|^2}\right)^{-1} \widehat{u}(\omega_j)\Delta\omega, \tag{3.24}$$

where $\widehat{K}^{T,N}(\omega) \stackrel{\text{def}}{=} \sum_{n=-N}^{N} K_n e^{it_n\omega} \Delta t$. Comparing (3.24) with (3.6), we see that if in the algorithm A_1 described in the previous section we choose the seed regularizer in the form

$$R_T(\omega) = \frac{\widehat{K}(\omega)}{\widehat{K}^{T,N}(\omega)} \frac{1}{1 + \alpha_T \dfrac{M(\omega)}{|\widehat{K}^{T,N}(\omega)|^2}}. \tag{3.25}$$

then $A_T = A_1(R_T)$. In principle, the analysis of the algorithm A_T can be performed similarly to the analysis of A_1. The additional complication is that now the seed regularizer depends on $\overline{\alpha} = (\Delta t, N^{-1}, \alpha_T)$, and not on the single parameter θ. However, for compactly supported kernels $K(t)$ (the only kernels that were considered in **[5]**) we can eliminate the dependence on N by taking a sufficiently large N:

$$N > N_K = T_K/\Delta t, \qquad \operatorname{supp} K(t) \subset [-T_K, T_K],$$

obtaining the formula

$$R'_T(\omega) = \frac{\widehat{K}(\omega)}{\widehat{K}^T(\omega)} \frac{1}{1 + \alpha_T \dfrac{M(\omega)}{|\widehat{K}^T(\omega)|^2}}. \tag{3.26}$$

Indeed, in this case $\widehat{K}^{T,N}(\omega) \equiv \widehat{K}^T(\omega)$.

In the case when the kernel $K(t)$ is not compactly supported, but only decreases ($K(t) = O(|t|^{-\varkappa})$ as $|t| \to \infty$, $\varkappa \geq 1 + \delta > 1$), several approaches can be used. The first approach consists in estimating the error caused by the replacement in $A_1(R)$ of the seed regularizer (3.25) by (3.26) (now these two regularizers do not coincide). This estimate is essentially based on the following elementary estimate for $\Delta\widehat{K}^T(\omega) \stackrel{\text{def}}{=} \widehat{K}^T(\omega) - \widehat{K}^{T,N}(\omega)$:

$$|\Delta\widehat{K}^T(\omega)| = \sum_{|n|>N} |K(t_n)e^{i\omega t_n}\Delta t| \leq C(\Omega/N)^{\varkappa-1}. \tag{3.27}$$

The second approach is based on the compactification of the original kernel, i.e., on replacing it by a compactly supported kernel. Here we use the observation that if we are interested in the solution (0.3) inside the interval $[-T_Z, T_Z]$, and $\operatorname{supp} u \subset [-t_u, T_u]$, then the behavior of the kernel for $|t| > T_Z + T_u$ is not essential. Therefore, we do not lose generality by analyzing only compactly supported functions $K(t)$.

In any event, we get rid of the dependence on N in the seed regularizer and reduce the problem to the analysis of $A_1(R'_T)$ with the seed regularizer (3.26). Here again we can estimate the difference between the solution given by the algorithm $A_1(R'_T)$ with R'_T from (3.26) and the solution obtained by RT-algorithm $A_0(\widetilde{R})$ with the regularizer

$$\widetilde{R}(\omega) = R'_T(\omega)\chi_\Omega(\omega) = \frac{\widehat{K}(\omega)}{\widehat{K}^T(\omega)} \frac{\chi_\Omega(\omega)}{1 + \alpha_T M(\omega)/|\widehat{K}^T(\omega)|^2}. \tag{3.28}$$

The regularizer $\widetilde{R}(\omega)$ itself depends on the kernel, so that we need explicit formulas for the kernel or, at least, rather detailed information about it. Note that we cannot apply Proposition 3.1 directly, since now both $\widetilde{R}(\omega)$ and $R'_T(\omega)$ depend on $\overline{\alpha} = (\Delta t, \alpha_T)$. However, the difference $Z_n^{A_1(R'_T)} - Z^{A_0(\widetilde{R})}(t_n)$ is small for all kernels that are interesting from the practical point of view. This remark shows that A_T converges for large N.

Finally, there is an approach to the analysis of A_T that is related to the construction of an efficient regularizer. Namely, an analog of Proposition 3.2 holds for

A_T, with the corresponding formal expression for an efficient regularizer (an analog of (3.21)) given by the formula

$$R^{\text{ef}}(A_T)(\omega) = \widehat{K}(\omega) \sum_{k=-N}^{N} \frac{1}{2N+1} \frac{\sin(((N+1)/2)(\omega-\omega_k)\Delta t)}{\sin(\frac{1}{2}(\omega-\omega_k)\Delta t)} \times \frac{1}{\widehat{K}^{T,N}(\omega_k)} \left(1+\alpha_T \frac{M(\omega_k)}{|\widehat{K}^{T,N}(\omega_k)|^2}\right)^{-1} \chi_\Omega(\omega). \tag{3.29}$$

Formula (3.29) can be analyzed using interpolation by trigonometric polynomials. For large N (when $\Omega/N \to 0$ sufficiently fast) $R^{\text{ef}}(A_T)$ is indeed a regularizer close to the regularizer $\widetilde{R}(\omega)$ given by (3.28).

The results below correspond to the approach when we first estimate the error caused by passing from A_T to $A_1(R'_T)$ and then from $A_1(R'_T)$ to $A_0(\widetilde{R})$ (where R'_T and $\widetilde{R}$ are given by (3.26) and (3.28) respectively).

PROPOSITION 3.3. *Let the kernel satisfy the following conditions:*
1) *$K(t)$ is a continuous function, and $K(t) = O(|t|^{\varkappa})$, $|T| \to \infty$, $\varkappa > 1$.*
2) *$\widehat{K}(\omega) \neq 0$, and $\widehat{L}(\omega) \equiv \widehat{K}^{-1}(\omega) \in \mathscr{L}(\Lambda)$.*
3) *The inequality*

$$|\overline{K}^T(\omega)/\widehat{K}(\omega)| \geq C_K^{-1} > 0, \qquad |\omega| \leq \Omega, \tag{3.30}$$

holds, where C_K is a positive constant that does not depend on Ω.

Let $\mathscr{D}^K_{(\Delta t, N^{-1})} \subset \mathbb{R}^+_2$ be a subset of the positive quadrant in the $(\Delta t, N^{-1})$-plane such that

$$\left|\frac{\Delta \widehat{K}^T(\omega)}{\widehat{K}(\omega)}\right| \leq C(\delta_K)\Omega^{-\delta_K} \quad \text{for } |\omega| \leq \Omega \tag{3.31}$$

for all (sufficiently small) $(\Delta t, N^{-1}) \in \mathscr{D}^K_{(\Delta t, N^{-1})}$ with positive constants $C(\delta_K)$, δ_K that do not depend on Ω and N; here $\Delta\widehat{K}^T(\omega) \stackrel{\text{def}}{=} \widehat{K}^T(\omega) - \widehat{K}^{T,N}(\omega)$. Let $u \in \mathscr{U}(U_M(\Lambda)$ be a compactly supported function with $\operatorname{supp} u \subset [-T_u, T_u]$.

Then for all admissible values of parameters from the region $\mathscr{D}_{\overline{\beta}} = \mathscr{D}^K_{(\Delta t, N^{-1})} \times \mathbb{R}^+_1$ (for sufficiently small Δt, N) we have

$$S_1 \stackrel{\text{def}}{=} \sup_n |Z_n^{A_T} - Z_n^{A_1(R'_T)}| \leq C\Omega^{-\delta_K}, \tag{3.32}$$

where C is an explicitly computable constant that depends on $\widetilde{Z}$ (1.8) and $\|u(t)\|_{L^1}$ but not on Ω, N, α_T; $Z_n^{A_T}$ and $Z_n^{A_1(R'_T)}$ are the solutions obtained by using, respectively, the algorithm A_T and the algorithm A_1 with the seed regularizer (3.26).

PROOF. Formulas (3.24), (3.6), and (3.26), which hold under the conditions of the proposition, imply that

$$S_1 \leq \frac{1}{2\pi} \sum_{j=-N}^{N} |\widehat{u}^T(\omega_j)| \Delta\omega A(\omega_j),$$

where

$$A(\omega) = \left| \frac{\widehat{K}^{T,N^*}(\omega)}{|\widehat{K}^{T,N}(\omega)|^2 + \alpha_T M(\omega)} - \frac{\widehat{K}^{T^*}(\omega)}{|\widehat{K}^T(\omega)|^2 + \alpha_T M(\omega)} \right|.$$

Since $M(\omega)$ is nonnegative, we have

$$A \le \frac{3|\Delta \widehat{K}^T|}{|\widehat{K}^{T,N}|^2} + \frac{|\Delta \widehat{K}^T|^2}{|\widehat{K}^{T,N}|^2 |\widehat{K}^T|} + \frac{|\Delta \widehat{K}^T|}{|\widehat{K}^T|^2}.$$

If Ω is sufficiently large (so that $C(\delta_K)\Omega^{-\delta_K} \le \frac{1}{2}C_K^{-1}$), (3.31) implies

$$|\widehat{K}^{T,N}/\widehat{K}| \le \tfrac{1}{2}C_K^{-1}.$$

Therefore,

$$A \le 12C_K^2 \frac{|\Delta \widehat{K}^T|}{|\widehat{K}|^2} + 4C_K^2 \frac{|\Delta \widehat{K}^T|^2}{|\widehat{K}|^3}.$$

Now for S_1 we have

$$S_1 \le C'\Omega^{-\delta_K} \frac{1}{2\pi} \sum_{j=-N}^{N} |\Lambda(\omega_j)\widehat{u}^T(\omega_j)|\Delta\omega,$$

where we again used (3.31) and the fact that Ω is sufficiently large. It remains to show that

$$\frac{1}{2\pi} \sum_{j=-N}^{N} |\Lambda(\omega_j)\widehat{u}^T(\omega_j)|\Delta\omega \le C'' < \infty.$$

This follows from inequalities (3.15) and (3.16), obtained in the proof of Proposition 3.1; these inequalities hold for $u \in \mathscr{U}_M(\Lambda)$. □

Condition (3.31) is rather rough. In fact, (3.32) holds in a much wider region.

PROPOSITION 3.4. *Let the kernel and the right-hand side satisfy the conditions of Proposition* 3.3 *and let the condition* (3.8) *be satisfied. Also, at least for large* Ω, *let*

$$\left|\frac{d}{d\omega}\frac{1}{\widehat{K}^T(\omega)}\right| \le C'|\omega|^{\rho'}\Lambda(\omega), \qquad \rho' \ge 0, \quad C' > 0, \tag{3.33}$$

for $|\omega| \le \Omega$. *Assume that* $M_Z \ge \rho' + 1 + \delta$, $N \ge T_u\Delta t > 3$, *and* $\alpha_T < \infty$. *Then for* $|n| \le N_Z < N$ *the following estimate holds*:

$$|Z_n^{A_1(R'_T)} - Z^{A_0(\widetilde{R})}(t_n)| \le C\Omega/N, \tag{3.34}$$

where C *is an explicitly computable constant that depends on* $\widetilde{Z}$ (1.8), $\widetilde{Z}^1$, $\widetilde{Z}^1$ (3.8), $\|u(t)\|_{L^1}$, T_u, *and* T_Z, *but not on the parameters* α_T, Ω, N. *Here* $Z_n^{A_1}$ *and* $Z^{A_0}(t_n)$ *are the solutions obtained, respectively, by the algorithm* A_1 *with the seed regularizer* (3.26) *and the RT-algorithm* A_0 *with the seed regularizer* (3.26).

PROOF. The only difference from the proof of Proposition 3.1 is in the method used to obtain the bound (3.14) for the absolute value of the derivative of the integrand

$$f(\omega) = e^{-i\omega t_n} \frac{1}{\widehat{K}^T(\omega)} \left(1 + \alpha_T \frac{M(\omega)}{|\widehat{K}^T(\omega)|^2}\right)^{-1} \widehat{u}^T(\omega)$$

in (0.10) for $Z^{A_0(\widetilde{R})}(t_n)$. Using the conditions of the proposition (in particular, (3.30), (3.33), and the inequality $M(\omega) \geq 0$), we easily get (at least, for sufficiently large Ω)

$$\left|\frac{1}{\widehat{K}^T(\omega)}\right| \leq C_K \Lambda(\omega), \qquad \left|\frac{d}{d\omega}\frac{1}{\widehat{K}^T(\omega)}\right| \leq C'|\omega|^{\rho'}\Lambda(\omega),$$

$$\left|\left(1 + \alpha_T \frac{M(\omega)}{|\widehat{K}^T(\omega)|^2}\right)^{-1}\right| \leq 1, \qquad \left|\frac{1}{\widehat{K}^T(\omega)}\left(1 + \alpha_T \frac{M(\omega)}{|\widehat{K}^T(\omega)|^2}\right)^{-1}\right| \leq C_K \Lambda(\omega).$$

Using once more (3.30), (3.33), and properties of $\widehat{K}(\omega)$ and $M(\omega)$, we obtain

$$|f'(\omega)| \leq (C_1 + C_2|\omega|^{\rho'}) \left|\Lambda(\omega)\sum_n \widehat{u}(\omega + 2n\Omega)\right| + C_3 \left|\Lambda(\omega)\sum_n \widehat{u}^{(1)}(\omega + 2n\Omega)\right|$$

for sufficiently large Ω, i.e., (3.14). The rest of the proof is the same as for Proposition 3.1. □

Now we can easily prove the following result.

THEOREM 3.2. *Let the kernel and the right-hand side satisfy the conditions of Propositions* 3.3 *and* 3.4 (*in particular, conditions* (3.30), (3.33), (3.8)). *Furthermore, let the kernel satisfy the Poisson formula*

$$\widehat{K}^T(\omega) = \sum_n \widehat{K}(\omega + 2n\Omega).$$

Then the algorithm A_T converges uniformly on the described class of right-hand sides inside any set of parameter values $\mathscr{D}_{\overline{\beta}}$ with a large number N of nodes, i.e., such that

1) $\mathscr{D}_{\overline{\beta}} \subset \mathscr{D}^K_{(\Delta t, N^{-1})} \times [0, \overline{\alpha}_T]$ (*this guarantees* (3.31));
2) $\Omega/N \to 0$, $|\overline{\beta}| \to 0$, $\overline{\beta} \in \mathscr{D}_{\overline{\beta}}$.

PROOF. Since the conditions of the theorem imply the estimates (3.32) and (3.34), it suffices to prove the convergence of the algorithm $A_0(\widetilde{R})$. But this follows readily from the fact that under the condition of Theorem 3.2 the regularizer $\widetilde{R}$ defined by (3.28) belongs to $\mathscr{R}(\Lambda)$ and satisfies the Nyquist condition. □

Now let us discuss when the conditions of the theorem are satisfied. To satisfy (3.30), it is sufficient that $K(t)$ be an even function with $\widehat{K}(\omega) \neq 0$. Indeed, in this case $\widehat{K}(\omega)$ is real and does not change sign, so that $|\widehat{K}^T(\omega)| \geq |K(\omega)|$ and we have (3.30) with $C_K = 1$. Condition (3.33) is an analog of condition (3.7); it is satisfied in most cases and its verification usually is quite easy. As for condition (3.8), we have already mentioned that it follows from smoothness and decrease properties of the exact solution $Z(t)$. The Poisson formula follows from the condition $K(t) = O(|t|^{-\varkappa})$ with $\varkappa > 1$ and the boundedness of the variation of $K(t)$. The size of the convergence area guaranteed by the theorem depends on (3.31), and the convergence region is usually much smaller than the region $\Omega/N \leq$ const, which is interesting from the practical point of view. The only exception is the class of compactly supported kernels such that $\Delta K^T \equiv 0$ for $N > T_K/\Delta t$ (i.e., $\operatorname{supp} K(t) \subset [-T_K, T_K]$). For such kernels Theorem 3.2 proves the convergence in regions with $\Omega/N \to 0$, which is very close to practically interesting cases. To ensure (3.31) for non-compactly-supported kernels one usually needs $N \gtrsim \Omega^{1+\delta}$, with the minimal possible δ depending on the form of the kernel. In the framework of our approach, the results can be strengthened by replacing the rough condition (3.31) with a more subtle condition that ensures (3.32) in Proposition 3.3.

Consider some examples. Let $K(t) = e^{|-t/t_0|}$, $\widehat{K}(\omega) = 2t_0(1 + (\omega/\omega_0)^2)^{-1}$, $\omega_0 = 1/t_0$. One can easily see that all conditions of Theorem 3.2, including (3.33), are satisfied:

$$|\Delta\widehat{K}^T(\omega)| \leq \sum_{|n|\geq N+1} e^{-|\Delta t_n/t_0|}\Delta t = 2e^{\Delta t(N+1)/t_0}\frac{\Delta t/2t_0}{\sinh(\Delta t/2)t_0} \leq 2e^{-(\pi\omega_0 N/\Omega)}.$$

The condition (3.31) is satisfied provided that

$$e^{-(\pi\omega_0 N/\Omega)}\Omega^2 \leq C(\delta_K)\Omega^{-\delta_K}.$$

It is clear that the last condition is satisfied if $N \geq C\Omega^{1+\delta}$ with an arbitrarily small δ. The convergence region described by this inequality is sufficiently large.

Now let us consider $\widehat{K}(\omega) = (1 + |\omega/\omega_0|^p)^{-1}$, $p > 1$. The conditions of Theorem 3.2 are satisfied, and $K(t) = O(|t|^{-[p]-1})$, $|t| \to \infty$; hence we have the bound (3.27):

$$|\Delta\widehat{K}^T(\omega)| \leq C(\Omega/N)^{[p]}.$$

To satisfy (3.31) we need to have $(\Omega/N)^{[p]}\Omega^p \leq C(\delta_K)\Omega^{-\delta_K}$, i.e., $N \geq C\Omega^{1+p/[p]+\delta}$, with an arbitrarily small $\delta > 0$. Let us consider the fast-growing kernel of the form

$$K(t) = e^{-(t/t_0)^2}, \qquad \widehat{K}(\omega) = \sqrt{\pi}t_0 e^{-i(\omega/\omega_0)^2}, \qquad \omega_0 = 2/t_0.$$

Estimating ΔK^T, we have

$$|\Delta K^T(\omega)| \leq \sum_{|n|\geq N+1} e^{-(n\Delta t/t_0)^2}\Delta t \leq 2t_0\int_{N\Delta t/t_0}^{\infty} e^{-x^2}\,dx \leq \frac{2t_0^2}{\pi\sqrt{\pi}}\frac{\Omega}{N}e^{-(\pi N/t_0\Omega)^2}$$

(the last inequality in this sequence is true for $\pi N/t_0\Omega \geq 1$). Therefore, to satisfy (3.31) we need to have

$$\frac{N}{\Omega}e^{-(\pi N/t_0\Omega)^2+(\Omega/\omega_0)^2} \leq C\Omega^{-\delta_K},$$

i.e.,

$$N \geq \frac{2}{\pi}\Omega^2/\omega_0^2.$$

Here we have $\delta_K = 1$.

In conclusion, let us mention once more the approach related to the analysis of the formal expression (2.29) for an efficient regularizer. The above results show that when the number N of nodes is large we have $R^{\mathrm{ef}} = \widetilde{R}$ (here $\widetilde{R}$ is given by (2.28)). In this case we can use $\widetilde{R}$ to estimate the noise and the resolution of the algorithm. Moreover, it is clear that the convergence of the algorithm results from the fact that the efficient regularizer is cut off at the Nyquist frequency, which is related to the passage to the lattice. Therefore, the passage to the lattice is, in a sense, a regularization procedure; this is quite clear and natural from the point of view of general theory.

References

1. F. Natterer, *The mathematics of computerized tomography*, Teubner, Stuttgart, and Wiley, New York, 1986.
2. A. N. Tikhonov and V. A. Arsenin, *Methods for solving ill-posed problems*, 2nd ed., "Nauka", Moscow, 1979; English transl. of 1st ed., Wiley, New York, 1977.
3. C. W. Groetsch, *The theory of Tikhonov regularization for Fredholm equations of the first kind*, Res. Notes in Math., vol. 105, Pitman, Boston, MA, 1984.
4. V. A. Morozov, *Regular methods for solving ill-posed problems*, 2nd ed., "Nauka", Moscow, 1987; English transl. of 1st ed., Springer-Verlag, Berlin, 1984.
5. A. N. Tikhonov et al., *Numerical methods for solving ill-posed problems*, " Nauka", Moscow, 1990. (Russian)
6. *Mathematical problems of computerized tomography*, Proc. IEEE **74** (1983), no. 3.
7. T. S. Huang (ed.), *Picture processing and digital filtering*, Topics in Appl. Phys., vol. 6, Springer-Verlag, Berlin, 1975.
8. N. I. Akhiezer, *Lectures on the therory of approximation*, 2nd ed., "Nauka", Moscow, 1965; English transl. of 1st ed., Ungar, New York, 1956.
9. D. A. Popov and D. V. Sushko, *On the convergence of algorithms for the numerical solution of convolution equations*, Dokl. Akad. Nauk SSSR **315** (1990), no. 2, 309–313; English transl. in Soviet Math. Dokl. **42** (1991).
10. D. A. Popov, *On the application of smooth regularizers for the computation of the convolution*, Dokl. Akad. Nauk SSSR **276** (1984), no. 1, 38–42; English transl. in Soviet Math. Dokl. **29** (1984).
11. V. I. Arnol′d, A. N. Varchenko, and S. M. Guseĭn-Zade, *Singularities of differentiable mappings*. Vol. 2, "Nauka", Moscow, 1984; English transl., Birkhäuser, Basel, 1988.
12. A. N. Varchenko, *On the number of integral points in a family of homothetic regions in* $\mathbb{R}^n$, Funktsional. Anal. i Prilozhen. **17** (1983), no. 2, 1–6; English transl. in Functional Anal. Appl. **17** (1983).
13. R. S. Varga, *Functional analysis and approximation theory in numerical analysis*, SIAM, Philadelphia, PA, 1971.
14. E. C. Titchmarsch, *Introduction to the theory of Fourier integrals*, Clarendon Press, Oxford, 1937.
15. ______, *The theory of functions*, 2nd ed., Oxford Univ. Press, Oxford, 1939.
16. G. M. Fihtengol′ts, *A course in differential and integral calculus*. Vol. 3, 2nd ed., Fizmatgiz, Moscow, 1960; German transl., VEB Deutscher Verlag Wiss., Berlin, 1966.
17. N. Wiener, *The Fourier integral and certain of its applications*, Cambridge Univ. Press, Cambridge, 1933; reprint, Dover, New York, 1959.
18. S. M. Nikolskiĭ, *Quadrature formulas*, 2nd ed., "Nauka", Moscow, 1974; English transl. of 1st ed., Hindustan, Dehli, 1964; Spanish transl. of 4th ed., "Mir", Moscow, 1990.
19. A. Erdélyi et al., *Higher transcendental functions*. Vol. 1, McGraw-Hill, New York, 1953.
20. N. N. Bogolyubov and D. V. Shirkov, *Introduction to quantum field theory*, 3rd ed., " Nauka", Moscow, 1976; English transl., Wiley, New York, 1980.
21. N. S. Bakhvalov, *Numerical methods*, "Nauka", Moscow, 1973; English transl. of later ed., "Mir", Moscow, 1977.

Amer. Math. Soc. Transl.
(2) Vol. **162**, 1994

Mathematical Models in Two-dimensional Radon Tomography

D. A. Popov, E. B. Sokolova, and D. V. Sushko

Contents

INTRODUCTION

In the Introduction we want to explain what we mean by a mathematical model in tomography, and why we need these models at all when we have the Radon inversion formula. To answer this question, let us consider a very simple model. First we recall the inversion formula, introducing the necessary notation and explaining the terminology. Let us consider the plane $\mathbb{R}^2$ (the plane of the tomogram) with a distinguished point O (the scanning center), which will be considered as the origin of a Cartesian coordinate system (x, y), $\vec{r} = (x, y)$. Consider the class $\{\mu\}$ of functions $\mu(\vec{r})$ of the form

$$\mu(\vec{r}) = \sum_{i=1}^{I} g_i(\vec{r})\chi_{\mathscr{D}_i}(\vec{r}), \tag{0.1}$$

where $g_i(\vec{r})$ are smooth functions ($g_i \in C^\infty$), and $\chi_{\mathscr{D}}(\vec{r})$ is the characteristic function

0065-9290/94/\$1.00 + \$.25 per page

of a region $\mathscr{D}$ with the piecewise smooth boundary $\partial\mathscr{D}$,

$$\chi_{\mathscr{D}}(\vec{r}) = \begin{cases} 1, & \vec{r} \in \mathscr{D}, \\ 0, & \vec{r} \notin \mathscr{D}. \end{cases} \tag{0.2}$$

The functions $\mu(\vec{r})$ are the objects we want to analyze; we assume that the class $\{\mu\}$ is sufficiently large to describe practically interesting objects. By specifying $\mu(\vec{r})$, we define a model of the object we want to reconstruct from its *Radon transform* $\mathscr{R}\mu$. To define $\mathscr{R}\mu$, we introduce *canonical coordinates* (φ, q) in the space of straight lines in $\mathbb{R}^2$. In these coordinates a line is defined by the equation

$$\langle \vec{r}, \vec{\eta} \rangle = q \qquad (\vec{\eta} = (\cos\varphi, \sin\varphi)), \tag{0.3}$$

where $\langle\ ,\ \rangle$ is the inner product in $\mathbb{R}^2$. By definition,

$$\begin{aligned} \mathscr{R}\mu(\varphi, q) \equiv J(\varphi, q) &= \int_{(\varphi,q)} \mu(\vec{r})\, ds \\ &= \int_{-\infty}^{\infty} \mu(q\cos\varphi - t\sin\varphi, q\sin\varphi + t\cos\varphi)\, dt. \end{aligned} \tag{0.4}$$

Since $J(\varphi + \pi, -q) = J(\varphi, q)$, we will mostly use a single-valued parameterization, assuming that

$$-\infty < q < +\infty, \qquad 0 \leq \varphi \leq \pi - 0 \tag{0.6}$$

On the class $\{\mu\}$ we have the *projection theorem*

$$\widehat{J}(\varphi, \lambda) = \widehat{\mu}(\lambda\cos\varphi, \lambda\sin\varphi). \tag{0.7}$$

where $\widehat{f}$ denotes the *Fourier transform* of the function f, and

$$\widehat{J}(\varphi, \lambda) = \int J(\varphi, q) e^{i\lambda q}\, dq, \qquad \widehat{\mu}(\lambda\cos\varphi, \lambda\sin\varphi) = \iint \mu(e^{i\lambda\langle\vec{r},\vec{\eta}\rangle} d^2\vec{r}. \tag{0.8}$$

Whenever summation or integration limits are omitted, we assume the summation or integration is from $-\infty$ to $+\infty$, and is undestood in the sense of principal value. The projection theorem (0.7) implies that in the class $\{\mu\}$ we have the inversion formula

$$\mu(\vec{r}) = \frac{1}{4\pi^2} \int_0^{\infty} d\varphi \int |\lambda| e^{-i\lambda\langle\vec{r},\vec{\eta}\rangle}\, d\lambda \int e^{i\lambda q} J(\varphi, q)\, dq. \tag{0.9}$$

Now we can say that we have described a mathematical model with $\{\mu\}$ as the class of *analyzed objects*, $J(\varphi, q)$ as the *array of* (experimental) *data*, and formula (0.9) as the *reconstruction algorithm*.

Now let us discuss the physical assumptions that form the basis for the above model, and whether or not this model is realistic. Let us have a point radiation source M and a point detector D. The measurement of $J(\varphi, q)$ corresponds to the case when both the source and the detector lie on the line (φ, q) with the radiation propagating along this line. The above model corresponds to an infinite number of measurements (all (φ, q)) performed without error by a point detector. It is clear that these conditions are not satisfied in practice, since there are no error-free point detectors and infinitely many measurements require an infinite time. Attempts to take into account these considerations lead to the notion of the *basic mathematical model* (BMM). We will distinguish BMM without statistical errors (noise), to be denoted

BMM below, and the model with the noise (BMMΔ). In both models we preserve the just-described model of the object. In the BMM we assume that the quantities

$$I_{jk} = \int \Pi(q_j - q) J(\varphi_k, q)\, dq \tag{0.10}$$

are known. Here $\Pi(q)$ is the *apparatus function*, which we do not fix. This function defines a phenomenological *model of the measurement channel* and, in particular, indicates the nonpreciseness of the detector. By definition, φ_k and q_j are given by

$$\varphi_k = k\Delta\varphi, \quad q_j = j\Delta q + \delta \qquad (0 \le \delta < \Delta q), \tag{0.11}$$

and we have

$$|j| \le N_q, \qquad k = 0, 1, \dots 2N_\varphi - 1, \qquad \Delta\varphi = \pi/N_\varphi. \tag{0.11}$$

The sampling interval k is chosen in such a way that even even if $\delta \neq 0$ and $\Pi(q) \neq \Pi(-q)$, the cycle condition

$$I_{j,2N_\varphi} = I_{j0} \tag{0.13}$$

is satisfied. Moreover, if

$$\Pi(q) = \Pi(-q), \qquad \delta = 0 \text{ or } \Delta q/2, \tag{0.14}$$

it suffices to take

$$k = 0, 1, \dots N_\varphi - 1. \tag{0.15}$$

It is assumed that

$$\mu(\vec{r}) = 0 \quad \text{for } r = |\vec{r}| > R_H \tag{0.16}$$

and the region of $\vec{r}$'s considered (the *reconstruction region*) lies inside the circle

$$r < R_b, \qquad R_b > \sqrt{2} R_H. \tag{0.17}$$

The function $\Pi(q)$ is assumed to be *local*,

$$\Pi(q) = 0 \quad \text{for } |q| > q_\Pi, \tag{0.18}$$

and N_q are assumed to satisfy the completeness condition.

$$R_b = N_q \Delta q > R_H + q_\Pi. \tag{0.19}$$

In BMMΔ everything is the same, but instead of I_{jk} we are given

$$I_{jk}^\Delta = I_{jk} + \Delta I_{jk}, \tag{0.20}$$

where the ΔI_{jk} are random variables with given properties. In BMMΔ it is assumed that the ΔI_{jk} are independent normal random variables with zero mean and the given covariance matrix $\sigma_J^2(j.k)$, i.e.

$$\mathbb{E}(\Delta I_{jk}) = 0, \qquad \mathbb{E}(\Delta I_{jk} \cdot \Delta I_{j'k'}) = \sigma_J^2(j,k)\delta_{kk'}\delta_{jj'}. \tag{0.21}$$

Here and later $\mathbb{E}(v)$ is the *expectation* of a random variable v.

Hence, we have defined the *data array* $[I_{jk}]$ (or $[I_{jk}^\Delta]$) that is used to reconstruct μ in the BMM (or BMMΔ). Denote by $\{I_{jk}\}$ the class of all arrays corresponding to various $\mu \in \{\mu\}$. A given data array $[I_{jk}]$ depends on the choice of $\Delta\varphi$, Δq, δ, and the apparatus function $\Pi(q)$. Models with all these parameters chosen compatibly appear to be most interesting. These *compatibility conditions*, which further specify the class of models under investigation, will be discussed in §1.1.

The next step in constructing a BMM is to define a *reconstruction algorithm* A. Since the only difference between a BMM and a BMMΔ is that I_{jk} is replaced by I_{jk}^{Δ}, below we restrict ourselves to models without noise.

A reconstruction algorithm (for a BMM) is a mapping

$$A : \{I_{jk}\} \to \{\mu^A(\vec{r})\}, \qquad A[I_{jk}] = \mu^A(\vec{r}) \tag{0.22}$$

that associates to the data array $[I_{jk}]$ corresponding to an object μ the *tomogram* $\mu^A(\vec{r})$ of this object.

Since $\mu^A(\vec{r}) \neq \mu(\vec{r})$, we come to the question of estimating the reconstruction quality. The formulation of the *performance criterion* completes the description of a BMM (or BMMΔ). We will not define the algorithm A and the quality criterion here in the Introduction (see Chapters 2 and 3), but remark only that we will restrict our analysis to the class of *convolution and backprojection algorithms*, which are most closely related to the Radon inversion formula. As for quality criteria, their definition includes such notions as the noise level of the tomogram, the spatial resolution, etc. All these notions will be discussed in Chapter 3.

In constructing a BMM we took into account the discretization (finiteness of the number of measurements), aperture (finite size of the detector in the tomogram plane, and statistical error. These parameters are absolutely essential, and should be taken into account in any model. The basic model is the minimal (the simplest) model that takes into account all these parameters.

In the example of a BMM we described the main steps in the construction of any model and the principal components of a model. Therefore, any model must include model of the object, a model of measurement procedure, an algorithm for the computation of the data array, a reconstruction algorithm, and a family of quality criteria together with algorithms for their estimation. Then the described model can be analyzed both numerically and theoretically. From the theoretical point of view, one of the main ingredient is the estimation of quality criteria depending on parameters (including functional parameters) describing the model. Even the simplest BMM is rather complicated from the theoretical point of view, and its theory cannot be considered to be complete. One of the goals of this paper is to describe theoretical and numerical results related to a BMM and to pose some questions that remain to be answered. These questions deal, mostly, with the construction of an algorithm A that is optimal with respect to a given quality criterion.

The second goal of the paper is to present several examples that show how a model should be modified when we take into account certain physical phenomena that are not included in a BMM. Here the BMM serves not only as a "zero order" approximation, but also as a reference model that enables us to "see" the influence of particular physical factors on the quality of the tomogram.

Obviously, we cannot even pretend that we have described all physical phenomena that are relevant in tomography. We mention right now that we will not consider models that take into account nonlinearity of radiation propagation (like scattering effects for X-ray radiation, or refraction and reflection for ultrasound radiation). Also, we will not consider models and algorithms with incomplete data, when we do not know the Radon transform in a large region in the space of lines. On the other hand, we will show how the model should be modified to take into account various geometric and dynamic factors, nonlinearity, detector delays, spectral parameters of the X-ray radiation, etc.

As we have defined it, the BMM is not specific to a given type of tomographs. However, from the point of view of the geometry of the line array (φ_k, q_j) (see (0.11)) that carries the data I_{jk}, this model can be considered as the model of a first generation tomograph. To describe tomographs of subsequent (second to fourth) generations one must first describe the array of lines (φ_{mn}, q_{mn}) (numbered by two indices n, m) that carries measurements. The dependence of φ, q on n, m is determined by the geometry of the scanning system. This is an example of what we call a geometric factor, and in this case the consideration of geometric factors requires a modification of the reconstruction algorithm. Another example of the geometric factor is the finiteness of the detector size in the direction perpendicular to the tomogram plane. This finiteness requires a change of the object model and the replacement of the function $\mu(\vec{r})$ by a function $\mu(\vec{r}, z)$ of three variables.

One might think that the basic model becomes practically useless when we pass to tomographs of the third and fourth generations. One of the goals of this paper is to show that this is far from being true. We emphasize that this statement is based on results of numerical experiments, and that the authors are unaware of any explicit results about the models that are more complicated than the basic model. Of course, one can define the notion of a basic model for each geometric scanning scheme. We will not do it (although such models will in a sense be constructed below). Instead, we want to emphasize that the BMM constructed above is sufficiently universal. Nongeometric factors (nonlinearity, delay, etc.) can, of course, change reconstruction results completely, and it is reasonable to consider these factors only under the assumption that they are small. To find out what "small" means from the point of view of quality criteria is yet another goal of this paper.

Mathematical model of two-dimensional Radon tomography have been considered in a large number of publications, and we do not intend to review them. To justify this we can only say that almost any theoretical paper on tomography is related to the topic of this paper. We mention **[1–7]**, with their extensive bibliographies. Mathematical analysis of the BMM was performed in **[8]**. Based on results of that paper, we present (see Chapter 3) analytical estimates of all the main quality reconstruction parameters for a BMM.

We hope that this paper can serve as a short introduction to tomography for applied mathematicians and engineers.

The authors' level of understanding of tomography problems reflected in this paper is based on experience gained in working with a software package for modelling tomography systems. The major part of that package was written by L. P. Svyadosz, and we would like to acknowledge sincerely her contribution.

We number formulas consecutively in each chapter, and the first digit in the tag is the chapter number. Sections are numbered in the same way. The first digit 0 indicates the Introduction, and 4 the Conclusion.

Chapter 1. Data Array

§1.1. General remarks

In this chapter we describe a *model of an object* and a *model of measurement*. Let us begin by making the BMM more precise, so that we can narrow the class of models under consideration. A model of an object for a BMM was given earlier (see (0.1)). A model of a measurement is an algorithm (operator) that enables us to construct from a model of an object, an array of initial data that will be used in the reconstruction. In particular, for a BMM this operator (denoted below by $\mathcal{J}$) is of the form

$$\mathcal{J}:\{\mu\}\to\{I_{jk}\},\quad \mathcal{J}\mu=[I_{jk}], \tag{1.1}$$

where the array I_{jk} is given by (0.10). Let us note that although (0.10) defines $\mathcal{J}$, it does not give an algorithm for the computation of I_{jk}. To define such an algorithm we must provided an algorithm for the computation of the Radon transform $\mathcal{R}\mu(\varphi,q)$ and an algorithm for the (numerical) computation of the integral (0.10).

To make the BMM completely precise we must fix δ, $\Delta\varphi$, Δq, and the apparatus function $\Pi(q)$. It is clear that not every choice of these parameters defines a model that is interesting from the practical point of view. Let us note first that Δq is always assumed to be small. This means that

$$\Delta q \ll R_b \qquad (N_q\gg 1). \tag{1.2}$$

The parameters $\Delta\varphi$ and Δq must be chosen to be compatible. The *compatibility condition* has a simple geometrical meaning and can be written in the form

$$\Delta\varphi R_b \le C\Delta q. \tag{1.3}$$

Here and later C denotes a constant *of order* 1 that does not depend on parameters like $\Delta\varphi$ and Δq, which are called *small*. The same latter C in different formulas can denote different constants. Condition (1.3) can be written in the form

$$N_\varphi = CN_q. \tag{1.4}$$

By definition, the apparatus function $\Pi(q)$ satisfies the normalization condition

$$\widehat{\Pi}(0)=\int \Pi(q)\,dq = 1. \tag{1.5}$$

As a typical example one can consider

$$\Pi(q)=\begin{cases} d^{-1}, & |q|<d/2,\\ 0, & |q|>d/2.\end{cases} \tag{1.6}$$

Then (see (0.10))

$$I_{jk}=d^{-1}\int_{q_i-d/2}^{q_i+d/2} J(\varphi_k,q)\,dq$$

and d can be interpreted as the aperture of the detector. The function $\Pi(q)$ defines a regularization of the delta function $\delta(q)$ (since $\Pi(q)\to\delta(q)$ as $d\to 0$). Usually it is an even function taking its maximal value at 0, and the parameter d characterizes the effective size of the support of $\Pi(q)$:

$$\Pi(0)d = C. \tag{1.8}$$

The parameters d and Δq are *compatible*,

$$d = C\Delta q. \tag{1.9}$$

Therefore, a model depends on parameters $\Delta\varphi$, Δq, d that are assumed to be *small* and satisfy the *compatibility conditions* of the form (1.3), (1.9). A specific BMM is determined by the choice of constants $C \sim 1$ in these formulas. In analyzing the mathematical theory of a BMM one studies the asymptotics of $\mu^A(\vec{r})$ as the small parameters $\Delta\varphi$, Δq, d tend to zero, and the compatibility conditions (1.3), (1.9) specify the limiting process.

Let us try to explain (to some extent) the meaning of these compatibility conditions. They are necessary in order that the data array can enable us to reconstruct details of size h on the tomogram:

$$h = C\Delta q. \tag{1.10}$$

The parameter h is called the *spatial resolution* of the tomograph. We do not give a precise definition, since compatibility conditions can be considered as the definition of the class of models under consideration and h is used only in the arguments explaining why a particular definition is natural. Problems related to the precise definition of spatial resolution require the knowledge of the algorithm A and will be considered below (see §2.2). Here we only remark that if D is the diameter of the support of $\mu(\vec{r})$ and $D \ll \Delta q$, then h characterizes the size of the support of $\mu^A(\vec{r})$. The possibility of satisfying (0.10) is not self-evident and imposes additional conditions on the algorithm A, separating the *class of high-resolution algorithms* (see §2.2). If h is assumed to be given, then compatibility conditions can be considered as the requirement that the number of measurements be minimal. The next remark shows that even for $\Delta\varphi = 0$ we cannot expect relations of the form

$$h = C\Delta q^\alpha, \qquad \alpha > 1. \tag{1.11}$$

Indeed, let $J(\varphi, q_j)$ be given. Introduce the function

$$J_\Omega(\varphi, q) = \sum_{|j| \le N_q} J(\varphi, q_j) \frac{\sin(\Omega(q - q_j))}{\Omega(q - q_i)}. \tag{1.12}$$

The parameter Ω is called the *Nyquist frequency*. It is defined by

$$\Omega = \pi/\Delta q. \tag{1.13}$$

We mention that

$$\begin{aligned} J_\Omega(\varphi, q_j) &= J(\varphi, q_j), \\ \widehat{J}_\Omega(\varphi, \lambda) &= \sum_{|j| \le N_q} e^{i\lambda q_j} J(\varphi, q_j)\chi_\Omega(\lambda)\Delta q, \end{aligned} \tag{1.14}$$

where χ_Ω is the characteristic function of the *Nyquist interval*

$$\chi_\Omega(\lambda) = \begin{cases} 1, & |\lambda| < \Omega, \\ 0, & |\lambda| > \Omega. \end{cases} \tag{1.15}$$

Substituting $J_\Omega(\varphi, q)$ in the inversion formula (0.9), we obtain $\mu_\Omega(\vec{r})$. The function

$\mu_\Omega(\vec{r})$ is an entire function of exponential type Ω, and the Bernstein inequality implies the following estimates for its derivatives:

$$|\nabla \mu_\Omega(\vec{r})| \le C\Omega. \tag{1.16}$$

Therefore, in our case

$$h \ge C\Delta q. \tag{1.17}$$

Now we come to the analysis of data array $[I_{jk}]$. Quantities similar to I_{jk} are called *local functionals on the space of Radon transforms* $\{\mathscr{R}\mu\}$. A functional (not necessarily linear) is said to be *local and supported on the line* (φ_0, q_0) if it depends only on values of $J(\varphi, q)$ at points from the subset

$$|q - q_0| \le C\Delta q, \qquad |\varphi - \varphi_0| \le C\Delta\varphi \tag{1.18}$$

of this line. Therefore, a data array $[I_{jk}]$ in a BMM is a collection of local functionals supported on lines (φ_k, q_j). We will denote this as follows:

$$I_{jk} \simeq \mathscr{R}\mu(\varphi_k, q_j). \tag{1.19}$$

This notation means not only that

$$I_{jk} \to J(\varphi_k, q_j) \qquad (\Delta q \to 0), \tag{1.20}$$

but also that I_{jk} is interpreted as $\mathscr{J}(\varphi_j, q_k)$ in the reconstruction algorithm. The family of lines (φ_j, q_k) defined by (0.11), (0.12) is called *canonical* and denoted $[P^1_{jk}]$. Therefore, in a BMM we assume that a family of lines $[P^1_{jk}]$ satisfying the compatibility condition (1.3) and a data array $[I_{jk}]$ are given. This array is a collection of local functionals supported on the corresponding lines of the family.

Let us describe a somewhat more general scheme, which, as examples show, is sufficient for the majority of applications. Let (u, v) be certain coordinates in the space of straight lines intersecting a disk $\mathscr{D}_b$ (defined by $r \le R_b$). We assume that these coordinates are chosen in such a way that any line intersecting $\mathscr{D}_b$ satisfies

$$|u| \le u_b, \qquad |v| \le v_b, \tag{1.21}$$

$$\mathscr{R}\mu(u, v) = 0, \qquad |u| > u_H, \quad |v| > v_H. \tag{1.22}$$

Let us consider the *lattice of lines* $[P_{nm}]$ defined as follows. The line P_{nm} has the coordinates $(n\Delta u, m\Delta v)$, and

$$|n| \le N_u, \qquad |m| \le N_v \qquad N_u = \left[\frac{u_b}{\Delta u}\right], \qquad N_v = \left[\frac{v_b}{\Delta v}\right]. \tag{1.23}$$

Here $[\cdot]$ denotes the integral part of a number. The relation between the coordinates (u, v) and (φ, q) is given by the functions

$$\varphi = \varphi(u, v), \qquad q = q(u, v), \tag{1.24}$$

which are smooth and invertible in the region (1.21). Tomographic measurements are assigned to lines from $[P_{nm}]$ with coordinates $(n\Delta u, m\Delta v)$.

The specific form of the coordinates (u, v) is prescribed by the geometry of the scanning system (see below). Local functionals I_{nm} supported on lines P_{nm} are measured under the assumption that there is no noise. Therefore in the two-dimensional linear model we have

$$I_{nm} = \iint \mathscr{K}_{nm}(u, v) \mathscr{R}\mu(u, v)\, du dv, \tag{1.25}$$

$$\mathscr{K}_{nm}(u, v) = 0, \qquad |u - n\Delta u| > C\Delta u, \quad |v - m\Delta v| > C\Delta v. \tag{1.26}$$

To take into account the main statistical errors we must replace I_{nm} by I_{nm}^{Δ}, where the I_{nm}^{Δ} are random variables that will be described later (see §1.5). To simplify the exposition we will formulate all statements for noiseless models. Functions $\mathscr{K}_{nm}(u, v)$ are called *apparatus functions*; in the majority of models

$$\mathscr{K}_{nm}(u, v) = \mathscr{K}(u - n\Delta u, v - m\Delta v). \tag{1.27}$$

Of course, we assume the normalization conditions

$$\iint \mathscr{K}_{nm}(u, v)\, du dv = 1 \tag{1.28}$$

to be satisfied. In the general case (in particular, when we want to model *nonlinearity effects*) we introduce a function $F(\mathscr{J})$ with the inverse function F^{-1} and assume that

$$I_{nm} = F^{-1}\left\{\iint \mathscr{K}_{nm}(u, v) F(\mathscr{R}\mu(u, v)\, du dv\right\}. \tag{1.29}$$

The function F is assumed to be known. If we want to consider effects related to the fact that F is unknown or not known precisely, we must omit taking the inverse function in (1.29). In the general case F can depend on the number of the measurement. Then in (1.29) we must replace F by F_{nm}.

To describe three-dimensional effects or effects similar to beam hardening **[2, 4, 9]**, we must consider certain generalizations of the above scheme. Examples of such generalizations are considered below (see §2.1). Here we only remark that in these cases we essentially have an analog of $\mathscr{R}\mu$ that depends on certain additional parameters. In the measurement process we average over these parameters, again obtaining something similar to I_{nm}. Formulas of the type (1.25), (1.29) define the model of measurement (see (1.1))

$$\mathscr{J} : \{\mu\} \to \{I_{jk}\}, \qquad \mathscr{J}\mu = [I_{jk}]. \tag{1.30}$$

Using the locality of functionals (in the same sense as in (1.19)) we can write, in both the linear and the nonlinear case,

$$I_{nm} \simeq \mathscr{R}\mu(n\Delta u, m\Delta v). \tag{1.31}$$

Let us note that the assumption about the uniformity of steps (Δu and Δv) in the coordinates u and v is not essential, and we use it only to simplify the exposition. On the other hand, it is the assumption that in the coordinates u, v measurements are made at equal intervals $\Delta u, \Delta v$ that distinguishes a natural (for this measurement process) coordinate system in the space of lines. Let us consider analogs of *compatibility conditions* (3.1) in the general case (in doing so it is useful to keep in mind the corresponding set of examples; see §1.3). Given a lattice $[P_{nm}]$, $|n| \leq n_H$, $|m| \leq m_H$, one can associate to it several parameters with the dimension of length. The lattice density is characterized by

$$d_0 = \max_{\vec{r} \in \mathscr{D}_H} d(\vec{r}, [P_{nm}]), \tag{1.32}$$

where $d(\vec{r}, M)$ is the distance between $\vec{r}$ and a set $M \subset \mathbb{R}^2$, so that d_0 is the distance between $\vec{r}$ and the set $[P_{nm}] \subset \mathbb{R}^2$. Next we can consider

$$d_1 = \max(d_u, d_v), \tag{1.33}$$

where d_u and d_v are defined as follows:

$$d_u = \max_{\vec{r} \in P_{nm}} d(\vec{r}, P_{n+1,m}), \qquad d_v = \max_{\vec{r} \in P_{nm}} d(\vec{r}, P_{n,m+1}), \tag{1.34}$$

so that d_u and d_v are the distances between neighboring (in terms of the coordinates u, v) lines. Finally,

$$d_2 = (R_H^2 / n_H m_H)^{1/2}. \tag{1.35}$$

The example of the canonical lattice $[P^1_{jk}]$ shows that as an analog of condition (1.3) one can take

$$d_u = C d_v. \tag{1.36}$$

Let us remark that, similarly to the canonical lattice, we have

$$d_1 = C \Delta q. \tag{1.37}$$

The above remarks about the reconstruction with $\Delta\varphi = 0$ show that of the three parameters d_0, d_1, d_2 only d_1 can be taken as a measure of spatial resolution in the reconstruction from $[I_{nm}]$. A lattice $[P_{nm}]$ is said to be *equivalent to the canonical lattice* $[P^1_{jk}]$ if

$$d_1([P^1_{jk}]) = c d_1([P_{nm}]). \tag{1.38}$$

For such a lattice it is natural to assume that in the reconstruction from $[I_{nm}]$ one again gets (1.10), and local functionals I_{nm}, considered as functions on the space of lines, can be interpolated to the equivalent canonical lattice without noticeable loss of spatial resolution. These qualitative arguments agree with numerical experiments and show how to select (up to a constant) the small parameters $\Delta\varphi, \Delta q$ in the interpolation.

§1.2. A model of an object

As we mentioned in the Introduction, a model of an object depends on the choice of those physical factors that we want to take into account. In this section we clarify this choice by giving several examples. However, first we return to the BMM. Here the model of an object (0.1) uses nonsmooth functions. These nonsmooth functions are even more necessary because the reconstruction of discontinuous functions is a main criterion determining the general quality of reconstruction. To formulate reconstruction quality criteria, it suffices to consider regions $\mathscr{D}_i$ of two types only: disks and rectangles. Below we denote by $\mathscr{D}(b, \vec{a})$ the disk of radius b centered at a point $\vec{a} \in \mathscr{D}_H$, and by $\chi_{b,\vec{a}}$ its characteristic function. By χ_b we denote the characteristic function of the disk of radius b centered at the origin. Let us introduce the terminology used in estimating the reconstruction quality. Leaving aside effects similar to beam hardening (see below), this terminology directly corresponds to the physics of the process. A function $\mu(\vec{r})$ (object of investigation) is called a *phantom*. A homogeneous phantom $\mu_0(\vec{r})$ is a function of the form

$$\mu(\vec{r}) = \mu_0\chi_B(\vec{r}), \qquad B \simeq R_b. \tag{1.39}$$

To estimate the quality it suffices to consider phantoms of the form

$$\mu(\vec{r}) = \mu_0(\vec{r}) + \Delta\mu \sum_{i=1}^{I} \chi_i(\vec{r}), \tag{1.40}$$

where $\chi_i(\vec{r})$ are the characteristic functions of either disks or rectangles lying inside the circle of radius B. Hence, a phantom is a homogeneous object with several round or rectangular inclusions. The parameter $\Delta\mu$ is called the *contrast*. One can consider more general phantoms of the form

$$\mu(\vec{r}) = \sum_i \mu_i \chi_{\mathscr{D}_i}(\vec{r}), \tag{1.41}$$

where the $\mathscr{D}_i$ are disks, ellipses, or rectangles. Functions $\mu(\vec{r})$ of such a form are rather convenient, because their Radon transforms $\mathscr{R}\mu(\varphi, q)$ can be computed explicitly:

$$\mathscr{R}\mu(\varphi, q) = \sum_i \mu_i l_{\mathscr{D}_i}(\varphi, q), \tag{1.42}$$

where $l_{\mathscr{D}}(\varphi, q)$ is the length of the segment of the line (φ, q) that lies inside $\mathscr{D}$. For the above regions, $l_{\mathscr{D}}(\varphi, q)$ can be computed using simple explicit formulas. For example, if $\mathscr{D} = \mathscr{D}(b, \vec{a})$ (the disk of radius b centered at $\vec{a}$), we have

$$l_{\mathscr{D}}(\varphi, q) = \begin{cases} 2[b^2 - (q - \langle \vec{a}, \vec{\eta} \rangle^2]^{1/2}, & b > |q - \langle \vec{a}, \vec{\eta} \rangle|, \\ 0, & b < |q - \langle \vec{a}, \vec{\eta} \rangle|. \end{cases} \tag{1.43}$$

We do not give similar formulas for ellipses and rectangles.

Let us emphasize once again that in discussing modeling algorithms we assume that $\mathscr{R}\mu(\varphi, q)$ can be computed explicitly. This restriction has, however, one serious drawback. All the regions $\mathscr{D}$ mentioned above have a convex boundary; thus they do not allow us to reproduce artifacts that occur on tomograms at the lines passing through the points of the boundary $\partial\mathscr{D}$ where the boundary become flat (i.e., points with curvature $\kappa = 0$). All the above applies to the BMM. Let us discuss how we must change the model if we want to consider, for example, *three-dimensional effects*, like the finiteness of the detector size in the direction perpendicular to the tomogram plane, or the noncoincidence of the detection plane with the plane in which the source moves (for a fourth generation tomograph); see §1.4. These changes reduce to consideration of objects $\mu(\vec{r}, z)$ (a function on $\mathbb{R}^3$) of the same type (1.41), where now the $\mathscr{D}_i$ are balls, ellipsoids, cylinders, or tetrahedra in $\mathbb{R}^3$. In all these cases the length $l_{\mathscr{D}}$ of the segment inside $\mathscr{D}$ of the line joining a point of the source with a point of the detector can again be computed explicitly. Let us emphasize that nowhere below do we consider reconstruction of a function $\mu(\vec{r}, z)$ in three variables, assuming instead that during the measurement process we average with respect to the variable z (see §1.4). Therefore this variable is necessary only on the stage of modeling, and we reconstruct a function $\mu^A(\vec{r})$, $\vec{r} \in \mathbb{R}^2$, averaged in z.

As a second example of a change of a model of an object let us consider the case when $\mu(\vec{r})$ depends on an additional parameter ε. In the X-ray case ε is the energy in the spectrum of X-ray radiation, $\mu(\vec{r},\varepsilon)$ is the absorption coefficient at the point $\vec{r}$ for energy ε, and effects related to the dependence of μ on ε are called *beam hardening effects* [**2, 4, 9**]. Similarly to the modeling of three-dimensional effects, the variable ε is necessary only on the modelling stage, and what we reconstruct is the result of a certain averaging with respect to ε (see §1.5). Depending on the model, ε can run over a continuous spectrum $0 \leq \varepsilon \leq \varepsilon_M$ or over a discrete spectrum $\varepsilon = \varepsilon_p$, $p = 1, \ldots, P$. Usually we know $\mu(\vec{r},\varepsilon)$ only at certain points ε_p, and in the numerical averaging over the continuous spectrum we actually again have the discrete case. Therefore we can assume that the object is defined by a family

$$(1.44) \qquad \mu_p(\vec{r}) = \mu(\vec{r},\varepsilon_p), \qquad p = 1, \ldots P,$$

where, similarly to (1.41),

$$(1.45) \qquad \mu_p(\vec{r}) = \sum_i \mu_{ip}\chi_{\mathscr{D}_i}(\vec{r}).$$

Let us briefly describe how μ_{ip} is specified in the case of X-ray tomography. Here i is the index that specifies the substance filling the region $\mathscr{D}_i$, and for this substance we have $\mu_{ip} = \mu_i(\varepsilon_p)$. The parameters $\mu_i(\varepsilon_p)$ are determined experimentally. One can also use tables containing mass coefficients $(\mu/\rho)_k(\varepsilon_p)$ for various elements k. In this case, with the density of the substance i being equal to ρ_i and the relative concentration of the element k in the substance i being equal to $C_k(i)$ (so that $\sum_k C_k(i) = 1$), we have

$$(1.46) \qquad \mu_{ip} = \mu_i(\varepsilon_p) = \rho_i \sum_k C_k(i)(\mu/\rho)_k(\varepsilon_p).$$

§1.3. Scanning geometry and lattices of lines

Let us discuss practical realization of observation along the lattice of lines $[P_{nm}]$. The form of the lattice and the choice of coordinates (u, v) is determined by the construction of the scanning system. To be able to use physical terminology, in this section we assume that the detector and the source are points and all measurements are instantaneous, so that the line P_{nm} corresponds to a measurement at the moment when the detector and the source are on this line. One can design a lot of constructions of scanning systems with lattices $[P_{nm}]$ satisfying the general conditions formulated in §1.1. However, we consider only those scanning systems that correspond to tomographs of the first four generations.

In passing to nonpoint detectors (sources) and noninstantaneous measurements the lattice $[P_{nm}]$ plays the roles of lattices consisting of lines to which we ascribe these measurements.

The scanning scheme of a *tomograph of the first generation* is shown in Figure 1. In this scheme the source M and the detector D are rigidly connected and move along the rails $M'M''$, $D'D''$ with relative position determined by the angle φ_k. The measurements are made at times when q is given by (0.11). After the source and the detector move from the initial position $M_A D_A$ to the final position $M_B D_B$ the rails turn by an angle $\Delta\varphi$ around the scanning center O, and the process starts anew. It is clear that for an appropriate choice of the initial position $M_A D_A$ and the final position $M_B D_B$ we obtain a lattice of lines $[P^i_{jk}]$ from the BMM that is determined by equation

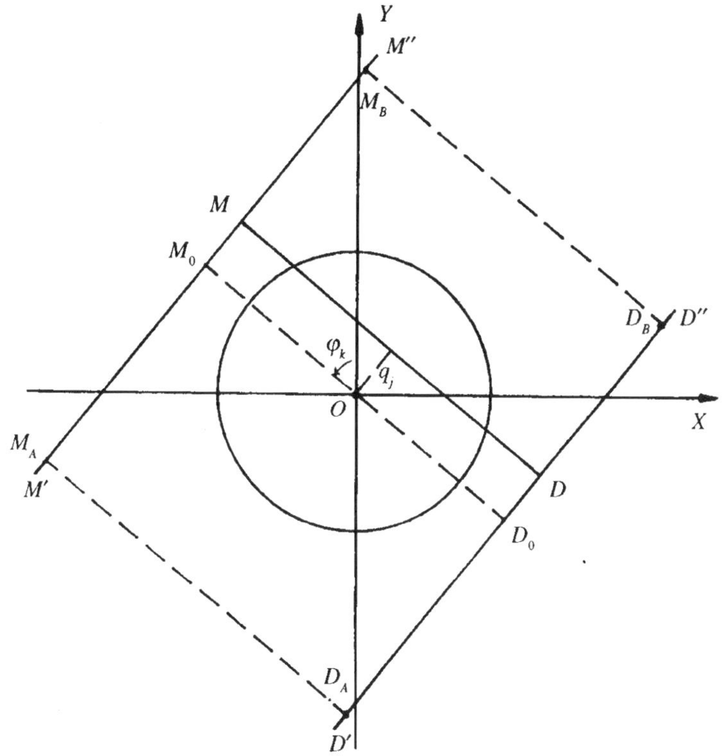

FIGURE 1

(0.11). Furthermore, the completeness condition (0.9) will be satisfied. Therefore, in this case the canonical coordinates (φ_k, q_j) of lines are directly related to measurement process. Actually this means that measurements are made in equal intervals $\Delta\varphi, \Delta q$. A first generation scheme can be realized in a tomograph with several detectors if we assume that the source M is "moved away to ∞", i.e., we have a parallel radiation beam. The *second generation scheme* is usually realized when we have several (few) detectors. This scheme is illustrated in Figure 2, where the geometric meaning of the coordinates (α, β, t) is also shown. Now detectors D_j are located on an arc of radius MD_0. The angle of view Δ of the detector arc from the point M is small, so that the disk $\mathscr{D}_H$ is not covered by the circular sector M_0AB. The scanning is similar to that in a first generation detector with the only difference that now the entire detector arc moves along $D'D''$. Measurements are made for a fixed $\alpha = \alpha_k$ by all detectors simultaneously at the moments when the variable t take values $t_p = p\Delta t$. After that the entire system rotates by the angle $\Delta\alpha$. The coordinates (φ, q) and (α, β, t) are related as follows:

$$\varphi = \alpha + \beta, \qquad q = R_M \sin\beta + t\cos\beta. \tag{1.47}$$

Here and later

$$R_M = d(0, M_0), \qquad R_D = d(0, D_0), \tag{1.48}$$

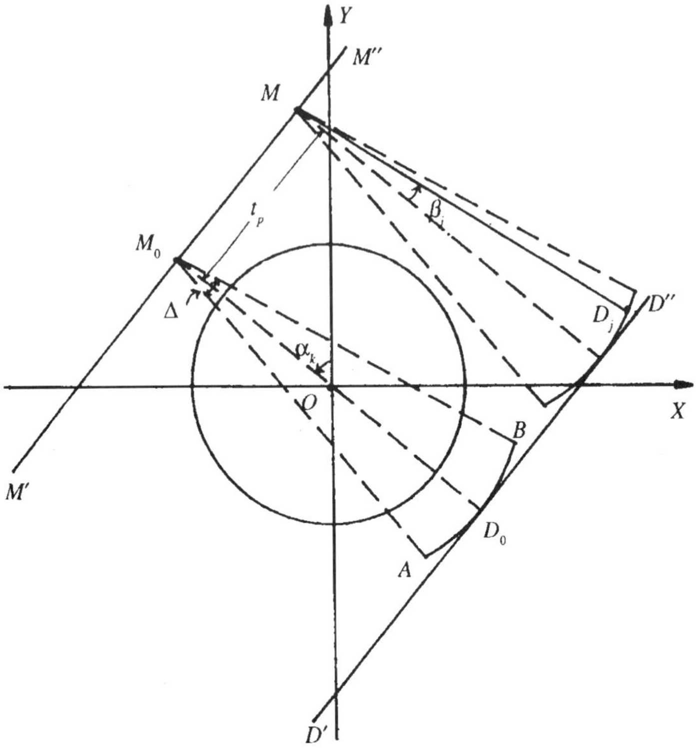

FIGURE 2

so that if a measurement corresponds to a line M_0D_0 passing through the scanning center O, then R_D (respectively, R_M) is the distance between the detector D_0 (respectively, the source M_0) and the scanning center. If the distance between neighboring detectors equals $\Delta\beta$, then the lattice of lines $[P^2_{kjp}]$ is given by equations

$$\alpha_i = i\Delta\alpha, \qquad \beta_j = j\Delta\beta, \qquad t_p = p\Delta t. \tag{1.49}$$

Here α, β, t vary in the intervals

$$\begin{gathered} -\Delta/2 \leq \beta \leq \Delta/2, \qquad -\Delta/2 \leq \alpha \leq \pi + \Delta/2, \\ |t| \leq t_M = \frac{R_M \sin(\Delta/2) + R_H}{\cos(\Delta/2)}. \end{gathered} \tag{1.50}$$

For

$$\Delta\alpha = \Delta \tag{1.51}$$

we get a lattice equivalent to $\lfloor P^1_{jk} \rfloor$ with $\Delta\varphi = \Delta\beta$, $\Delta q = \Delta t$. This means that by decreasing the number of detectors we can increase the rotation angle of the scanning system. Conditions (1.50) guarantee the completeness (1.25) of the data array.

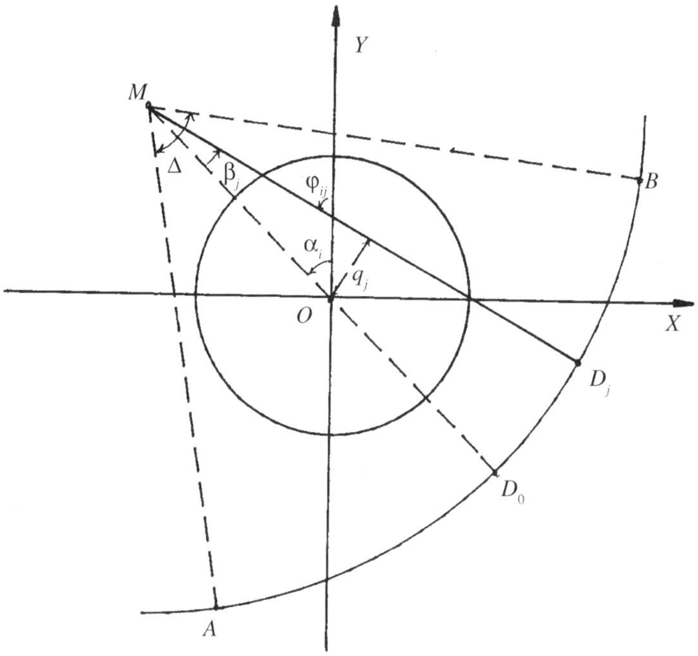

FIGURE 3

Assuming in the previous example that the opening angle Δ is sufficiently large, i.e.,

$$R_H < R_M \sin(\Delta/2), \tag{1.52}$$

we can make t fixed. Taking $t = 0$, we obtain the scanning system of a *third generation tomograph* (see Figure 3). Therefore, in such a system detectors lie on an arc $S = D'D''$ of radius $R_M + R_D$, are rigidly connected with the source M, and rotate together with it around the point O. Measurements are made by all detectors simultaneously at the time moments when $\alpha = \alpha_i$. Natural coordinates of lines are the angles (α, β),

$$\varphi = \alpha + \beta, \qquad q = R_M \sin\beta. \tag{1.53}$$

If the angular coordinates of detectors are

$$\beta_j = j\Delta\beta, \tag{1.54}$$

then (sufficient) *completemess conditions* are of the form

$$-\Delta/2 \leq \beta_j \leq \Delta/2, \qquad -\Delta/2 \leq \alpha_i \leq \pi + \Delta/2. \tag{1.55}$$

We can take

$$\alpha_i = \frac{\Delta}{2} + (i-1)\Delta\alpha, \qquad 1 \leq i \leq N_\alpha, \quad N_\alpha = \left[\frac{\pi + \Delta}{\Delta\alpha}\right] \tag{1.56}$$

We obtain a lattice of lines $[P^3_{ij}]$ specified by the relations

$$\varphi_{ij} = \alpha_i + \beta_j, \qquad q(\beta_j) = R_M \sin\beta_j. \tag{1.57}$$

One of the canonical lattices $[P^1_{jk}]$ equivalent to $[P^3_{ij}]$ can be obtained, for example, by taking

$$\Delta q = R_M \sin \Delta\beta, \qquad \Delta\varphi = \Delta\alpha \tag{1.58}$$

and in this case the compatibility conditions take the form

$$R_b \Delta\alpha = C R_M \sin \Delta\beta. \tag{1.59}$$

According to (1.52), we can assume that

$$|j| \leq j_M, \qquad j_M = [\Delta/2\Delta\beta]. \tag{1.60}$$

Let us note that instead of (1.56) we can choose, say, Δq in such a way that

$$\Delta q R_M \sin(\Delta/2)/j_M. \tag{1.61}$$

In the case of a *fourth generation tomograph* the source moves along a circle of radius R_M and stationary detectors lie on a circle of radius R_D. Therefore, contrary to the other schemes, now the source moves and the detectors are stationary. Measurements are made by all detectors simultaneously at the moment when $\alpha = \alpha_i$. This scheme, together with the geometric meaning of the natural coordinates (α, ψ)

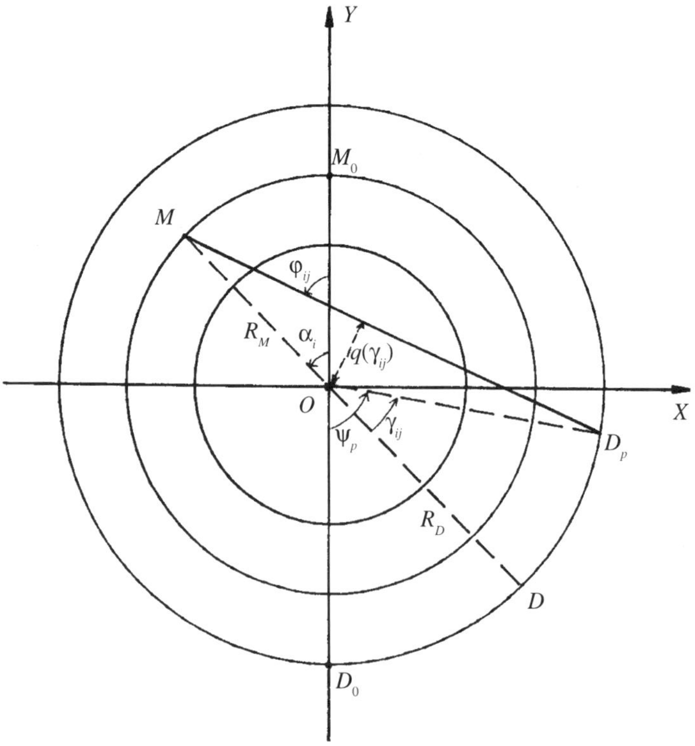

FIGURE 4

and the coordinates (α, γ), is shown in Figure 4. The angular coordinates of the detector D_p are given by

$$\psi_p = p\Delta\gamma, \qquad p = 0, 1, \dots N_D - 1, \tag{1.62}$$

where p is the detector index and N_D is the total number of detectors,

$$\Delta\gamma = 2\pi/N_D. \tag{1.63}$$

Assuming that

$$\alpha_i = \alpha_0 + i\Delta\alpha, \qquad i = 0, 1, \dots N_\alpha - 1, \tag{1.64}$$

we obtain a lattice of lines $[P^4_{ip}]$ with $\alpha = \alpha_i$, $\psi = \psi_p$.

Together with the coordinates (α, ψ), it is sometimes convenient to use the coordinates (α, γ). Then

$$\begin{aligned} \psi &= \alpha + \gamma, \\ \gamma &= \arcsin \frac{q}{R_D} + \arcsin \frac{q}{R_M}, \\ \varphi &= \alpha + \arcsin \frac{q}{R_M}. \end{aligned} \tag{1.65}$$

If

$$N(i) = \left[\frac{(\alpha_i + \Delta\gamma/2) \pmod{2\pi}}{\Delta\gamma} \right] \tag{1.66}$$

is the index of the detector closest to the point D and

$$p = (N(i) + j) \pmod{N_D}, \tag{1.67}$$

then the line (α_i, ψ_p) has the coordinates (α_i, γ_{ij}), where

$$\gamma_{ij} = j\Delta\gamma + \frac{1}{2}\Delta\gamma - \left\{ \frac{(\alpha_i + \Delta\gamma/2) \pmod{2\pi}}{\Delta\gamma} \right\} \Delta\gamma. \tag{1.68}$$

In (1.66) and (1.68), $[x]$ and $\{x\}$ denote the integral and the fractional parts of x.

Let us consider completeness conditions for the lattice $[P^4_{ij}]$ of lines (α_i, γ_{ij}) (if the condition (1.67) is satisfied, the lattice $[P^4_{ij}]$ coincides with $[P^4_{ip}]$). Note first that we can confine ourselves to the case

$$\begin{aligned} |j| &\leq j_M, \\ j_M &= \left[\Delta^{-1}(\arcsin(R_H/R_M) + \arcsin(R_H/R_D)) \right] + j_0, \end{aligned} \tag{1.69}$$

where j_0 is the parameter that determines the number of detectors such that the lines joining them with M do not intersect the disk $\mathscr{D}_b$. In this case we can assume that for a given α_k we have

$$N_T = 2j_M + 1 \tag{1.70}$$

measurements. Completeness conditions can be taken in the form

$$\begin{aligned} N_\alpha \Delta\alpha &\geq \pi + \Delta, \\ \Delta &= 2 \arcsin \left(\frac{\sin(\Delta\gamma N_T/2)}{\left[1 + (R_M/R_D)^2 + 2(R_M/R_D)\cos(\delta\gamma N_T/2) \right]^{1/2}} \right). \end{aligned} \tag{1.71}$$

An equivalent canonical lattice $[P^1_{ij}]$ can be defined by the same relations (1.58) or

(1.61) as for third generation tomographs. Therefore for models of tomographs of each generation (from first to fourth) we have defined a lattice of lines $[P^1_{ij}]$, $[P^2_{ijp}]$, $[P^3_{ij}]$, $[P^4_{ip}]$ to which measurements are assigned. Below these lattices will be used for the indication of the model under consideration.

§1.4. Examples of apparatus functions

In this section we illustrate the influence of various factors determining the measurement procedure on the specific form of apparatus functions by formulas similar to (1.25) and (1.29). In addition, we briefly discuss three-dimensional effects that cannot be modeled with these formulas. For more details, see **[10]**.

We begin with the simplest case of *two-dimensional models* of first generation tomographs. After that the passage to tomographs of the third and fourth generations is easy; it will be illustrated by several examples. To indicate the geometry (generation) to which a given formula refers, we will add to it the symbol of the corresponding lattice of lines. The lattices $[P^1_{jk}]$, $[P^3_{ij}]$, and $[P^4_{ip}]$ were defined in §1.3. Sometimes instead of $[P^4_{ip}]$ we will use the lattice $[P^4_{ij}]$. For the first generation tomograph ($[P^1_{jk}]$) we consider the simplest model with the nonpoint source. If the detector size along the line $D'D''$ equals d (see Figure 1), and $d \ll R_M$ (R_M is defined by (1.48)), then for a *point pulse source* radiating at time moments when $q = q_j$, we have, in the simplest case,

$$I_{jk} = d^{-1} \int_{q_i - d/2}^{q_i + d/2} J(\varphi_k, q)\, dq \qquad [P^1_{jk}], \tag{1.72}$$

This corresponds to the apparatus function (1.6) in the BMM. If the point source is moving and radiates permanently, and the measurement refers to the interval $[q_j - \Delta q/2, q_j + \Delta q/2]$, then instead of (1.72) we must take

$$I_{jk} = (\Delta q d)^{-1} \int_{q_i - \Delta q/2}^{q_i + \Delta q/2} dq \int_{q - d/2}^{q + d/2} J(\varphi_k, q')\, dq' \qquad [P^1_{jk}]. \tag{1.73}$$

The corresponding apparatus function in the BMM is

$$\Pi(q) = (d\Delta q)^{-1} \chi_{\Delta q}(q) \underset{q}{\otimes} \chi_d(q). \tag{1.74}$$

Here and later

$$\chi_a(q) = \begin{cases} 1, & |q| < a/2, \\ 0, & |q| > a/2, \end{cases} \tag{1.75}$$

and $\otimes_q$ means the convolution with respect to q.

Now we consider the *nonpoint pulse source* of size m along the line $M'M''$. For $m \ll R_M$ we have

(1.76)
$$I_{jk} = (md)^{-1} \int_{-m/2}^{m/2} dt \int_{-d/2}^{d/2} ds\, J\left(\varphi_k + \frac{s - t}{R_M + R_D}, q_j + \frac{R_M s + R_D t}{R_M + R_D}\right) \qquad [P^1_{jk}].$$

Strictly speaking, this case cannot be considered in the framework of the BMM.

Let us consider numerical realization for the simplest formula (1.72). To compute the corresponding integral we must apply a quadrature formula. As a result, we obtain relations of the form

$$I_{jk} \simeq \sum_p C_p J(\varphi_k, q_i + \delta_p), \qquad \delta_p = p\delta q, \qquad \delta q \ll d/2, \tag{1.77}$$

with

$$\sum_p C_p = 1, \qquad \delta_p \leq d/2. \tag{1.78}$$

Therefore the application of a quadrature formula is equivalent to the replacement of the nonpoint detector by a weighted sum of point detectors inside the aperture. Formulas of this form can be considered as basic formulas in the modeling of various effects. Numerical realization of formulas (1.73), (1.76) can be done similarly.

Now we consider *detector delay* effect. Earlier we actually assumed (without saying so explicitly) that the detector reacts to the change of the signal $J(t) = J(\varphi, q)$ instantaneously (in the scanning process q and φ are functions of the time t). Each actual measurement system has a delay, i.e., the response $I(t)$ to the signal $\mathscr{J}(t)$ has the form

$$I(t) = \int_{-\infty}^{t} K(t-t')J(t')\,dt' \tag{1.79}$$

with

$$\int_0^{\infty} K(t)\,dt = 1. \tag{1.80}$$

Usually the following approximation is made:

$$K(t) = A^{-1}\sum_p C_p e^{-t/\pi_p}, \qquad A = \sum_p C_p \tau_p. \tag{1.81}$$

For a first generation tomograph the inclusion of delay is equivalent to the introduction of the following apparatus function:

$$\Pi_\tau(q) = \begin{cases} K(q/v)v^{-1}, & q > 0, \\ 0, & q < 0, \end{cases} \tag{1.82}$$

where v is the linear scanning speed. We emphasize that this apparatus function is not an even function. For example, to include delay in the case (1.73) it suffices to replace the apparatus function $\Pi(q)$ (1.74) by the function

$$\Pi(q) = \chi_{\Delta q} \underset{q}{\otimes} \Pi_\tau \otimes \chi_d. \tag{1.83}$$

Then instead of (1.73) (in the case (1.81)) we obtain

$$\begin{aligned} I_{jk} = \sum_p \frac{C_p}{\Delta q \cdot d \cdot A \cdot v} \int_{q_j - \Delta q/2}^{q_j + \Delta q/2} dq \\ \times \int_{-\infty}^{q} e^{-(q-q'/\tau_p v)}\,dq' \int_{q'-d/2}^{q'+d/2} J(\varphi, q'')\,dq'' \qquad [P^1_{jk}]. \end{aligned} \tag{1.84}$$

Let us consider how these formulas should be modified for tomographs of the third and the fourth generations. An analog of (1.72) for a third generation tomograph has the form

$$I_{ij} = (\delta\beta)^{-1} \int_{\beta_j - \delta\beta/2}^{\beta_j + \delta\beta/2} J(\alpha_i, \beta)\, d\beta \qquad [P^3_{ij}], \tag{1.85}$$

and for a fourth generation tomograph

$$\begin{aligned} I_{ip} &= (\delta\gamma)^{-1} \int_{\psi_p - \delta\gamma/2}^{\psi_p + \delta\gamma/2} J(\alpha, \psi)\, d\psi \qquad [P^4_{ip}], \\ I_{ij} &= (\delta\gamma)^{-1} \int_{\gamma_{ij} - \delta\gamma/2}^{\gamma_{ij} + \delta\gamma/2} J(\alpha, \gamma)\, d\gamma \qquad [P^4_{ij}]. \end{aligned} \tag{1.86}$$

Here $\delta\beta$ and $\delta\gamma$ are angular apertures of the corresponding detectors. An analog of (1.73) that takes into account the tomograph motion for a fourth generation tomograph has the form

$$I_{ij} = (\delta\gamma \cdot \Delta\alpha)^{-1} \int_{\alpha_i - \Delta\alpha/2}^{\alpha_i + \Delta\alpha/2} d\alpha \int_{\gamma_{ij}(\alpha) - \delta\gamma/2}^{\gamma_{ij} + \delta\gamma/2} J(\alpha, \gamma)\, d\gamma \qquad [P^4_{ij}], \tag{1.87}$$

where $\gamma_{ij}(\alpha) = \gamma_{ij} + \alpha_i - \alpha$. The corresponding formula for the lattice $[P^3_{ij}]$ is quite similar:

$$I_{ij} = (\delta\beta \cdot \Delta\alpha)^{-1} \int_{\alpha_i - \Delta\alpha/2}^{\alpha_i + \Delta\alpha/2} d\alpha \int_{\beta_j - \delta\beta/2}^{\beta_j + \delta\beta/2} J(\alpha, \beta)\, d\beta \qquad [P^3_{ij}]. \tag{1.88}$$

Now we modify the model corresponding (1.88) so that to include the case of a nonpoint source. This can be done similarly to (1.77) and results in the following modification of (1.88):

$$\begin{aligned} I_{ij} &= (\delta\beta \cdot \Delta\alpha)^{-1} \sum_p C_p \int_{\alpha_i + \delta_p - \Delta\alpha/2}^{\alpha_i + \delta_p + \Delta\alpha/2} d\alpha \int_{\beta_j - \delta\beta/2}^{\beta_j + \delta\beta/2} J(\alpha, \beta)\, d\beta \qquad [P^3_{ij}], \\ &\sum_p C_p = 1, \qquad |\delta_p| = |p\delta\alpha| < \Delta\alpha, \quad \delta\alpha \ll \Delta\alpha. \end{aligned} \tag{1.89}$$

Here we actually replace a continuous nonpoint source by a weighted sum of point sources, and the coefficient C_p characterize the intensities of these point sources. Inclusion of nonpoint sources into the model (1.87) can be done similarly.

Let us discuss also how we can take into account the delay for a fourth generation tomograph. If the ith measurement fills the time interval $[t_i - \Delta t/2, t_i + \Delta t/2]$, so that

$$t_i = i\Delta t + t_0, \tag{1.90}$$

and a point source moves with the angular speed ω, then

$$\alpha = \omega(t - t_0) + \alpha_0, \qquad \alpha_i = \alpha(t_i), \qquad \Delta\alpha = \omega\Delta t. \tag{1.91}$$

In the case of a linear model we assume that we measure

(1.92)

$$I_{ip} = \frac{1}{\Delta t \cdot \delta\gamma \cdot A} \int_{t_i - \Delta t/2}^{t_i + \Delta t/2} dt \int_{t_i - T_H}^{t} K(t - t')\, dt' \int_{\psi_p - \delta\gamma/2}^{\psi_p + \delta\gamma/2} J(\alpha', \psi)\, d\psi \qquad [P^4_{ip}],$$

where $\alpha' = \omega(t' - t) + \alpha_0$. We assume that

$$\omega T_H > \Delta\alpha/2 \tag{1.93}$$

and the parameter T_H characterizes the time of signal accumulation. Changing variables from t, t' to α, α' we obtain

$$\begin{aligned} I_{ip} = {} & \frac{1}{\Delta\alpha \cdot \delta\gamma \cdot A \cdot \omega} \int_{\alpha_i - \Delta\alpha/2}^{\alpha_i + \Delta\alpha/2} d\alpha \int_{\alpha_i - \omega T_H}^{\alpha} d\alpha' \Pi(\alpha - \alpha') \\ & \times \int_{\psi_p - \delta\gamma/2}^{\psi_p + \delta\gamma/2} J(\alpha', \psi)\, d\psi \qquad [P_{ip}^4] \end{aligned} \tag{1.94}$$

and if $K(t)$ is of the form (1.81), then

$$\Pi(\alpha) = \sum_p C_p e^{-\alpha/\omega\tau_p}. \tag{1.95}$$

Note that, exchanging the order of integration with respect to α and α', we can make (1.84) a two-dimensional integral.

Let us consider now *two-dimensional nonlinear models.* According to (1.29), to define such a model we must specify an invertible function $F(J)$. This corresponds to the assumption that we measure not the Radon transform, but a function F in it. The inclusion of nonlinearity effects in any of the above formulas is made by a direct use of (1.29), i.e., by replacing J by $F(J)$ under the integral sign and applying F^{-1} after the integration. The choice of an appropriate function F is determined by physical properties of the problems, and, for example, to model the exponential absorption low in the X-ray case (see §1.5) we can take

$$F(J) = e^{-J} \qquad (F^{-1} = -\log). \tag{1.96}$$

Consider, for example, modifications that occur in this case in the simplest formula (1.79). According to (1.29), we get

$$I_{jk} = -\log \frac{1}{d} \int_{q_j - d/2}^{q_j + d/2} e^{-J(\varphi_k, q)}\, dq \qquad [P_{jk}^1]. \tag{1.97}$$

Similarly, one can include nonlinearity in any of the above cases.

Formula (1.97) shows that in the model under consideration nonlinearity effects disappear as $d \to 0$. This is related to the fact that the function F is assumed to be known. If we want to perform the phenomenological analysis of effects of an unknown nonlinearity, we must make a simple change

$$I_{jk} \to \widetilde{I}_{jk} = I_{jk} + \alpha I_{jk}^2, \tag{1.98}$$

with further analysis of the dependence of quality criteria on α.

Let us discuss briefly the modeling of *three-dimensional phenomena.* All the models we have considered up to now had the property that they are completely described by parameters defined in the tomogram plane x, y, so that these models can be called two-dimensional models. This is an approximation to the real situation where we ignore finite size of the source and of the detector in the direction of the axis z perpendicular to the plane x, y. As an example we consider the influence of the finiteness of the detector aperture δ_z along the axis z assuming the source to be point-like. The influence of the finiteness of the source size is considered similarly. Let

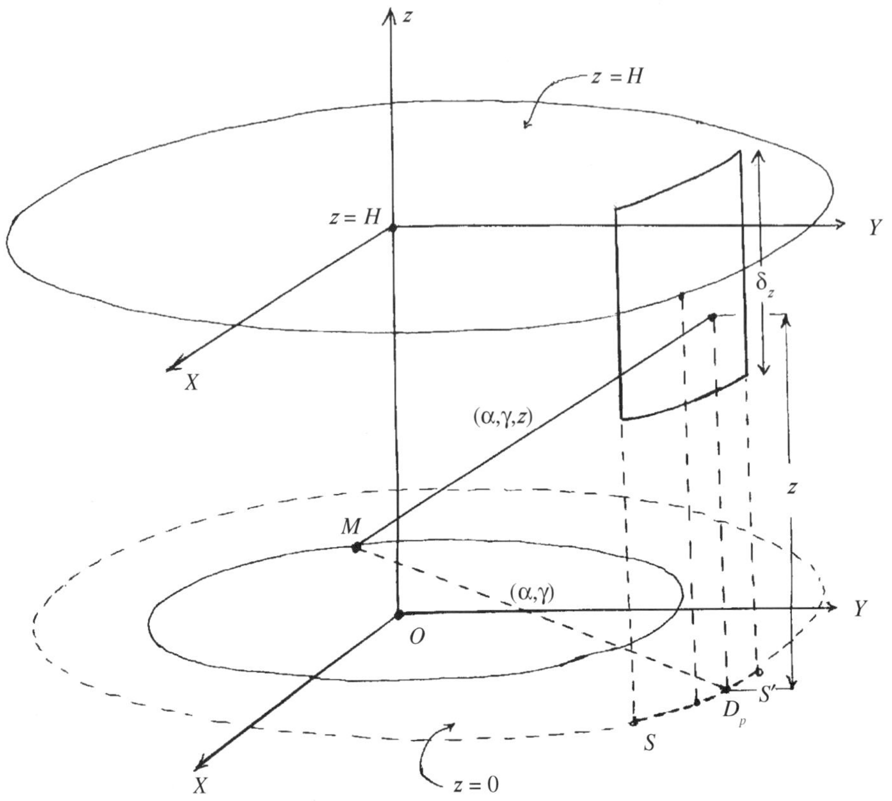

FIGURE 5

us consider one of the two-dimensional models we discussed earlier, for example, the model $[P_{ij}^4]$ (see (1.86)). Construct a cylinder passing through the "one-dimensional" detector SS' and perpendicular to the plane x, y (see Figure 5).

In the general case, the centers of detectors D' lie on the plane $z = H$. The "one-dimensional" detector SS' is the projection of the two-dimensional detector onto the plane $z = 0$. The line (α, γ) joining the source M and the detector SS' coincides with the projections of lines (α, γ, z) joining M and the two-dimensional detector. So, we have defined the coordinates of lines in the three-dimensional case. To study three-dimensional phenomena it is sufficient to replace $J(\alpha, \gamma)$ with $J(\alpha, \gamma, z)$ in (1.86) and to average with respect to z over the interval $[H - \delta_z/2, H + \delta_z/2]$. As a result, we replace (1.86) with the following formula:

$$I_{ij} = (\delta_\gamma \cdot \delta_z)^{-1} \int_{\gamma_{ij}-\delta\gamma/2}^{\gamma_{ij}+\delta\gamma/2} d\gamma \int_{H-\delta_z/2}^{H+\delta_z/2} J(\alpha, \gamma, z)\, dz \qquad [P_{ij}^4]. \tag{1.99}$$

Here $J(\alpha, \gamma, z)$ is the integral of the function $\mu(\vec{r}, z)$ over the line (α, γ, z) in $\mathbb{R}^3$ joining the source and the detector (see Figure 5). Modifications of other models are performed similarly and reduce to a certain averaging with respect to z. Let us only remark that for tomographs of the first, second, and third generations we can take $H = 0$. For fourth generation tomographs the plane of source motion and the plane of detector centers usually do not coincide (for technical reasons), so that

$H \neq 0$. In this case it is more natural to associate the data I_{ij} not to the plane $z = 0$ (as we did earlier), but to the plane $z = H/2$, i.e., to assume that the tomogram plane is the plane $z = H/2$.

Although in this section we have mostly considered specific examples, these examples should make it clear to the reader what set of operators should be applied to known Radon transforms $\mathscr{R}\mu$ in order to incluee a given collection of nonlocality and nonlinearity effects into a single model. Modeling of statistical errors and of beam hardening effects will be discussed later.

Let us also remark that up to now we have not used special features of the scanning radiation.

§1.5. Statistical errors and X-ray tomography

Phenomenological statistical error can be included into any of the models $[P_{nm}]$, $[I_{nm}]$ by assuming that we observe not the data $[I_{nm}]$, but the modified data

$$I_{nm}^{\Delta} = I_{nm} + \Delta I_{nm}, \tag{1.100}$$

where ΔI_{nm} are random variables with known statistical properties. To formulate quality criteria, it suffices to specify the expectations $\mathbb{E}(\Delta I_{nm})$ and the covariance $\mathbb{E}(\Delta I_{nm} \cdot \Delta I_{n'm'})$. Let us consider specific models of the noise; this permits us to separate noises of various natures and to determine their properties. First of all, note that the above models contain a number of parameters. Each of these parameters can be looked upon as a random parameter, leading to diffirent models of statistical errors. Let us discuss some examples. Consider the model (1.88) $[P_{ij}^3]$. Replacing α_i by $\alpha_i + \Delta\alpha_i$, where the $\Delta\alpha_i$ are independent Gaussian random variables with zero means and variances σ_α^2 (we denote this by $\Delta\alpha_i \in G(\sigma_\alpha^2)$), we obtain a model that takes into account the nonstability of the speed at which the source is moving. Replacing the parameter δ_p by $\delta_p + \Delta\delta_{ip}$ in $[P_{ij}^3]$ (1.89) and assuming that $\Delta\delta_{ip} \in G(\sigma_\alpha^2)$, we obtain a model that takes into account the nonstability of the shape of the source. Similarly one can "randomize" parameters in other models. The analysis of the influence of this noise on the reconstruction quality allows us to obtain reasonable technical requirements on the stability of the corresponding parameters.

Up to now we have not taken into account the specific physical nature of the radiation. Now we consider the most important example of *X-ray tomography*. In this case there is a nonremovable noise related to the quantum nature of the measurement process. We consider this noise, constructing at the same time the model for the analysis of beam hardening effects (see §1.2) and clarifying to some extent the origin of phenomenological formulas like (1.29) for nonlinear effects.

Measurements and quantum noise in X-ray tomography. The following two facts are essential in X-ray tomography.

1. For X-rays we can ignore diffraction and refraction phenomena, assuming that radiation propagates along straight lines.

2. X-ray quanta absorption satisfies the exponential law. This means that if ε_p is the energy of a quantum and N_p^0 is the number of quanta in the incident stream, then the number of quanta passing an object along a straight line is given by the formula

$$N_p = N_p^0 \exp\left(-\int \mu_p(\vec{r})\,ds\right), \tag{1.101}$$

where $\mu_p(\vec{r})$ is the absorption coefficient and the integral is taken over the line in question. Here $\mu_p(\vec{r}) = \mu_p(\varepsilon_p, \vec{r})$ (see §1.2). Phenomena related to the existence of several functions $\mu_p(\vec{r})$, $p = 1, 2, \dots, P$, are called *beam hardening phenomena.*

In the case of X-ray radiation we assume that the actual radiation spectrum is replaces by a step function, where ε_p is the middle point of the step and $\Delta\varepsilon_p$ is its width, $0 < \varepsilon_p < \varepsilon_M$. Let us consider the measurement along a fixed line with indices j, k (the (j,k)-measurement). Below the meaning of the indices j, k is not important, but for completeness we will have in mind the model (1.72) with the lattice $[P^1_{jk}]$. Let us consider first the noiseless model, so that we are interested in formula (1.97) and certain modifications that take beam hardening phenomena into account. During the (j,k)-measurement the source radiates the following energy towards the detector:

$$\mathscr{E}^0_{jk} = \sum_p N^0_{p,jk}\varepsilon_p. \tag{1.102}$$

Here $N^0_{p,jk}$ is the number of quanta with energy ε_p, and the sum over p from 1 to P is the sum over the spectrum. According to (1.101), we have

$$\mathscr{E}_{jk} = \sum_{p=1}^{P} \varepsilon_p N_{p,jk}, \qquad N_{p,jk} = N^0_{p,jk}\eta_{p,jk}, \tag{1.103}$$

where $\eta_{p,jk}$ is the average (over the aperture) attenuation coefficient. For example, in the case of the model (1.72) we have

$$\eta_{p,jk} = d^{-1}\int_{q_j-d/2}^{q_j+d/2} e^{-J_p(\varphi_k,q)}\,dq, \qquad J_p(\varphi_k, q) = \int_{(\varphi_k,q)} \mu_p(\vec{r})\,ds. \tag{1.104}$$

We assume that in addition to $\mathscr{E}_{jk}$, we perform independent measurements of the parameters $\mathscr{E}^0_{jk}$. Then the model that includes beam hardening phenomena can be described as follows:

$$I_{jk} = -\log\frac{\mathscr{E}_{jk}}{\mathscr{E}^0_{jk}} = -\log\sum_p S_{jk}(p)\eta_{p,jk}, \tag{1.105}$$

$$S_{jk}(p) = \frac{N^0_{p,jk}\varepsilon_p}{\sum_p \varepsilon_p N^0_{p,jk}}. \tag{1.106}$$

These formulas can be considered as modifications of (1.72) that take account of beam hardening phenomena. The above example makes it clear how one should modify other models, in particular those that correspond to other forms of nonlinearity. The simplest model is obtained under the assumption

$$N^0_{p,jk} = N^0_p, \tag{1.107}$$

which corresponds to a stable isotropic source. In this case

$$S_{jk}(p) = S^0(p) = \frac{N_p\varepsilon_p}{\sum_p N^0_p\varepsilon_p} \tag{1.108}$$

and

$$I_{jk} = -\log \sum_p S^0(p)\eta_{p,jk}, \tag{1.109}$$

$$\sum_p S^0(p) = 1. \tag{1.110}$$

Under the assumption

$$\mu_p(\vec{r}) \equiv \mu(\varepsilon_p, \vec{r}) = \mu(\vec{r}) \tag{1.111}$$

we again obtain (1.97). Similar formulas are obtained for the pointlike spectrum $S^0(p) = \delta_{pp_0}$ with $\mu(\vec{r}) = \mu_{P_0}(\vec{r})$. To make a model more precise, we must specify the *normalized spectral function* $S^0(p)$ of the source. In the X-ray case one can use as an example the function $S^0(p)$ obtained from the formula

$$N_p^0 = a(\varepsilon_M - \varepsilon_p)\Delta\varepsilon_p. \tag{1.112}$$

The functions $S^0(p)$ are parameters of the model, and on randomizing these functions, i.e., replacing them by

$$S_{jk}^{\Delta}(p) = S^0(p) + \Delta S_{jk}(p), \tag{1.113}$$

where $\mathbb{E}(\Delta S_{jk}) = 0$, we obtain a model that includes nonstability of the source. Let us note that here the normalization condition

$$\sum_p S_{jk}^{\Delta}(p) = 1 \tag{1.114}$$

must be preserved.

To obtain a model that includes the *quantum noise* we must replace $N_{p,jk}$ by

$$N_{p,jk}^{\Delta} = N_{p,jk} + \Delta N_{p,jk}, \tag{1.115}$$

where the $\Delta N_{p,jk}$ are independent Poisson random variables with

$$\mathbb{E}(\Delta N_{p,jk}) = 0, \qquad \mathbb{E}((\Delta N_{p,jk})^2) = N_{p,jk}. \tag{1.116}$$

Usually one assumes that $N_{p,jk} \gg 1$, and then the $\Delta N_{p,jk}$ can be assumed to be Gaussian random variables. Defining I_{jk}^{Δ} from the relation

$$I_{jk}^{\Delta} = -\log \frac{\sum_p \varepsilon_p N_{p,jk}^{\Delta}}{\sum_p \varepsilon_p N_{p,jk}^0}. \tag{1.117}$$

and using the assumption $N_{p,jk} \gg 1$, we obtain from (1.105)

$$I_{jk}^{\Delta} = I_{jk} + \Delta I_{jk}, \tag{1.118}$$

and, in accordance with (0.21),

$$\mathbb{E}(\Delta I_{jk}) = 0, \qquad \mathbb{E}(\Delta I_{jk} \cdot \Delta I_{j'k'}) = \sigma_J^2(j,k)\delta_{jj'}\delta_{kk'}. \tag{1.119}$$

Here

$$\sigma_J^2(j,k) = \frac{\sum_p \varepsilon_p^2 N_{p,jk}}{\left(\sum_p \varepsilon_p N_{p,jk}\right)^2}. \tag{1.120}$$

Hence, the I_{jk}^{Δ} are Gaussian random variables with zero means and variances $\sigma_J^2(j,k)$.

Ignoring beam hardening and assuming that conditions (1.107) and (1.111) are satisfied, we obtain from (1.120) that

$$\sigma_J^2(j,k) = (N_0 \eta_{jk})^{-1}. \tag{1.121}$$

For the model (1.72) considered here, we have

$$\eta_{jk} = d^{-1} \int_{q_j - d/2}^{q_j + d/2} e^{-J(\varphi_k, q)}\, dq. \tag{1.222}$$

and N_0 is the effective number of quanta emitted by the source during one measurement,

$$N_0 = \frac{(\sum_p \varepsilon_p N_p^0)^2}{\sum_p \varepsilon_p N_p^0}. \tag{1.123}$$

Since the attenuation coefficient η_{jk} is determined by integral characteristics of the object, whose diameter is much larger than d, in (1.121) we can use the approximation

$$\eta_{jk} = e^{-J(\varphi_k, q_j)}. \tag{1.124}$$

Formulas (1.118), (1.119), (1.121) will be used for the definition of *noise in the BMM*, and N_0 plays the role of an additional parameter of the model. Let us remark that in the absence of noise the BMM is linear, so that it does not have an internal scale for μ. This scale is defined by the parameter N_0.

In all other models the quantum noise can be defined similarly. For example, in $[P_{ij}^3]$ (1.85) the parameters I_{ij}^{Δ} can be defined again by (1.109) with the appropriate change of indices, and (1.124) can be replaced by

$$\eta_{ij} = e^{-J(\alpha_i, \beta_j)}. \tag{1.125}$$

We mention that sometimes it is more convenient to take another approximation of the form

$$\eta_{ij} = e^{-I_{ij}}. \tag{1.126}$$

Chapter 2. Reconstruction Algorithms

We start with general definitions. Let us assume that we are given a complete data array $[I_{nm}]$ (or $[I_{nm}^{\Delta}]$), which, according to (1.31), will be interpreted in this chapter as the Radon transform of a certain function along straight lines from a certain lattice $[P_{nm}]$ with coordinates $(n\Delta u, m\Delta v)$. Sometimes we will use the more detailed notation $[I_{nm}, P_{nm}(\Delta u, \Delta v)]$. By $[I_{jk}]$ (or $[I_{jk}, P_{jk}^1(\Delta\varphi, \Delta q)]$) we will always denote an array obtained from the canonical lattice P_{jk}^1. A *reconstruction algorithm* A is a mapping

$$A : \{I_{nm}, P_{nm}\} \to \{\mu^A(\vec{r})\}, \qquad A[I_{nm}] = \mu^A(\vec{r}). \tag{2.1}$$

Hence, this mapping is defined on the square K_b:

$$|x| \le x_M, \quad |y| \le x_M, \qquad x_M = R_b/\sqrt{2}. \tag{2.2}$$

Let us note that the square K_b contains the support of μ ($\mathscr{D}_\mu \subset K_b$). Although we have assumed that the function $\mu^A(\vec{r})$ is defined for all $\vec{r}$, in practical applications an algorithm reconstructs the values $\mu^A(\vec{r}_{\alpha\beta})$ for points of a square lattice with, for example,

$$(2.3) \qquad \begin{aligned} &\vec{r}_{\alpha\beta} = (x_\alpha, y_\beta), \qquad x_\alpha = \alpha\Delta x, \qquad y_\beta = \beta\Delta x, \\ &|\alpha| \le \alpha_M, \qquad |\beta| \le \alpha_M, \qquad \alpha_M = [x_M/\Delta x] \end{aligned}$$

The choice of Δx is determined by the expected spatial resolution, so that usually

$$(2.4) \qquad \Delta x = Cd_1,$$

where d_1 is defined in (1.33). In this case (provided that the lattice $[P_{nm}]$ satisfies the compatibility conditions (1.36)) the number N_x^2 of points on the tomogram ($N_x = 2\alpha_M$) is of the same order as the number of lines in the lattice $[P_{nm}]$ (see (1.23)),

$$(2.5) \qquad N_x^2 = CN_uN_v.$$

In this chapter we will describe a certain class of algorithms $\{A\}$. We do not intend to review and evaluate various algorithms. Instead, our goal is to indicate the main points in the construction of algorithms and to present examples of algorithms for the cases $[I^1_{jk}, P^1_{jk}]$, $[I_{ij}, P^3_{ij}]$, $[I_{ip}, P^4_{ip}]$ described in Chapter 1. Let give a general description of the *class of algorithms under consideration*. An algorithm A is the superposition of the *preliminary processing algorithm* $\mathscr{P}$ and of the *main reconstruction algorithm* A_0, applied consecutively,

$$(2.6) \qquad A = A_0 \circ \mathscr{P}.$$

The main algorithm A_0 is a version of the numerical realization of the Radon inversion formula. If the initial array $[I_{nm}, P_{nm}]$ refers to coordinates (u, v) in the space of lines, we can consider main algorithms based on the Radon inversion formula expressed in coordinates (u, v). Examples of such algorithms can be found in **[2, 5]**. However, we will not consider general algorithms of this type, restricting ourselves to basic *filtered backprojection algorithms* (FBPA), which use the inversion formula (0.9), i.e., the inversion formula in canonical coordinates (φ, q). The general theory of FBPA is discussed in **[1, 8]**. In this case the preliminary processing algorithm can be defined as a mapping

$$(2.7) \qquad \mathscr{P} : \{I_{nm}, P_{nm}\} \to \{I_{jk}, P^1_{jk}\}, \qquad \mathscr{P}[I_{nm}] = [I_{jk}],$$

and the main algorithm A_0 gives, in accordance with (2.6),

$$(2.8) \qquad A_0 : \{I_{jk}, P^1_{jk}\} \to \{\mu^A(\vec{r})\}, \qquad A_0[I_{jk}] = \mu^A(\vec{r}).$$

With this definition the algorithm $\mathscr{P}$ can include the "*beam straightening*" algorithm, i.e., an interpolation algorithm that allows us to obtain the values of the function $\mathscr{R}_\mu$ at points (φ_k, q_j) from its values at points $(n\Delta u, m\Delta v)$. Here we come to the problem of choosing $\Delta\varphi$ and Δq, which was already considered in Chapter 1. Let us note that it makes sense to introduce $\mathscr{P}$ even for the basic model. In this case the preliminary processing is reduces to filtration (deconvolution). At the same time, for a BMM it makes sense to consider algorithms without preliminary processing, i.e., those with $\mathscr{P} = \mathbf{1}$ (where $\mathbf{1}$ is the identity mapping) and $A = A_0$.

§2.1. Preliminary processing algorithms

In this section $[I_{nm}, P_{nm}]$ is an arbitrary data array (not necessarily the initial one). Denote by B a beam straightening algorithm, i.e., a mapping of the form

$$B : \{I_{nm}, P_{nm}(\Delta u, \Delta v)\} \to \{I_{jk}, P^1_{jk}\}, \qquad B[I_{nm}] = [I_{jk}]. \tag{2.9}$$

A sufficiently generic preliminary processing algorithm has the form

$$\mathscr{P} = Q_2 \circ B \circ Q_1, \tag{2.10}$$

where the algorithms (mappings) Q_1, Q_2 are superpositions of certain simpler algorithms, among which we distinguish *filtration*, *compression*, and *correction* algorithms.

Let us briefly describe these algorithms. By definition, a filtration algorithm is a mapping Φ of the form

$$\Phi : \{I_{nm}, P_{nm}(\Delta u, \Delta v)\} \to \{I^{\Phi}_{nm}, P_{nm}(\Delta u, \Delta v)\}, \qquad \Phi[I_{nm}] = [I^{\Phi}_{nm}], \tag{2.11}$$

which usually is a convolution in one or both variables. For example, in the case of one variable this algorithm takes the form

$$I^{\Phi}_{nm} = \sum_p \Phi_{n-p} I_{pm} \tag{2.12}$$

with

$$\Phi_k = 0 \quad \text{for } |k| \geq k_0, \qquad \sum_k \Phi_k = 1. \tag{2.13}$$

As an example we present the simplest algorithm that is used to decrease the noise. For this algorithm,

$$\Phi_k = 1/(2k_0 + 1). \tag{2.14}$$

Similarly one can describe algorithms with a two-dimensional convolution. This applies to deconvolution type algorithms that can be used, for example, in the BMM in the case when the support of $\Pi(q)$ is too large. Nonlinear filtrations, like, for example, the median filtration, are also possible. The outline and the analysis of such algorithms is not among our goals in this paper; we remark only that these and other similar algorithms are widely used in practical image processing [**11**]. In our language, filtration algorithms are characterized by the condition that they do not change the lattice of lines to which the data (2.11) is assigned.

Compression algorithms change the steps Δu and Δv in the above lattice. They have the form

$$\begin{gathered} C_{N_1,N_2} : \{I_{nm}, P_{nm}(\Delta u, \Delta v)\} \to \{I^C_{nm}, P_{nm}(\Delta u', \Delta v')\}, \\ \Delta u' = N_1 \Delta u, \qquad \Delta v' = N_2 \Delta v. \end{gathered} \tag{2.15}$$

These algorithms cut down the data array and can be used, for example, in the case when the compatibility conditions (1.36) are violated. The simplest algorithm of this type is a simple screening algorithm (discarding "redundant" data)

$$I^C_{nm} = I_{nN_1,mN_2}. \tag{2.16}$$

As our second example, we consider the compression algorithm in one variable with averaging. This refers to the algorithm of the form (2.15) with $N_2 = 1$ such that

$$I^C_{nm} = \left(2[N_1/2]+1\right)^{-1} \sum_{i=N_1n-[N_1/2]}^{N_1n+[N_1/2]} I_{im}. \tag{2.17}$$

Similarly to filtration algorithms, *correction algorithms* K do not change the lattice of lines. They have the form

$$K : \{I_{nm}, P_{nm}(\Delta u, \Delta v)\} \to \{I^k_{nm}, P_{nm}(\Delta u, \Delta v)\}, \qquad K[I_{nm}] = [I^k_{nm}]. \tag{2.18}$$

The majority of correction algorithms used in practice are connected with the transfer of the operator F^{-1} in formula (1.29) to the preliminary processing stage. Following our definitions, we will not consider such algorithms, restricting ourself to *algorithms for the correction of beam hardening phenomena* (see **[9]**). A model that includes beam hardening was described in §1.5. Since formula (1.109) includes averaging over the spectrum, we cannot hope to recover even a single function $\mu_p(\vec{r})$ describing the object from the data $[I_{nm}]$. This raises the question of what we actually recover from the data $[I_{nm}]$ and what are the requirements we can impose on the tomogram $\mu^A(\vec{r})$. Let us consider an object described by functions $\mu_p(\vec{r})$, $p = 1, \dots, P$, of the form (1.45). In this case the region $\mathcal{D}_i$ is filled with the homogeneous substance i ($\mu_i(\varepsilon_p) = \mu_{ip}$). A natural requirement on the algorithm A would be that in this case the function $\mu^A(\vec{r})$ has the form (at least approximately)

$$\mu^A(\vec{r}) \simeq \sum_i \mu_i \chi_{\mathcal{D}_i}(\vec{r}), \tag{2.19}$$

where μ_i are unknown constants satisfying the conditions of the form

$$|\mu_i - \mu_j| = C \max_p \left(|\mu_{ip} - \mu_{jp}| S^0(p)\right). \tag{2.20}$$

This means that the homogeneous regions remain almost homogeneous on the tomogram $\mu^A(\vec{r})$, with contrast lines preserved. Algorithms for correcting beam hardening phenomena are introduced to satisfy these requirements. All such algorithms have a limited area of applications (beam hardening should not be too high) and require a priori information about the object. Below we present the simplest example of such an algorithm.

Consider an object $\mu(\vec{r})$ of the form

$$\mu(\vec{r}) = \sum_i \mu_i \chi_{\mathcal{D}_i}(\vec{r}). \tag{2.21}$$

In this case

$$\mathcal{R}\mu(n\Delta u, m\Delta v) = \sum_i \mu_i l^i_{nm}, \tag{2.22}$$

where l^i_{nm} is the length of the segment of the line $(n\Delta u, m\Delta v)$ inside the region $\mathscr{D}_i$. To fulfill the above requirements, the algorithm K should satisfy the conditions

$$K[I_{nm}] = [I^k_{nm}], \tag{2.23}$$

$$I^k_{nm} \simeq \sum_i \mu_i l^i_{nm}, \tag{2.24}$$

where the μ_i are unknown.

Suppose we know that the analyzed object is mainly (except for small inclusions) composed of a known substance (indexed below by the subscript 0) or of certain substances whose properties are close to those of the substance 0. We consider samples of various length x made of the substance 0 and measure the parameters $I^0(x)$ (analogs of I_{nm}) under the same conditions (with the same apparatus functions) that were used in measuring I_{nm}. Then we draw the line

$$T(x) = \mu_0 x \tag{2.25}$$

on the graph $(x, I^0(x))$ that is close to $I^0(x)$. The exact value of μ_0 is irrelevant. Let x_{nm} be the solution of the equation

$$I_{nm} = I^0(x). \tag{2.26}$$

Then, by definition, in (2.18) we take

$$I^k_{nm} = T(x_{nm}) = \mu_0 x_{nm}. \tag{2.27}$$

The main property of this algorithm is formulated as follows. Let all substances i under consideration satisfy the condition

$$(\mu/\rho)_i(\varepsilon) = f(\varepsilon), \tag{2.28}$$

where (μ/ρ) is the mass absorption coefficient (see (1.46)). If we ignore the influence of the aperture, then the parameters I^k_{nm} satisfy the condition (2.24) exactly, so in (2.24) we can take the equality sign.

This completes the description of algorithms Q in (2.10). These algorithms are superpositions of mappings C, K, Φ in an arbitrary order, i.e.,

$$Q = Q^3 \circ Q^2 \circ Q^1, \tag{2.29}$$

where Q^i is either one of the algorithms C, K, Φ or the identity transformation $\mathbf{1}$.

It remains to consider *beam straigtening algorithms* B of the form (2.9). Since I_{nm} and I_{ij} are interpreted as the values of the same function $\mathscr{R}\mu$ at points $(n\Delta u, m\Delta v)$ and (φ_k, q_j) respectively, B is a certain interpolation algorithm for a function of two variables. Therefore, any algorithm for two-dimensional interpolation defines a mapping B. In practical problems one generally uses interpolation algorithms of a special form, when one interpolates first with respect to one of the variables and then with respect to the remaining variable. We consider only such algorithms, and introduce some notation that will be used below. Let $f(s)$ be a sufficiently smooth function (defined on the whole real axis) and let its samples $f_n = f(s_n)$ at points $s_n = n\Delta s$ be given. A *local interpolation* is an operator

$$V : \{f_n\} \to \{Vf\} \tag{2.30}$$

determined by the *interpolation function* $V(s)$ according to the formula

$$(Vf)(s) = \sum_n V(s - s_n) f_n \Delta s. \tag{2.31}$$

It is assumed that $V(s)$ is a piecewise smooth function satisfying the conditions

$$V(s) = V(-s), \qquad \widehat{V}(0) = \int V(s)\, ds = 1, \qquad V(s) = 0, \qquad |s| > r\Delta s. \tag{2.32}$$

In this case we will say that $V \in \{V\}$. Let us note the similarity between the properties of $V(s)$ and of $\Pi(q)$. The last condition in (2.32) expresses the *locality requirement*. Here r is an integer. Let us immediately mention that although the mapping is called an interpolation, in general we do not require the interpolation conditions

$$(Vf)(s_n) = f_n \tag{2.33}$$

to be satisfied, and a better name for V would be approximation. The dependence of V on Δs sometimes will be indicated explicitly, and in these cases we will write $V_{\Delta s}$. Ususally, the function $V_{\Delta s}(s)$ has the form

$$V_{\Delta s}(s) = \Delta s^{-1} F(s/\Delta s). \tag{2.34}$$

Let us present some examples. The most often used interpolation is the interpolation by B-splines of order k. In this case we write

$$V = B_{\Delta s}^{(k)} \qquad (V(s) = B_{\Delta s}^{(k)}(s)). \tag{2.35}$$

By definition,

$$B_{\Delta s}^{(k)} = B_{\Delta s}^{0} \otimes \cdots \otimes B_{\Delta s}^{0}, \tag{2.36}$$

$$B_{\Delta s}^{0} = \Delta s^{-1} \begin{cases} 1, & |s| < \Delta s/2, \\ 0, & |s| > \Delta s/2. \end{cases} \tag{2.37}$$

The mappings

$$V^0 = B_{\Delta s}^{0} = B_{\Delta s}^{(1)}, \qquad V^1 = B_{\Delta s}^{2} \tag{2.38}$$

are called, respectively, the *piecewise constant* and the *linear* interpolation. Let us note that although they satisfy conditions (2.33), these conditions are violated already for $k = 4$. Formula (2.36) immediately implies that

$$\widehat{B}^{(k)}_{\Delta s}(\lambda) = \left(\frac{\sin(\lambda\Delta s/2)}{\lambda\Delta s/2}\right)^k. \tag{2.39}$$

Let us consider *superposition of interpolations*. For a function $g(s) = (Vf)(s)$ we know its samples $g'_n = g(s'_n)$ (where $s'_n = n\Delta s'$), so that for $V' \in \{V\}$ the function

$$(V'g)(s) = \sum_n g'_n V'_{\Delta s'}(s - s'_n)\Delta s \tag{2.40}$$

is defined. If

$$\Delta s = k\Delta s', \qquad k = 1, 2, 3, \dots, \tag{2.41}$$

we can write

$$(V'g)(s) = \sum_n W_{\Delta s}(s - s_n) f_n \Delta s, \tag{2.42}$$

$$W_{\Delta s}(s) = \sum_n V'(s - n\Delta s')V(n\Delta s')\Delta s', \tag{2.43}$$

and

$$\widehat{W}_{\Delta s}(\lambda) = \widehat{V}'(\lambda)\sum_p \widehat{V}\left(\lambda + \frac{2\pi pk}{\Delta s}\right). \tag{2.44}$$

The function $W_{\Delta s}$ belongs to $\{V\}$ provided that

$$\sum_{p\neq 0} \widehat{V}\left(\frac{2\pi kp}{\Delta s}\right) = 0. \tag{2.45}$$

For the B-spline interpolation this condition is clearly satisfied. In practice, the mapping B (2.9) is constructed using the operators V^0, V^1 (2.38), i.e., the two-dimensional interpolation operator B is constructed from simple one-dimensional operators with respect to each variable. Let us give explicit formulas for the operators V^0 and V^1:

$$(V^0 f)(s) = f(s_n), \qquad s_n - \Delta s/2 \le s < s_n + \Delta s/2 \tag{2.46}$$

and

$$(V^1 f)(s) = f(s_n) + \frac{f(s_{n+1}) - f(s_n)}{\Delta s}(s - s_n), \qquad s_n \le s \le s_n + \Delta s. \tag{2.47}$$

Up to now we have considered the case $s_n = n\Delta s$. It is clear that (2.46) defines a zero order interpolation operator V^0_s even without this assumption. For a general sequence s_n, the linear interpolation operator V^1_s is given by

$$\begin{gathered}(V^1_s f)(s) = f(s_n) - \frac{f(s_{n+1}) - f(s_n)}{\Delta s_n}(s - s_n),\\ s_n \le s \le s_n + \Delta s_n, \qquad \Delta s_n = s_{n+1} - s_n.\end{gathered} \tag{2.48}$$

Keeping these remarks in mind, let us give examples of beam straightening algorithms for the lattices $[P^3_{ij}]$, $[P^4_{ip}]$. We begin with the construction of an algorithm B for a third generation tomograph:

$$B : \{I_{ij}, P^3_{ij}\} \to [I_{jk}, P^1_{jk}], \tag{2.49}$$

where the lattice $[P^3_{ij}]$ is given by (1.57). In §1.3 we have already discussed how to choose $\Delta\varphi$ and Δq from the point of view of the equivalence of lattices $[P^3_{ij}]$ and $[P^1_{jk}]$. This equivalence shows the order of magnitude of $\Delta\varphi$ and Δq under the assumption that the lattice $[P^3_{ij}]$ is compatible (1.59). Below we assume that we have chosen some $\Delta\varphi$ and Δq.

We recall that

$$I_{ij} \simeq \mathscr{R}\mu(\alpha_i, \beta_j) \qquad [P^3_{ij}], \tag{2.50}$$

in the sense of (1.31). On the other hand, we can write

$$I_{ij} \simeq \mathscr{R}\mu(\alpha_i, q(\beta_j)). \tag{2.51}$$

Depending on whether we consider the I_{ij} as samples of $\mathscr{R}\mu(\alpha, \beta)$ (2.50) or as samples of $\mathscr{R}\mu(\alpha, q)$, we obtain different interpolation operators. In both cases the first step is to obtain from I_{ij} an array that can be thought of as $\mathscr{R}\mu(\alpha_i, q_j)$. Later in this section we will consider only linear interpolation. However, our notation indicates possible modifications of algorithms. If we start with (2.50), then the first step is to construct the array

$$[I^1_{ij}] = B^1_\beta[I_{ij}] \simeq \mathscr{R}\mu(\alpha_i, q_j). \tag{2.52}$$

To define B^1_β, let us consider I_{ij} for a given i as samples $f(\beta_j)$ of a function $f(\beta)$. By definition, set

$$\begin{gathered} I^1_{ij} = (V^1_{\Delta\beta} f)(\beta q_j)), \\ I^1_{ij} = I_{in} + (I_{i,n+1} - I_{in})\Delta\beta^{-1}(\beta(q_j) - \beta_n). \end{gathered} \tag{2.53}$$

In this formula $n = n(j)$ is determined from the condition

$$\beta_n \le \beta(q_j) < \beta_{n+1}, \qquad \beta(q) = \arcsin q/R_M. \tag{2.54}$$

If we start with (2.51), then, similarly,

$$\begin{gathered} I^2_{ij} = B^1_q[I_{ij}] \simeq \mathscr{R}\mu(\alpha_i, q_j), \\ I^2_{ij} = I_{ip} + \frac{I_{i,p+1} - I_{ip}}{q(\beta_{p+1}) - q(\beta_p)}(q_j - q(\beta_p)). \end{gathered} \tag{2.55}$$

Now $p = p(j)$ is determined from the condition

$$q(\beta_p) \le q_j < q(\beta_{p+1}) \qquad (q(\beta) = R_M \sin\beta). \tag{2.56}$$

Each of the arrays I^t_{ij}, $t = 1, 2$, can again be interpreted in two ways:

$$I^t_{ij} \simeq \mathscr{R}\mu(\alpha_i, q_j), \qquad I^t_{ij} \simeq \mathscr{R}\mu(\varphi(\alpha_i q_j), q_j). \tag{2.57}$$

Similarly to the above, we get

$$[I^{1,t}_{jk}] = B^1_\alpha[I^t_{ij}] \simeq [\mathscr{R}\mu(\varphi_k, q_j)], \qquad [I^{2,t}_{jk}] = B^1_\varphi[I^t_{ij}] \simeq [\mathscr{R}\mu(\varphi_k, q_j)]. \tag{2.58}$$

Here the operators B^1_α and B^1_φ of linear interpolation with respect to α and φ are given by

$$I^{1,t}_{jk} = I^t_{ij} + \frac{I^t_{i+1,j} - I^t_{ij}}{\Delta\alpha}(\alpha(\varphi_k, q_j) - \alpha_i), \tag{2.59}$$

where $i = i(k, j)$ is determined from the condition

$$\alpha_i \leq \alpha(\varphi_k, q_j) < \alpha_{i+1}, \qquad \alpha(\varphi, q) = \varphi - \beta(q), \tag{2.60}$$

and, respectively,

(2.61)
$$I^{2,t}_{ij} = I^t_{ij} + \frac{I^t_{i+1,j} - I^t_{ij}}{\varphi(\alpha_{i+1}, q_j) - \varphi(\alpha_i, q_j)}(\varphi_k - \varphi(\alpha_i q_j)), \qquad \varphi(\alpha, q) = \alpha + \beta(q),$$

where $i = i(j, k)$ is determined from the condition

$$\varphi(\alpha_i, q_j) \leq \varphi_k < \varphi(\alpha_{i+1}, q_j). \tag{2.62}$$

Formulas (2.58) and (2.60) give the required data arrays $[I_{jk}, P^1_{jk}]$. We remark that since in the case under consideration we have a linear dependence on $\varphi(\alpha)$, both operators B^1_α and B^1_φ coincide. Therefore, we have constructed two straightening operators B (2.47) for the lattice $[P^3_{ij}]$:

$$B = B^1 = B^1_\varphi \circ B^1_\beta, \qquad B = B^2 = B^1_\varphi \circ B^1_q. \tag{2.63}$$

Using other interpolation techniques, one can similarly construct other examples of the operator B for $[P^3_{ij}]$.

Let us consider now one specific example of the straightening operator B:

$$B : \{I_{ip}, P^4_{ip}\} \to \{I_{ik}, P^1_{jk}\}. \tag{2.64}$$

for a fourth generation tomograph. Earlier (in §1.3) it was shown that on applying the renumbering (1.67) to the array $[I_{ip}, P^4_{ip}]$, we obtain the array $[I_{ij}, P^4_{ij}]$ such that

$$I_{ij} \simeq \mathcal{R}\mu(\alpha_i, \gamma_{ij}). \tag{2.65}$$

The convenience of coordinates (α, γ) is related to the fact that, similarly to third generation tomographs, (1.65) shows that for these coordinates we have $\gamma = \gamma(q)$. Therefore, we have a complete similarity with the case of third generation tomographs considered above, and on replacing β by γ in (2.54) and (2.60) we obtain the operator B (2.64) of the form

$$B = B^1_\varphi \circ B^1_\gamma. \tag{2.66}$$

Here

$$B^1_\gamma[I_{ij}] = [I^1_{il}], \qquad I^1_{il} = I_{ij} + \frac{I_{i,j+1} - I_{ij}}{\Delta\gamma}(\gamma(q_j) - \gamma_{ij}), \tag{2.67}$$

where $j = j(i, l)$ is determined from

$$\gamma_{ij} \leq \gamma(q_l) < \gamma_{i,j+1}. \tag{2.68}$$

Finally,

$$I_{jk} = B[I_{ij}] = B^1_\varphi[I^1_{il}],$$

(2.69)
$$I_{jk} = I^1_{ij} + \frac{I^1_{i+1,j} - I^1_{ij}}{\varphi(\alpha_{i+1}, q_j) - \varphi(\alpha_i, q_j)}(\varphi_k - \varphi(\alpha_i, q_j)),$$

where $\varphi(\alpha, q)$ is given by (1.65) and $i = i(k, j)$ is determined from the relation

(2.70)
$$\varphi(\alpha_i, q_j) \leq \varphi_k < \varphi(\alpha_{i+1}, q_j).$$

This closes the discussion of lattice straightening algorithms B and preliminary processing algorithms $\mathscr{P}$ (2.7).

§2.2. The main algorithm

In this section we complete the description of the reconstruction algorithm A (2.1) by constructing the main algorithm A_0 (2.8). We start with an array $[I_{jk}, P^1_{jk}]$ satisfying conditions (1.19). The main algorithm A_0 will be constructed for an example of the BMM data array (0.9) for which

(2.71)
$$I_{jk} = J^\Pi(\varphi_k, q_j) \equiv J^\Pi(k\Delta\varphi, j\Delta q + \delta).$$

Here $J^\Pi(\varphi, q)$ is determined by the relation

(2.72)
$$J^\Pi(\varphi, q) = \int \Pi(q - q')R(\varphi, q')\,dq'.$$

and φ_k, q_j are determined from (0.11), (0.12). We assume that the apparatus function $\Pi(q)$ is piecewise smooth, decreases rapidly, and satisfies the normalization conditions (1.5). As we already mentioned in the Introduction, we restrict ourself to the class $\{A_0\}$ of *filtered backprojection algorithms* (FBPA). The theory of such algorithms was described in **[1, 8]**. Here we repeat the main steps of the construction of these algorithms in a somewhat more general situation, but without excessive rigor. We present several main arguments that allow us to separate a class of FBPA that are interesting for applications, namely the class of *high-resolution algorithms*. From the practical point of view, these algorithms are algorithms with the spatial resolution h satisfying $h = C\Delta q$. It might be useful to compare the arguments below with those from §1.1.

To construct the algorithms A_0 we are interested in, we introduce the class of functions $\{R\}$ called *regularizers*. We say that $R \in \{R\}$ if $R(\lambda)$ is an even bounded piecewise smooth function that satisfy the conditions

(2.73)
$$R(0) = 1, \qquad |R(\lambda)| \leq C\lambda^{-2}$$

and are continuous in some neighborhoods of the points $\lambda = 2n\Omega$. Recall that $\Omega = \pi/\Delta q$ (see 1.13)) is called the Nyquist frequency, and the spatial frequency interval $[-\Omega, \Omega]$ is called the Nyquist interval. The inversion formula (0.8) suggests that it is useful to consider the function

$$\mu_{R\Pi}(\vec{r}) = (8\pi^2)^{-1} \int_0^{2\pi} d\varphi \int |\lambda| e^{-i\lambda\langle\vec{r},\vec{\eta}\rangle} J(\lambda)\, d\lambda \int e^{i\lambda q} R^{\Pi}(\varphi, q)\, dq. \tag{2.74}$$

Then $\mu_{R\Pi}(\vec{r})$ can be expressed as a *filtered backprojection* (a superposition of the convolution and the backprojection),

$$\mu_{R\Pi}(\vec{r}) = \frac{1}{2} \int_0^{2\pi} d\varphi \int H_R(\langle\vec{r},\vec{\eta}\rangle - q) J^{\Pi}(\varphi, q)\, dq, \tag{2.75}$$

where the function $H_R(s)$, called the *kernel*, is defined by

$$H_R(s) = (4\pi^2)^{-1} \int |\lambda| e^{-i\lambda s} R(\lambda)\, d\lambda. \tag{2.76}$$

Formula (2.75) is the first step in the construction of A_0. On the other hand, we can say that (2.75) defines a *continuous BMM* corresponding to the original data array $J^{\Pi}(\varphi, q)$. First, let us consider properties of this model. This permits us to recognize interesting classes of regularizers and of apparatus functions. Furthermore, we will see later that the continuous BMM is useful in the analysis of the original BMM.

In applications one usually considers monotone regularizers. Typical examples are

$$R(\lambda) = \left(1 + (\lambda/\Lambda)^4\right)^{-1}, \qquad R(\lambda) = e^{-\lambda^2/\Lambda^2}. \tag{2.77}$$

Therefore, a regularizer depends (in addition to λ) on a parameter Λ^{-1}, called the *regularization parameter.* Below we will consider only *homogeneous regularizers* of the form

$$R(\lambda) = S_R(\lambda/\Lambda). \tag{2.78}$$

Examples show that apparatus functions are usually of the form

$$\Pi(\lambda) = S_{\Pi}(\lambda d), \tag{2.79}$$

where d is a parameter playing the role of the detector aperture. Introducing the function

$$\mu_R(\vec{r}) = \frac{1}{2} \int_0^{2\pi} d\varphi \int H_R(\langle\vec{r},\vec{\eta}\rangle - q) J(\varphi, q)\, dq, \tag{2.80}$$

one can easily see that

$$\mu_{R\Pi}(\vec{r}) = \mu_{R_{\Pi}}(\vec{r}), \tag{2.81}$$

$$R_{\Pi}(\lambda) = R(\lambda)\widehat{\Pi}(\lambda), \tag{2.82}$$

and, in the case (2.78), (2.79),

$$R_{\Pi}(\lambda) = S_R(\lambda/\Lambda)\, S_{\Pi}(\lambda d). \tag{2.83}$$

Therefore,

$$\begin{aligned} R_{\Pi}(\lambda) &\simeq S_R(\lambda/\Lambda), & \Lambda &\ll d^{-1}, \\ R_{\Pi}(\lambda) &\simeq S_{\Pi}(\lambda d), & \Lambda &\gg d^{-1}. \end{aligned} \tag{2.84}$$

Therefore for a given d it is reasonable to take

$$\Lambda = Cd^{-1}. \tag{2.85}$$

Back in §1.1 we presented arguments that suggest the compatibility condition $d = C\Delta q$ (1.9). In this case we obtain

$$R(\lambda) = S_R(\lambda/\Omega), \qquad \widehat{\Pi}(\lambda) = S_\Pi(\lambda/\Omega). \tag{2.86}$$

Conditions (2.86) are called *homogenuity conditions*; below we usually assume them to be satisfied. To complete the arguments we must show that at least in the model (2.80) with the condition (2.78) the spatial resolution (see §1.1) satisfies

$$h = C\Lambda^{-1}. \tag{2.87}$$

Recall that we still have not defined h (see §1.1). Introduce the notion of the *spatial resolution* h_R *of the regularization* R in the model (2.80). This can be done in several ways. The first is based on the relations

$$\mu_R(\vec{r}) = \mu(\vec{r}) \underset{\vec{r}}{\otimes} \delta_R(r) \qquad (r = |\vec{r}|), \tag{2.88}$$

$$\delta_R(r) = (2\pi)^{-1} \int_0^\infty \lambda r(\lambda) J_0(\lambda r)\, d\lambda. \tag{2.89}$$

Here and later, $J_\nu(z)$ is the Bessel function. The function $\delta_R(r)$ is called the *point image function*. It is the result of reconstructing the function $\mu(\vec{r}) = \delta(\vec{r})$ using formula (2.80) (so that $R(\varphi, q) = \delta(q)$). The inversion formula for the Bessel transform (for (2.89)) gives

$$R(0) = 1 = (2\pi)^{-1} \int_0^\infty r\delta_R(r)\, dr. \tag{2.90}$$

Define $h_R = h_R^\delta$ from the condition

$$(2\pi)^{-1}\delta_R(0) \int_0^{h_R^\delta} r\, dr = 1. \tag{2.91}$$

The condition (2.90) shows that h_R^δ is the essential size of the support of the function $\delta_R(r)$. Since

$$\delta_R(0) = \frac{\Lambda^2}{2\pi} \int_0^\infty \xi S_R(\xi)\, d\xi, \tag{2.92}$$

we have

$$h_R^\delta = \Lambda^{-1}\pi 8^{-1/2} \left[\int_0^\infty \xi S_R(\xi)\, d\xi\right]^{-1} = C\Lambda^{-1}. \tag{2.93}$$

Another definition of $h_R = h_R^P$ is based on the definition of h_R as the width of the image of the jump of $\mu(\vec{r})$ under the regularization. To introduce h_R^P we consider

$$\mu(\vec{r}) = \chi_b(\vec{r}) \tag{2.94}$$

(recall that $\chi_b(\vec{r})$ is the characteristic function of the disk of radius b centered at the origin). Then

$$\mu_R(\vec{r}) = \mu_R^b(r) = b \int_0^\infty R(\lambda) J_0(\lambda r) J_1(\lambda b)\, d\lambda. \tag{2.95}$$

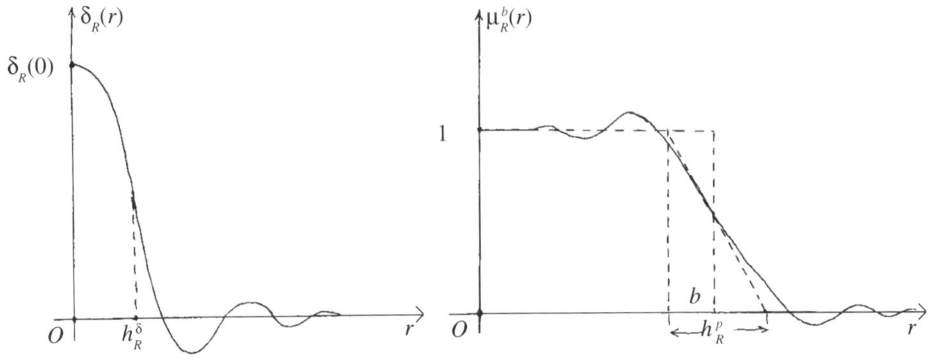

FIGURE 6

For $b\Lambda \gg 1$ formula (2.95) implies the asymptotic relation

$$\frac{d\mu_R}{dr}\Big|_{r=b} \simeq \frac{1}{\pi}\int_0^\infty R(\lambda)\,d\lambda. \tag{2.96}$$

Defining

$$h_R^P = \left|\frac{d\mu_R}{dr}\Big|_{r=b}\right|^{-1} \qquad (\Lambda b \gg 1) \tag{2.97}$$

we obtain

$$h_R^P = \pi\left[\int_0^\infty R(\Lambda)\,d\Lambda\right]^{-1} = \pi\Lambda^{-1}\left[\int_0^\infty S_R(\xi)\,d\xi\right]^{-1} = C\Lambda^{-1}. \tag{2.98}$$

The geometric meaning of h_R^δ and of h_R^P is clear from Figure 6. Therefore, both definitions of h give (2.87), and under the homogeneity condition (2.86) (with $\Lambda = \Omega$) we have

$$h_R^\delta = C\Delta q, \qquad h_R^P = C\Delta q. \tag{2.99}$$

This implies that if both homogeneity conditions in (2.86) are satisfied, then (2.99) holds in the continuous model (2.75) as well, in full conformity with (1.10). Regularizers satisfying (2.99) are called *high-resolution regularizers*; only such regularizers will be considered below. Our discussion above showed only that in the homogeneous case (2.86) are high-resolution conditions satisfied.

The general theory of regularization was mainly developed using as an example the convolution equation [**12**]. All problems in tomography related to the choice of regularizers have analogs for convolution equations. Although in constructing algorithms based on some regularization, *high-resolution* requirements are always taken into account, the explicit formulation of these requirements as one of the main conditions used in the construction algorithms was first given in [**13**]. The general theory of high-resolution algorithms for convolution equations was presented in [**14**]. Further restrictions to the class $\{R\}$, implied, in particular, by the results of this paper, will be formulated below.

Let us begin with the construction of algorithms. Below we construct two classes of algorithms, denoted as $A_0 = A_\infty(R)$ (algorithm without interpolation) and $A_0 = A_\alpha(R, V)$ (algorithm with interpolation). Note that in the construction we do not use any restrictions on the regularizer (other than the existence of the kernel $H_R(s)$; see (2.76)).

Let us recall that the BMM satisfies (2.71), and rewrite (2.75) in the form

$$\mu_{R\Pi}(\vec{r}) = \frac{1}{2}\int_0^{2\Pi} \Psi_{R\Pi}(\langle \vec{r}, \vec{\eta}\rangle, \varphi)\, d\varphi, \tag{2.100}$$

$$\Psi_{R\Pi}(a, \varphi) = \int H_R(a - q - \delta) J^{\Pi}(\varphi, q + \delta)\, dq \tag{2.101}$$

Then the simplest version of the principal algorithm $A_0 = A_\infty(R)$ is obtained by applying the trapezoid quadrature formula to the integrals (2.100) and (2.101). It is given by the formula

$$A_\infty(R)[I_{jk}] = \mu_R^T(\vec{r}), \tag{2.102}$$

where

$$\mu_R^T(\vec{r}) = \frac{1}{2}\sum_{k=0}^{2N_\varphi - 1} \Psi_R^T(\langle \vec{r}, \vec{\eta}_k\rangle, \varphi_k)\Delta\varphi \qquad (\vec{\eta}_k = (\cos\varphi_k, \sin\varphi_k)), \tag{2.103}$$

$$\Psi_R^T(a, \varphi_k) = \sum_{|j| \le N_q} H_R(a - j\Delta q - \delta) I_{jk} \Delta q. \tag{2.104}$$

We emphasize that this defines an algorithm for an arbitrary array $[I_{jk}, P_{jk}^1]$, and not only for a BMM.

In this paper, we will not consider principal algorithms based on the application of more complicated quadrature formulas to integrals of the form (2.100), (2.101). There are several reasons for this. First, as $N_\varphi \to \infty$ and $N_q \to \infty$, any quadrature formula without a weight based on a local interpolation is a superposition of quadrature type formulas (2.103), (2.104) with steps that are multiples of $\Delta\varphi$, Δq. Second, trapezoidal (and rectangular) quadrature formulas are optimal for a wide class of periodic functions, and experiments show that algorithms based on these formulas yield rather satisfactory results.

Let us discuss the *complexity* of the algorithm $A_\infty(R)$. Here by the complexity of an algorithm we mean the asymptotic number of arithmetic operations needed for its realization. One can easily see that in order to reconstruct a tomogram at N_x^2 points from an array of size $N_\varphi N_q$ using the algorithm $A_\infty(R)$ (assuming that $N_\varphi \sim N_q \sim N_x \sim N$) we need $\sim N^4$ operations. Since there exist algorithms of complexity N^3, the algorithm $A_\infty(R)$ is almost never used in practical tomography.

Let us construct an algorithm of complexity N^3, which we will call the *algorithm with interpolation* and denote by $A_\alpha(R, V)$. This algorithm is described by the following sequence of operations:

(1) Fix an integer α and compute $\psi_R^T(n\Delta a, \varphi_k)$ with step $\Delta a = \Delta q/\alpha$ using formula (2.104).

(2) Next compute the discrete backprojection, with values of $\psi_R^T(a, \varphi_k)$ replaced by values of $(V\psi_R^T)(a, \varphi_k)$. Here V is any local interpolation operator (2.30).

Hence, the algorithm $A_\alpha(R, V)$

$$A_\alpha(R,V)[I_{jk}] = \mu^T_{R,V}(\vec{r}) \tag{2.105}$$

is given by the relations

$$\mu^T_{R,V}(\vec{r}) = \frac{1}{2}\sum_{k=0}^{2N_\varphi - 1} (V\Psi^T_R)(\langle \vec{r}, \vec{\eta}_k\rangle, \varphi_k)\Delta\varphi, \tag{2.106}$$

$$(V\Psi^T_{R,V})(a,\varphi_k) = \sum_n V(a - n\Delta a)\Psi^T_R(n\Delta a, \varphi_k)\Delta a, \tag{2.107}$$

$$\Psi^T_R(n\Delta a, \varphi_k) = \sum_{|j|\le N_q} H_R(n\Delta a - j\Delta q - \delta)I_{jk}\Delta q. \tag{2.108}$$

These are precisely those reconstruction algorithms that are used in practical tomography. They depend on two functions R, V and on a positive integer α. Usually one takes

$$\alpha = 1. \tag{2.109}$$

As for the choice of the function V, as far as we know only the simplest functions $V = V^0$, $V = V^1$ (see (2.46), (2.47)) or their superposition have been used. Quite satisfactory results are obtained by using the linear interpolation algorithm

$$\alpha = 1 \qquad (\Delta a = \Delta q), \qquad V = V^1 = B^{(2)}_{\Delta q}, \tag{2.110}$$

which we denote by $A_1(R)$. To reduce the computation time the same algorithm with (see (2.43))

$$V(s) = \sum_n V^0\,(s + n\Delta a/r)\,V^1(\Delta a/r)(\Delta q/r). \tag{2.111}$$

is used to compute the backprojection. In this algorithm we compute $\psi^T_R(n\Delta q, \varphi_k)$ $(\alpha = 1)$. Then $(V\psi^T_R)(n\Delta q, \varphi_k)$, $\Delta a = \Delta q/r$, is computed using linear interpolation. Finally, to compute the backprojection, piecewise constant interpolation V^0 is used. For r between 4 and 8 this algorithm gives results that are close to those obtained by using $A_1(R)$. Let us note that for $V(s)$ given by (2.111) we have

$$\widehat{V}(\lambda) = \left(\frac{\sin(\lambda\Delta q/2r)}{\lambda\Delta q/2r}\right)\sum_p \left(\frac{\sin(\lambda\Delta q/2 + 2pr\Omega)}{\lambda\Delta q/2 + 2pr\Omega}\right)^2. \tag{2.112}$$

Let us consider the algorithm $A_\alpha(R, V)$. Formula (2.106) immediately implies that it can be rewritten in the same form as the algorithm without interpolation

$$\mu^T_{R,V}(\vec{r}) = \frac{1}{2}\sum_{k=0}^{2N_\varphi - 1} \Psi^T_{R,V}(\langle \vec{r}, \vec{\eta}_k\rangle, \varphi_k)\Delta\varphi, \tag{2.113}$$

$$\Psi^T_{R,V}(a, \varphi_k) = \sum_{|j|\le N_q} H_{R(V)}(a - j\Delta q - \delta)I_{jk}\Delta q. \tag{2.114}$$

In this formula

$$\widehat{H}_{R(V)}(s) = (VH_R)(s) = \sum_p V(s - p\Delta a)H_R(p\Delta a)\Delta a, \tag{2.115}$$

so that (see (2.44))

$$\widehat{H}_{R(V)}(\lambda) = \widehat{V}(\lambda) \sum_p \widehat{H}_R(\lambda + 2p\alpha\Omega). \tag{2.116}$$

Therefore, from the analytical point of view all filtered backprojection algorithms we have considered are of the same form as the algorithms $A_\infty(R)$, namely

$$A_0[I_{jk}] = \mu^A(\vec{r}), \tag{2.117}$$

$$\mu^A(\vec{r}) = \frac{1}{2} \sum_{k=0}^{2N_\varphi - 1} \Psi^A(\langle \vec{r}, \vec{\eta}_k \rangle, \varphi_k) \Delta\varphi, \tag{2.118}$$

$$\Psi^A(a, \varphi_k) = \sum_{|j| \le N_q} H_A(a - j\Delta q - \delta) I_{jk} \Delta q. \tag{2.119}$$

If symmetry conditions similar to (0.14) are satisfied, in (2.118) we can sum up to $N_\varphi - 1$ and omit the factor $1/2$. This is what is usually done in practice. However, one must take into account that the violation of symmetry can lead to substantial artificiality.

Formula (2.118) immediately yields several important consequences. Recall that

$$\widehat{H}_R(\lambda) = (2\pi)^{-1} |\lambda| R(\lambda). \tag{2.120}$$

First of all, it is evident that a necessary condition for the convergence of the algorithm A_0 is

$$\widehat{H}_A(\lambda) = (2\pi)^{-1} |\lambda| R_A(\lambda). \tag{2.121}$$

This statement can be proved rigorously, although we will not do it here (see **[8]**). The function $R_A(\lambda) \in \{R\}$ is called an *efficient regularizer*. For example, for $A_0 = A_\alpha(R, V)$ we have (see (2.116))

$$R_A(\lambda) = |\lambda|^{-1} \widehat{V}(\lambda) \sum_p |\lambda + 2p\alpha\Omega| R(\lambda + 2p\alpha\Omega). \tag{2.122}$$

To guarantee the condition $R_A(\lambda) \in \{R\}$ in the case $A_0 = A_\alpha(R, V)$, it is necessary that

$$\sum_{p=1}^{\infty} pR(2\alpha p\Omega) = 0. \tag{2.123}$$

This requirement immediately restricts the class of regularizers. In particular, it does not hold for positive regularizers of the form (2.77). On the other hand, (2.116) or (2.122) implies that it suffices to consider only compactly supported regularizers satisfying

$$R(\lambda) = 0, \qquad |\lambda| > \alpha\Omega, \tag{2.124}$$

for which the condition (2.123) is always satisfied.

In keeping with the above examples we will assume that $\widehat{V}(\lambda)$ satisfies the following analog of the homogeneity condition (2.86):

$$\widehat{V}(\lambda) = S_V(\lambda/\Omega). \tag{2.125}$$

Recall that we consider high-resolution algorithms. This condition automatically leads to the homogeneity condition for $R_A(\lambda)$ (an analog of the first condition in (2.86))

$$R_A(\lambda) = S_R^A(\lambda/\Omega), \tag{2.126}$$

which we will assume to be satisfied in the general case. Then

$$\widehat{H}_A(\lambda) = \Omega S_A(\xi) \qquad (\xi = \lambda/\Omega), \tag{2.127}$$

so that

$$\begin{aligned} S_A(\xi) &= (2\pi)^{-1}|\xi| S_R(\xi) \qquad (A_0 = A_\infty(R)), \\ S_A(\xi) &= (2\pi)^{-1} S_V(\xi) T(\xi) \qquad (A_0 = A_\alpha(R, v)); \end{aligned} \tag{2.128}$$

in the second formula in (2.128) we use the notation

$$T(\xi) = \sum_p |\xi + 2p\alpha| S_R(\xi + 2p\alpha). \tag{2.129}$$

Therefore, for $A_0 = A_\alpha(R, V)$ we have

$$S_R^A(\xi) = S_V(\xi) T(\xi) |\xi|^{-1}. \tag{2.130}$$

If the homogeneity conditions (2.125), (2.86) and the compatibility condition (1.3), which we write in the form

$$L\Delta\varphi = \Delta q, \tag{2.131}$$

are satisfied, then the reconstructed tomogram $\mu^A(\vec{r})$ depends on one small parameter Δq, and the *convergence conditions* for the algorithm A at a point $\vec{r} \in \mathscr{D}_b$ for $\mu \in \{\mu\}$ can be formulated as follows:

$$|\mu^A(\vec{r}) - \mu(\vec{r})| \leq C(\mu, R_b) \Delta q^{\sigma_A(\vec{r})}, \qquad \sigma_A(\vec{r}) > 0, \qquad \Omega > \Omega_0(\mu, R_b). \tag{2.132}$$

Of course, here we consider two-dimensional models without beam hardening phenomena, with the same class $\{\mu\}$ as for a BMM. The very existence of convergent high-resolution algorithms is not obvious even for smooth $\mu \in \{\mu\}$. The problem is that we essentially must construct convergent quadrature formulas for integrals of the form (2.101) in the case when the integrand (the function $H_R(s)$) has a singular dependence on the integration step.

It was shown in **[8]** that if $\mu \in \{\mu\}$ is smooth, necessary and sufficient conditions for the convergence of the algorithm $A_\infty(R)$ are of the form

$$R(2n\Omega) = 0, \qquad n = 1, 2, 3, \ldots, \tag{2.133}$$

and those for the algorithm $A_0 = A_\alpha(R, V)$ are of the form

$$\begin{aligned} &\sum_p (2p\alpha\Omega) R(2p\alpha\Omega) = 0, \\ &\widehat{V}(2n\Omega) \sum_p 2p\Omega R(2p\Omega) = 0, \qquad n = 1, 2, 3, \ldots, \\ &\widehat{V}(2n\alpha\Omega) = 0, \qquad n = 1, 2, 3, \ldots. \end{aligned} \tag{2.134}$$

These conditions are sufficient for the convergence on the entire class $\{\mu\}$ unless $\vec{r}$ belongs to the continuation of the straight part of the boundary $\partial\mathscr{D}_i$.

Let us present examples of regularizers that are most often used in practice. Let us note that quite often regularizers are called *spectral windows* (or simply windows), and that they have long been known in spectral analysis **[15, 16]**. We consider three windows $R_i(\lambda)$, $i = 1, 2, 3$, called the rectangular window (or the R-L window, for Ramachandran and Lakshminarayan), the Shepp-Logan (S-L) window, and the modified Shepp-Logan (MS-L) window respectively. These windows are given by the following formulas:

$$(2.135)\qquad R_1(\lambda) = \begin{cases} 1, & |\lambda| < \Omega, \\ 0, & |\lambda| > \Omega, \end{cases} \qquad H_j = \begin{cases} (4\Delta q^2)^{-1}, & j = 0, \\ 0, & j \text{ odd}, \\ -(\pi^2 j^2 \Delta q^2)^{-1}, & j \text{ even}; \end{cases}$$

$$(2.136)\qquad R_2(\lambda) = \begin{cases} \dfrac{\sin(\lambda\pi/2\Omega)}{\lambda\pi/2\Omega}, & \lambda < \Omega, \\ 0, & \lambda > \Omega, \end{cases} \qquad H_j = \frac{2}{\pi^2 \Delta q^2 (1 - 4j^2)};$$

$$(2.137)\qquad \begin{gathered} R_3(\lambda) = \begin{cases} \dfrac{\sin(\lambda\pi/\Omega)}{\lambda\pi/\Omega}, & \lambda < \Omega, \\ 0, & \lambda > \Omega, \end{cases} \\ H_j = \begin{cases} 0, & j \text{ odd}, \\ (\pi^2(1 - j^2)\Delta q^2)^{-1}, & j \text{ even}. \end{cases} \end{gathered}$$

Here the H_j are the corresponding samples of the kernel,

$$(2.138)\qquad H_j = H_R(j\Delta q).$$

We note that all these windows satisfy the condition

$$(2.139)\qquad \sum_j H_j = 0,$$

which is just another form of the condition (2.123) for $\alpha = 1$. It is proved using the Poisson summation formula.

In constructing the FBPA, we started with formula (2.73), which is essentially the inversion formula (0.9). As another starting formula we could take the classical Radon inversion formula **[3]**

$$(2.140)\qquad \mu(\vec{r}) = \int_0^\pi \Psi(\langle \vec{r}, \vec{\eta} \rangle, \varphi)\, d\varphi,$$

$$(2.141)\qquad \Psi(a, \varphi) = (2\pi^2)^{-1} \int_0^\infty t^{-2}[2J(a, \varphi) - J(\varphi, a - t) - J(\varphi, a + t)]\, dt,$$

although it cannot be applied to all functions from the class $\{\mu\}$. For simplicity, let

$$(2.142)\qquad \delta = 0, \qquad I_{j,k+N_\varphi} = I_{-j,k}.$$

To construct a quadrature formula for the integral (2.142) we break the integration interval into two intervals: $[0, r\Delta q]$ and $[r\Delta q, \infty]$, where r is an integer.

In the interval $[r\Delta q, \infty]$, which does not contain singularities of the integrand, one can use a quadrature formula, and in the interval $[0, r\Delta q]$ one can, for example, expand the expression in the square brackets in (2.141) in a Taylor series in t and integrate, replacing derivatives by their finite-difference analogs. This method results in a quadrature formula of the form

$$\Psi_B^T(a,\varphi_k) = \sum_j B_j I_{jk}\Delta q, \qquad |B_j| \le Cj^{-2}. \tag{2.143}$$

The discrete backprojection is computed in exactly the same way as we have just described. This algorithm $A_0 = A(B)$ fits in the framework of a general filtered backprojection algorithm with the function $H_R(s)$ replaced by

$$\begin{aligned} H_B(s) &= \sum_j B_j \frac{\sin((s-j\Delta q)\Omega)}{(s-j\Delta q)\Omega}, \\ \widehat{H}_B(\lambda) &= \sum_j B_j e^{-i\lambda j\Delta q}\chi_\Omega(\lambda), \end{aligned} \tag{2.144}$$

where $\chi_\Omega(\lambda)$ is the characteristic function of the Nyquist interval.

§2.3. Reconstruction error and analytic results

In this section we classify reconstruction errors and present results of their analytic investigation. We introduce the notion of the *basic analytic model* (BAM).

We start with the classification of reconstruction errors introducing incidentally several models that are useful in the analysis of the BMM.

Although in this section we confine ourself to the analysis of the BMM, some definitions can be easily generalized to more general models. For the BMM we assume that $A = A_0$. Then we can define the following parameters:

$$\widetilde{\Psi}_A(a,\varphi) = \int H_A(a-q)J^\Pi(\varphi,q)\,dq, \tag{2.145}$$

$$\widetilde{\mu}_A(\vec{r}) = \frac{1}{2}\int_0^{2\pi} \widetilde{\Psi}_A(\langle\vec{r},\vec{\eta}\rangle,\varphi)\,d\varphi, \tag{2.146}$$

$$\mu_\varphi^A(\vec{r}) = \frac{1}{2}\sum_{k=0}^{2N_\varphi-1} \widetilde{\Psi}_A(\langle\vec{r},\vec{\eta}_k\rangle,\varphi_k)\Delta\varphi, \tag{2.147}$$

$$\mu_q^A(\vec{r}) = \frac{1}{2}\int_0^{2\pi} \Psi_A(\langle\vec{r},\vec{\eta}\rangle,\varphi)\,d\varphi. \tag{2.148}$$

Direct computations show that

$$\widetilde{\mu}_A(\vec{r}) = \mu_{R_A(\Pi)}(\vec{r}), \tag{2.149}$$

where μ_R is defined by (2.80) and

$$R_A(\Pi) = \widehat{\Pi}(\lambda)R_A(\lambda). \tag{2.150}$$

Relations (2.146), (2.147), and (2.148) describe mathematical models. The most important for us is the model (2.146), which, by definition, describes the *basic analytic model* (BAM). This model is a convenient approximation in the analysis of the BMM. To describe it in all details we must also compute statistical errors. This will be done in Chapter 3.

The models μ_φ^A and μ_q^A can also be considered as approximations to the BMM. These models do not include, respectively, discretization errors with respect to q and with respect to φ. Now we can give a classification of reconstruction errors for the BMM. We call

$$\widetilde{\Delta\mu_A}(\vec{r}) = \widetilde{\mu}_A(\vec{r}) - \mu(\vec{r}) \tag{2.151}$$

the *regularization error* of the algorithm A, and

$$\Delta\mu_\varphi^A(\vec{r}) = \mu_\varphi^A(\vec{r}) - \widetilde{\mu_A}(\vec{r}), \tag{2.152}$$

$$\Delta\mu_q^A(\vec{r}) = \mu_q^A(\vec{r}) - \widetilde{\mu_A}(\vec{r}) \tag{2.153}$$

the *discretization errors* with respect to φ and with respect to q. The combined *reconstruction error* for the BMM, defined as

$$\Delta\mu^A(\vec{r}) = \mu^A(\vec{r}) - \mu(\vec{r}) \tag{2.154}$$

is the sum of the regularization error (2.151) and the *discretization error* $\Delta\mu_T^A$,

$$\Delta\mu_T^A(\vec{r}) = \mu^A(\vec{r}) - \widetilde{\mu_A}(\vec{r}), \tag{2.155}$$

$$\Delta\mu^A(\vec{r}) = \widetilde{\Delta\mu_A}(\vec{r}) + \Delta\mu_T^A(\vec{r}). \tag{2.156}$$

In its turn, the discretization error is the sum of the discretization error with respect to φ given by (2.152), the discretization error with respect to q given by (2.153), and the crossover term $\Delta\mu_L^A$ given by

$$\Delta\mu_T^A(\vec{r}) = \Delta\mu_\varphi^A(\vec{r}) + \Delta\mu_q^A(\vec{r}) + \Delta\mu_L^A(\vec{r}). \tag{2.157}$$

In principle, in the analytic approach each of these errors can be studied separately. This was done in **[8]**, and below we present some results from that paper. The tomogram itself allows us to evaluate the total reconstruction error (2.154). However, specific geometric behavior can sometimes tell us what kind of errors we are dealing with.

The regularization error is characterized by the property that it possesses the *translation invariance*

$$\widetilde{\mu}_A(\vec{r} \mid \vec{a}) = \widetilde{\mu}_A(\vec{r} - \vec{a}), \tag{2.158}$$

where we define

$$\mu(\vec{r} \mid \vec{a}) = \mu(\vec{r} - \vec{a}). \tag{2.159}$$

This enables us to separate the reconstruction error $\Delta\mu^A$ into the translation invariant part $\widetilde{\Delta\mu^A}$ and the translation noninvariant part $\Delta\mu_T^A$. Below the translation noninvariant part of the reconstruction error is called the *artifact*.

Reconstruction errors are clearly visible on tomograms only when we reconstruct discontinuous functions. In this case the regularization error is localized near the discontinuity and determines the spatial resolution of the tomograph (see Chapter 3). Near the discontinuity, i.e., for $\Omega d(\vec{r}, \partial\mathscr{D}) \sim 1$, where $d(\vec{r}, \partial\mathscr{D})$ is the distance from our point $\vec{r}$ to the discontinuity line $\partial\mathscr{D}$ of the function $\mu(\vec{r}) = \chi_{\mathscr{D}}(\vec{r})$, the above error $\widetilde{\Delta\mu^A}$ is of order 1 and decreases sufficiently fast as $\Omega d(\vec{r}, \partial\mathscr{D})$ increases. On the other hand, for a generic point $\vec{r}$ the discretization error is of order $\Omega^{-1/2}$ (if $\vec{r}$ does not depend on Ω) and is not localized near the discontinuity.

It is the behavior of $\mu^A(\vec{r})$ in the *close zone* ($\Omega d(\vec{r}, \partial\mathscr{D}) \sim 1$) that determines the *spatial resolution h_A of the algorithm A*. The definition of the spatial resolution of the algorithm A is absolutely similar to the definition for the regularizer. Applying this definition, we obtain h_A^δ, h_A^p that are similar to h_R^δ, h_R^p (we need only replace μ_R by μ^A in the definition of h_R). Although we gave the definition of a high-resolution algorithm, we have not yet claimed that such algorithms indeed have high resolution, i.e., that

$$h_A^\delta = C\Delta q, \qquad h_A^p = C\Delta q. \tag{2.160}$$

If the discretization error $\Delta\mu_T^A$ in the close zone is small (for example, is of order $\Omega^{-\sigma}$ with $\sigma > 0$), then the conditions (2.160) are satisfied. This can be easily deduced from the homogeneity conditions (2.125), (2.86). In the meantime the smallness of $\Delta\mu_T^A$ is proved only for algorithms without interpolation.

Now let us outline the results of the analytic investigation of reconstruction errors in the BMM. We consider the case

$$\mu = \chi_{\mathscr{D}} \tag{2.161}$$

with the smooth boundary $\partial\mathscr{D}$, and present only the simplest final expression, taken from **[8]**. In that paper it was shown in particular that in the case (2.161) the regularization error can be written in the form

$$\widetilde{\Delta\mu}_A(\vec{r}_0) = -2\pi \int_{\partial\mathscr{D}} ds \frac{[\vec{r}, \vec{l}\,]}{l^2} \int_0^\infty W_0^{(1)}(\xi) J_0(\Omega\cdot\xi\cdot l)\, d\xi. \tag{2.162}$$

Here $\vec{l} = \vec{l}(s) = \vec{r}(s) - \vec{r}_0$, $l = |\vec{l}(s)|$, and s is the natural parameter (length) on the curve $\partial\mathscr{D}$ defined by the function $\vec{r}(s)$ ($\vec{r}(s) \in \partial\mathscr{D}$). Furthermore,

$$W_0(\xi) = (4\pi^2)^{-1}(S_R^A(\xi)S_\Pi(\xi) - 1), \qquad [\vec{\tau}, \vec{l}\,] = \tau_x l_y - \tau_y l_x, \tag{2.163}$$

where $\vec{\tau}(s)$ is the tangent vector to $\partial\mathscr{D}$ (so that $\vec{\tau}(s) = d\vec{r}/ds$). The functions S_R^A and S_Π are defined in (2.126), (2.130), (2.86). Formula (2.162) immediately implies that $\widetilde{\Delta\mu}_A$ is translation invariant. Since the asymptotic behavior of $\widetilde{\Delta\mu}_A$ as $\Omega \to \infty$ is determined by the smoothness of $W_0(\xi)$, let us consider several examples of this function. In these examples we assume that

$$S_\Pi(\xi) = \frac{\sin(\pi\xi/2)}{\pi\xi/2}, \tag{2.164}$$

according to the apparatus function (1.6) at $d = \Delta q$. Furthermore, in these examples we consider algorithms of the form $A_1(R, V)$, i.e., algorithms with linear interpolation at $\alpha = 1$ (see (2.105)); for these algorithms we have

$$S_V(\xi) = \left(\frac{\sin(\pi\xi/2)}{\pi\xi/2}\right)^2. \tag{2.165}$$

As regularizers, we select the R-L window and the MS-L window. The corresponding functions are R_1 (see (2.135)) and R_3 (see (2.137)), so that

$$\begin{aligned} S_R(\xi) &= \begin{cases} 1, & |\xi| < 1, \\ 0, & |\xi| > 1 \end{cases} \qquad \text{(R-L window)}, \\ S_R(\xi) &= \begin{cases} \sin\pi\xi/\pi\xi, & |\xi| < 1, \\ 0, & |\xi| > 1 \end{cases} \qquad \text{(MS-L window)}. \end{aligned} \tag{2.166}$$

Since both regularizers are supported on the Nyquist interval, they satisfy

$$T(\xi) = (|\xi| S_R(\xi)) \pmod 2, \tag{2.167}$$

where $(f(\xi)) \pmod 2$ denotes the periodic (with period 2) continuation of a function $f(\xi)$ supported on $[-1,1]$. Therefore,

(2.168)
$$T(\xi) = (|\xi|) \pmod 2 \quad \text{(R-L window)}, \qquad T(\xi) = \frac{|\sin \pi\xi|}{\pi} \quad \text{(MS-L window)}.$$

and

(2.169)
$$S_R^A(\xi) = \left(\frac{\sin(\pi\xi/2)}{\pi\xi/2}\right) |\xi|^{-1}((|\xi|) \pmod 2) \quad \text{(R-L window)},$$
$$S_R^A(\xi) = \left(\frac{\sin(\pi\xi/2)}{\pi\xi/2}\right)^2 \frac{|\sin \pi\xi|}{|\pi\xi|}; \quad \text{(MS-L window)}.$$

In the cases we have just considered the function $W_0(\xi)$ is continuous, $W_0'(+0) = 0$, and $W_0'(\xi)$ is piecewise continuous with discontinuities of first kind at certain points ξ_p. Denote by

(2.170)
$$\Delta_p W_0^{(1)} = W_0^{(1)}(\xi_p + 0) - W_0^{(1)}(\xi_p - 0)$$

the jump of W_0' at the point ξ_p. Below the equality

(2.171)
$$f \underset{\Omega}{\simeq} f_0$$

means that f_0 is the first term in the asymptotic expansion of f as $\Omega \to \infty$.

It was shown in **[8]** that if $\vec{r}_0$ does not belong to the evolute of $\partial\mathscr{D}$, then for the class of functions $W_0(\xi)$ under consideration the following asymptotic formula holds:

(2.172)
$$\widetilde{\Delta\mu_A}(\vec{r}_0) \underset{\Omega}{\simeq} \operatorname{Im} 2^{5/2}\pi \sum_{\bar{s}} \frac{\varepsilon(\bar{s})\varepsilon'(\bar{s})e^{i\pi\varkappa(\bar{s})/4}}{(\Omega l(\bar{s}))^2|\varepsilon'(\bar{s})k(\bar{s})l(\bar{s}) + 1|^{1/2}} \times \sum_{p=1}^{\infty} \frac{\Delta_p W_0^{(1)}}{\xi_p} e^{i\Omega\cdot\xi_p\cdot l(\bar{s})}.$$

In this formula the value of $\bar{s}$ with $\varepsilon(\bar{s}) = \pm 1$, $\varepsilon'(\bar{s}) = \pm 1$, $\varkappa(\bar{s}) = \pm 1$, is defined from the relations

(2.173)
$$\vec{l}(\bar{s}) = \varepsilon'(\bar{s})l(\bar{s})\vec{\nu}(\bar{s}), \qquad \varepsilon(\bar{s}) = [\vec{\nu}(\bar{s}), \vec{\tau}(\bar{s})],$$
$$\varkappa(\bar{s}) = \operatorname{sgn}(\varepsilon'(\bar{s})k(\bar{s})l(\bar{s}) + 1),$$

where $\vec{\nu}(s)$ is the normal vector to $\partial\mathscr{D}$ and $k(s)$ is the curvature of $\partial\mathscr{D}$ at the point $\vec{r}(s)$, so that

(2.174)
$$d\vec{\tau}/ds = k(s)\vec{\nu}(s).$$

Therefore, when $\Omega d(\vec{r}_0, \partial\mathscr{D})$ increases, the regularization error $\widetilde{\Delta\mu_A}(\vec{r}_0)$ decreases as $(\Omega d(\vec{r}_0, \partial\mathscr{D}))^{-2}$. Hence, regularization errors on a tomogram (at least for standard algorithms) are usually suppressed by discretization errors (see below) everywhere except in the *close zone*, where

(2.175)
$$\Omega d(\vec{r}_0, \partial\mathscr{D}) = C.$$

To understand better the geometry of regularization errors, let us assume that $\partial\mathscr{D}$ is the circle centered at a point $\vec{a}$. Then $\widetilde{\Delta\mu_A}(\vec{r}_0)$ depends on $|\vec{r}_0 - \vec{a}|$ only, and the regularization errors (artifacts) form concentric circles centered at the point $\vec{a}$.

Now let us turn to the discussion of *discretization errors.* Again we consider the case (2.161). In this case (see **[8]**) the discretization error can be represented in the form

$$\Delta\mu_T^A(\vec{r}_0) = i\Omega \sum_{(n,m)\neq(0,0)} \int_0^{2\pi} d\varphi \int_0^{\infty} d\xi \int_{\partial\mathscr{D}} ds f_n e^{i\Omega\Phi_{nm}}. \tag{2.176}$$

In this formula,

$$\begin{gathered} f_n = f_n(\varphi,\xi,s) = \frac{S_A(\xi)S_\Pi(\xi+2n)}{2\pi(\xi+2n)}[\vec{\tau}\vec{\eta}], \\ \Phi_{nm} \equiv \Phi_{nm}(\varphi,\xi,s) = -2Lm\varphi + \langle \xi\vec{l}(s) + 2n\vec{r}(s), \vec{\eta}\rangle \end{gathered} \tag{2.177}$$

and the constant L is determined from the condition

$$L\Omega = N_\varphi. \tag{2.178}$$

Errors $\Delta\mu_\varphi^A$ (see (2.152)), $\Delta\mu_q^A$ (see (2.153)), and $\Delta\mu_L^A$ (see (2.157)) correspond to terms in the sum with $n = 0$, $m = 0$, and $n \neq 0$, $m \neq 0$ respectively. It was shown in **[8]** that $\mu_T^A(\vec{r}_0)$ attains its maximum in the region $T(\partial\mathscr{D})$ consisting of those $\vec{r}_0$ for which there exists a tangent line to $\partial\mathscr{D}$ passing through $\vec{r}_0$. For a generic point $\vec{r}_0 \in T(\partial\mathscr{D})$ (i.e., for a point not lying on a tangent line through a point $\vec{r} \in \partial\mathscr{D}$ with $k(\vec{r}) = 0$) we have the asymptotic formula

(2.179)
$$\Delta\mu_T^A(\vec{r}_0) \underset{\Omega}{\simeq} i\Omega\left(\frac{2\pi}{\Omega}\right)^{3/2} \sum_{(n,m)\neq(0,0)} \sum_{(\varepsilon_2,s_c)} \frac{f_n(z_c^{\varepsilon_2})^T \exp\left(i\Omega\Phi_{nm}(z_c^{\varepsilon_2}) + (i\pi/4)\varkappa_c^{\varepsilon_2}\right)}{l(s_c)k^{1/2}(s_c)|\xi_c^{\varepsilon_2} + 2n|^{1/2}}$$

$(z_c^{\varepsilon_2} = (\varphi_c^{\varepsilon_2}, \xi_c^{\varepsilon_2}, s_c))$. To determine s_c it suffices to draw tangent lines to $\partial\mathscr{D}$ through $\vec{r}_0$ ($r(s_c) \in \partial\mathscr{D}$ are the tangency points). Parameters $\varphi_c^{\varepsilon_2}$, $\xi_c^{\varepsilon_2}$, s_c are determined from the conditions

$$\begin{gathered} \vec{\eta}_c^{\varepsilon_2} = \varepsilon_2\vec{v}(s_c), \qquad \varepsilon_2 = \pm 1, \quad \varepsilon_c = \pm 1, \\ \vec{l}(s_c) = \varepsilon_c\vec{\tau}(s_c)l(s_c); \qquad \varepsilon = [\vec{v}\vec{\tau}](s_c); \\ \xi_c^{\varepsilon_2} = \varepsilon\varepsilon_2\varepsilon_c l^{-1}(s_c)(2Lm - 2n\varepsilon\varepsilon_2\langle\vec{r}(s_c), \vec{\tau}(s_c)\rangle). \end{gathered} \tag{2.180}$$

Here all parameters correspond to fixed values of n and m. The parameter $\varkappa_c^{\varepsilon_2}$ is the signature of the quadratic form of second derivatives $\Phi''_{nm}(z_c^{\varepsilon_2})$. We assume here that $k(s_c) \neq 0$ and the sum is taken over all s_c and $\varepsilon_2 = \pm 1$ such that

$$\xi_c^{\varepsilon_2} \geq 0. \tag{2.181}$$

Let us consider the case when *the number of samples is sufficiently large*, i.e.,

$$L > R_b. \tag{2.182}$$

In this case the function f_n is small at the point $\xi_c^{\varepsilon_2}$ with $|m| \geq 1$. This is related to the fact that the expression (2.177) for f_n contains the function $S_A(\xi)$ defined by (2.128) and the function $S_V(\xi)$ defined by (2.165), and both these functions decrease rapidly as ξ increases. Therefore, in this case the errors $\Delta\mu_\varphi^A$ and $\Delta\mu_L^A$ can be ignored in practical applications, and the main contribution to $\Delta\mu_T^A$ comes from $\Delta\mu_q^A$ (see 2.153)),

$$(2.183)\quad \Delta\mu_q^A(\vec{r}_0) \underset{\Omega}{\simeq} (i\Omega)\left(\frac{2\pi}{\Omega}\right)^{3/2} \sum_{|n|\geq 1}\sum_{(\varepsilon_2,s_c)} \frac{f_n(z_c^{\varepsilon_2})\exp\left(i\Omega\Phi_{n0}(z_c^{\varepsilon_2})+(i\pi/4)\varkappa_c^{\varepsilon_2}\right)}{l(s_c)k^{1/2}(s_c)|\xi_c^{\varepsilon_2}+2n|^{1/2}}$$

(m=0). Let us emphasize that $\Delta\mu_\varphi^A$ and $\Delta\mu_L^A$ have the same order in Ω as $\Delta\mu_q^A$, and the approximate equality

$$(2.184)\qquad \Delta\mu_T^A \simeq \Delta\mu_q^A$$

is nothing but a formula that is convenient in numerical estimates.

We remark that the analysis of the angular discretization error is rather simple and gives

$$(2.185)\quad \Delta\mu_\varphi^A(\vec{r}_0) \underset{\Omega}{\simeq} i\omega\left(\frac{2\pi}{\Omega}\right)^{3/2} \sum_{|m|\geq 1}\sum_{(\varepsilon_2,s_c)} \frac{f_0(z_c^{\varepsilon_2})\exp\left(i\Omega\Phi_{0m}(z_c^{\varepsilon_2})+(i\pi/4)\varkappa_c^{\varepsilon_2}\right)}{l(s_c)k^{1/2}(s_c)|\xi_c^{\varepsilon_2}|^{1/2}}.$$

In this case

$$(2.186)\qquad \xi_c^{\varepsilon_2} = 2Lml^{-1}(s_c).$$

Therefore, artifacts of angular discretization are translation invariant and their geometry coincides with the geometry of regularization artifacts. Comparison with the results of numerical experiments shows that under the condition (2.182) formulas (2.183) and (2.184) give a satisfactory description of discretization errors and of the geometry of artifacts. Since in the above examples the efficient regularizer (2.169) is small for $|\xi| > 2$, the artifact localization region can be determined from the condition

$$(2.187)\qquad 0 < \xi_c^{\varepsilon_2} < 2,$$

in agreement with the results of numerical experiments (see §3.4).

Chapter 3. Quality Criterion and Reconstruction Errors

The main problem discussed in this chapter is the choice of quantitative parameters describing the quality of a tomographic image. In practice, this problem is usually solved by choosing several basic quality criteria and describing the corresponding measurement methods. Theoretically, we speak about methods to describe the reconstruction error $\Delta\mu^A(\vec{r})$. Since $\Delta\mu^A(\vec{r})$ is a function with a complicated dependence on $\vec{r}$ and on the function μ, the only thing we can hope for is the possibility of choosing a small number of objects $\mu(\vec{r})$ (phantoms) and using their tomograms $\mu^A(\vec{r})$ to construct reasonable characteristics of the error $\Delta\mu^A(\vec{r})$ that allow us to obtain a sufficiently accurate description of the reconstruction quality for the entire class $\{\mu\}$.

One can raise the question about the completeness of a family of quality criteria, calling a family complete if it allows us to reconstruct $\Delta\mu^A(\vec{r})$ in principle for any $\mu \in \{\mu\}$. To achieve this in the BMM it is sufficient to "measure" the apparatus function $\Pi(q)$ and the numbers $\sigma_J^2(j,k)$ (see (0.21)). However, in formulating quality criteria we require that they be constructed using $\mu^A(\vec{r})$ only. This is related not only to the fact that in practice we never know the parameters of the measurement devices explicitly. Even the complete knowledge of the model does not free us from the necessity of formulating simple quality criteria that are directly related to the tomogram itself, do not depend on the choice of a model, and allow us to determine which algorithm is better (for example, in the BMM). In the general situation, the criteria should allow us to compare the quality of images obtained in various tomography systems using fast and clear methods.

The above remarks show that in choosing criteria there is, and always will be, some arbitrariness. We will not try to analyze the reasons behind the choice of a particular criterion. Instead, we will describe several main criteria that are used in practice. In essence, these criteria are borrowed from practical methods of quality estimation in linear optical systems.

The above-mentioned principal quality reconstruction criteria include such parameters as *noise level*, *constrast-dimension curve* (CD-*curve*), *and modulation transmission function* (MTF-*curve*). We define these criteria later. Furthermore, we introduce certain criteria that are convenient from the theoretical point of view and allow us to compute CD- and MTF-curves. It is important to emphasize that, as we will show later, all these criteria describe only the translation invariant part $\widetilde{\Delta\mu_A}$ of the reconstruction error (see (2.151)), and their theoretical analysis can be performed in the framework of the BAM, as described in the previous chapter. Moreover, these criteria make sense only if the discretization errors and the nonlinear effects are small, and this will be always assumed below.

To describe the translation noninvariant part $\Delta\mu_T^A$ of the reconstruction error, we introduce below an additional criterion called the *artifact level*. In analyzing these criteria we discuss both theoretical problems of how to compute them (in BMM or BAM) and what are the algorithms that construct them from tomograms. Essentially, we describe also methods to measure these criteria. This enables us to compare theoretical and experimental results. Let us recall that in theoretical investigation we deal, at best, with first terms of the asymptotics in BMM and BAM as the discretization step tends to zero.

§3.1. Noise level and contrast-dimension curve

To define the noise level let us consider a large homogeneous object, for example

$$\mu(\vec{r}) = \mu_0 \chi_{R_0}(\vec{r}), \qquad R_0 \lesssim R_b. \tag{3.1}$$

Inside this object and sufficiently far from its boundary let us separate a region (usually a square or a disk) that contains $N \gg 1$ points $\vec{r}_{\alpha\beta}$ in which the tomogram is reconstructed. Let $\langle \mu^A \rangle_{\mathscr{D}}$ be the "mean" value of μ^A in the region $\mathscr{D}$ on the tomogram

$$\langle \mu^A \rangle_{\mathscr{D}} = N^{-1} \sum_{\vec{r}_{\alpha\beta} \in \mathscr{D}} \mu^A_{\alpha\beta}. \tag{3.2}$$

Here and later we denote

$$\mu^A_{\alpha\beta} = \mu^A(\vec{r}_{\alpha\beta}), \tag{3.3}$$

where $\vec{r}_{\alpha\beta}$ is defined in (2.3). If $\langle (\mu^A - \langle \mu^A \rangle_{\mathscr{D}})^2 \rangle$ is the "mean square deviation"

$$\langle (\mu^A - \langle \mu^A \rangle_{\mathscr{D}})^2 \rangle_{\mathscr{D}} = N^{-1} \sum_{\vec{r}_{\alpha\beta} \in \mathscr{D}} (\mu^A_{\alpha\beta} - \langle \mu^A \rangle_{\mathscr{D}})^2, \tag{3.4}$$

then the noise level on the tomogram is defined as

$$\Sigma_{\mathscr{D}} = (\langle(\mu^A - \langle\mu^A\rangle_{\mathscr{D}})\rangle_{\mathscr{D}})^{1/2}. \tag{3.5}$$

These definitions constitute the essence of the practical method for determining the noise level. It is clear that $\Sigma_{\mathscr{D}}$ depends on the choice of the region $\mathscr{D}$, and in addition to the requirement $N \gg 1$ we need the diameter of $\mathscr{D}$ to be much larger than the noise correlation radius on the tomogram. In a real tomographic experiment there are contributions to $\Sigma_{\mathscr{D}}$ from various systematic errors (artifacts) that are difficult to separate from stochastic errors. The parameter $\Sigma_{\mathscr{D}}$ does indeed characterize the level of stochastic errors only in those cases when the level of artifacts is low. From the mathematical point of view, in the presence of stochastic errors each value $\mu^A_{\alpha\beta}$ becomes a random variable, and as the noise level at a point $\vec{r}_{\alpha\beta}$ it is natural to take its mean square deviation $\Sigma_{\alpha\beta}$. To use this approach for determining the noise level from the experiment, we need to perform a sufficiently large number of independent tomographic experiments. Therefore in practice this approach is hardly ever used. However, it is this approach that we use in the theoretical analysis. We will not discuss the relation between $\Sigma_{\mathscr{D}}$ and $\Sigma_{\alpha\beta}$, but just note that, under the natural assumptions made above, $\Sigma_{\mathscr{D}}$ and $\Sigma_{\alpha\beta}$ should be close, and the experiment supports this.

Now we discuss how to determine the noise level in a mathematical model. Contrary to the case of a real tomograph, in a mathematical model we can perform reconstruction in the absence of noise, excluding therefore the contribution from systematic errors. Let $\mu^A(\vec{r})$ be the result of reconstructing the object (3.1) in the absence of statistical errors, and $\mu^A_\Delta(\vec{r})$ the result of reconstructing in the presence of the noise ΔI_{nm} (see (1.100)). Then the parameter characterizing the noise level for the ideal tomogram is defined to be

$$\sum_{\mathscr{D}}^{A} = \left[N^{-1} \sum_{\vec{r}_{\alpha\beta}\in\mathscr{D}} ((\mu^A_\Delta)_{\alpha\beta} - \mu^A_{\alpha\beta})^2\right]^{1/2}. \tag{3.6}$$

Consider the basic mathematical model. We will assume that

$$I^\Delta_{jk} = J^\Pi(\varphi_k, q_j) + \Delta I_{jk}, \tag{3.7}$$

where the ΔI_{jk} are random variables satisfying (1.119). According to (1.121) and (1.126), we assume here that

$$\sigma^2_J(\varphi, q) = N^{-1}(\varphi, q), \qquad N(\varphi, q) = N_0 e^{-J^\Pi(\varphi, q)}. \tag{3.8}$$

Since $A = A_0$ for a BMM, we have

$$\mu^A_\Delta(\vec{r}) = A_0[I^\Delta_{jk}] = \mu^A(\vec{r}) + \delta\mu^A(\vec{r}), \tag{3.9}$$

and, by the linearity of the model,

$$\delta\mu^A(\vec{r}) = A_0[\Delta_{jk}]. \tag{3.10}$$

Using the Poisson formula and the definition of the algorithm $A = A_0$ (see (2.18)), we obtain

$$\mathbb{E}((\delta\mu^A(\vec{r}))^2) \equiv \sigma^2_\mu(\vec{r}) \underset{\Omega}{\simeq} \frac{\sigma^2_J(\vec{r})\Delta\varphi\Delta q}{4\pi^2} \int_0^\infty \lambda^2 R_A(\lambda)^2\, d\lambda, \tag{3.11}$$

where $R_A(\lambda)$ is the efficient regularizer (2.121) and

$$\sigma_J^2(\vec{r}) = \frac{1}{\pi}\int_0^{\pi} \sigma_J^2(\varphi, \langle \vec{r}, \vec{\eta}\rangle)\, d\varphi. \tag{3.12}$$

We can rewrite (3.12) in the form

$$\sigma_\mu^2(\vec{r}) \underset{\Omega}{\simeq} \frac{\sigma_J^2(\vec{r})\Delta\varphi}{\Delta q^2} C_\sigma(A). \tag{3.13}$$

The constant $C_\sigma(A)$ depends on the choice of the algorithm. In particular, for $A = A_0 = A_\alpha(R, V)$ we have

$$C_\sigma(A) = \frac{\pi}{4}\int_0^{\infty} S_V^2(\xi)\left[\sum_p |\xi + 2\alpha p| S_R(\xi + 2\alpha p)\right]^2 d\xi. \tag{3.14}$$

Therefore, for the BMM we can obtain the theoretical formula (as $\Omega \to \infty$) for the noise level. The comparison of (3.13) with the results of the model experiment used to define $\Sigma_{\mathscr{D}}^A$ by (3.6) will be considered in §3.2.

To illustrate the *constrast-dimension* curve ($\mathrm{CD}(b)$) we choose the simplest definition of this curve. Consider the homogeneous phantom with a round insertion of radius b and contrast $\Delta\mu$:

$$\mu(\vec{r}) = \mu_0(\vec{r}) + \mu_1(\vec{r}), \tag{3.15}$$

where $\mu_0(\vec{r})$ is defined by (3.7),

$$\mu_1(\vec{r}) = \Delta\mu\chi_{b,\vec{a}}(\vec{r}), \tag{3.16}$$

and $\chi_{b,\vec{a}}$ is the characteristic function of the disk of radius b centered at $\vec{a}$. We assume that $b \ll R_0$ and the point $\vec{a}$ is sufficiently far from the phantom boundary (for example, $|\vec{a}| < 0.5\, R_0$). Reconstructing $\mu(\vec{r})$, we obtain the tomogram $\mu(\vec{r})$, and in the linear approximation

$$\mu^A(\vec{r}) = \mu_0^A(\vec{r}) + \Delta\mu_{b,\vec{a}}^A(\vec{r}), \qquad \Delta\mu_{b,\vec{a}}^A(\vec{r}) = \Delta\mu\chi_{b,\vec{a}}^A(\vec{r}). \tag{3.17}$$

The functions $\chi_{b,\vec{a}}^A(\vec{r})$ are called the *disk image functions.*

Define the *constrast loss* function $C(b)$ by the formula

$$C(b) = \Delta\mu^{-1}\Delta\mu_{b,\vec{a}}^A(\vec{a}). \tag{3.18}$$

Then the contrast-dimension function $\mathrm{CD}(b)$ is defined from the relation

$$\mathrm{CD}(b) \cdot C(b) = \gamma\Sigma_{\mathscr{D}}, \tag{3.19}$$

where γ is a given number called the *detection level.* If we consider the value of $\mu_1^A(\vec{r})$ at the center of the inclusion μ_1 as the "signal" of this inclusion on the tomogram, then the $\mathrm{CD}(b)$ is the contrast value such that the corresponding signal is γ times more than the noise level. Since we consider only high-resolution algorithms, it is natural to expect that

$$C(b) \underset{\Omega}{\simeq} 1 \qquad (b\Omega \gg 1). \tag{3.20}$$

Therefore, in defining $C(b)$ it suffices to consider the case

$$b \leq C\Delta q. \tag{3.21}$$

In the case of BAM the function $C(b)$ can be easily computed, since (2.95) implies

$$C(b) = b \int_0^\infty \widehat{\Pi}(\lambda) R_A(\lambda) J_1(\lambda b)\, d\lambda. \tag{3.22}$$

Therefore, in this case the theoretical curve $\mathrm{CD}(b)$ takes the form

$$\mathrm{CD}(b) = \gamma \sqrt{\sigma_\mu^2 / C(b)}. \tag{3.23}$$

In this equality we take $\sigma_\mu^2 = \sigma_\mu^2(0)$, since the function $\sigma_{\vec{J}}^2(\vec{r})$ achieves its maximal value at $\vec{r} = 0$. One can give other, more complicated, definitions of the curve $\mathrm{CD}(b)$ that are based on a different definition of the signal or on a different choice of detection criteria. However, theoretically all these definition admit a complete description once we know $\sigma_\mu^2(\vec{r})$ and the disk image functions $\chi_{b,\vec{a}}^A(\vec{r})$. In the case (3.21) we are interested in the behavior of $\chi_{b,\vec{a}}^A(\vec{r})$ in the close zone

$$|\vec{a} - \vec{r}| \leq C\Delta q. \tag{3.24}$$

Therefore it makes sense to consider the function $T_b^0(r)$ defined as the result of reconstructing the disk with the unit contrast in the framework of the BAM. Formula (2.95) implies

$$T_b^0(r) = b \int_0^\infty \widehat{\Pi}(\lambda) R_A(\lambda) J_1(\lambda b) J_0(\lambda r)\, d\lambda. \tag{3.25}$$

If we assume that the discretization error in the near zone (i.e., near the discontinuity) is small (see §2.3), then

$$\mu_{b,\vec{a}}^A(\vec{r}) \underset{\Omega}{\simeq} \Delta\mu T_b^0(x), \qquad x = |\vec{r} - \vec{a}\,|. \tag{3.26}$$

This formula is in a good agreement (at least, for a BMM) with the results of the numerical experiment (see §3.2).

In the case when we can ignore translation-noninvariant and nonlinear phenomena, the disk image function $\chi_{b,\vec{a}}^A(\vec{r})$ takes the form

$$\chi_{b,\vec{a}}^A(\vec{r}) \underset{\Omega}{\simeq} T_b^A(x), \qquad x = |\vec{r} - \vec{a}\,|. \tag{3.27}$$

The method used to define $\chi_{b,\vec{a}}^A(\vec{r})$ is based on this assumption, and consists in the construction of the profile of the tomogram along the line that passes through the center of the disk. Below the disk image function is denoted $T_b^A(x)$.

§3.2. Spatial resolution and the MTF-curve

Problems related to the definition of spatial resolution have already been discussed; see §2.2. Arguments there show that this definition has a considerable amount of arbitrariness. Apparently, it is impossible to give a universal formal definition of a number that would characterize spatial resolution. Therefore, below we present several criteria, each characterizing these numbers at least to some extent. Let us remark, first of all, that one of the parameters characterizing spatial resolution is the contrast loss function $C(b)$ from (3.18), or more precisely, the function $\Delta\mu^A_{b,\vec{a}}(\vec{r})$ from (3.17). We will obtain various characterizations of spatial resolution considering the region (3.24) for small round inclusions (satisfying (3.21)) or the region

$$d(\vec{r}, \partial\mathscr{D}) \leq C\Delta q \tag{3.28}$$

for large inclusions ($b \gg \Delta q$); here $\partial\mathscr{D}$ is the boundary of the inclusion.

These introductory remarks being made, let us consider several examples. Following a tradition from optics, the main parameter characterizing spatial resolution used in application is the curve MTF(λ). Let us briefly describe a method used to construct this curve, keeping in mind that there are some criteria, to be described later, that are more convenient from the practical point of view.

The phantom used in the definition of MTF(λ) is given by the relation

$$\mu(\vec{r}) = \mu_0(\vec{r}) + \mu_1(\vec{r}), \tag{3.29}$$

where

$$\mu_1(\vec{r}) = \sum_{k=0}^{K} \Delta\mu\chi_{\vec{a}+2k\vec{l}} \qquad (|\vec{a} + 2k\vec{l}| < 0.5R_0). \tag{3.30}$$

In this equality, $\chi_{\vec{a}+2k\vec{l}}$ are the characteristic functions of identical disks or rectangles centered at points $\vec{a}+2k\vec{l}$. If we are using the disks, their diameters should be $l = |\vec{l}|$. In the case of rectangles the length of one of the sides (which is shorter than the other one and is directed along the vector $\vec{l}$) equals l. The length of the other side is $\gg l$. For simplicity, we consider the case $\Delta\mu = -\mu_0$. In this case it is natural to assume that $\mu_1^A(\vec{r})$ attains its maximum values at the points $\vec{r} = \vec{a} + (2k+1)\vec{l}$ and its minimum values at the points $\vec{r} = \vec{a} + 2k\vec{l}$. Denoting by $\overline{\mu^A_M}$ the average (with respect to k) value of $\mu^A(\vec{r})$ at maxima and by $\overline{\mu^A_m}$ the average at minima, we define MTF(λ) by the formula

$$\mathrm{MTF}(\lambda) = \frac{\overline{\mu^A_M} - \overline{\mu^A_m}}{\overline{\mu^A_M}}, \qquad \lambda = (2l)^{-1}. \tag{3.31}$$

If we ignore artifacts, then MTF(λ) will be a monotone decreasing function with MTF(0) = 1. If the function MTF(λ) is known, then we can define the following version of spatial resolution:

$$h = (2\lambda_{1/2})^{-1}, \tag{3.32}$$

where $\lambda_{1/2}$ is defined by the condition

$$\mathrm{MTF}(\lambda_{1/2}) = 1/2. \tag{3.33}$$

This definition is sometimes used in practical applications.

When round inclusions are used in the construction of the function $\mathrm{MTF}(\lambda)$, it can be reconstructed from $\Delta\mu^A_{\vec{a},b}$ (see (3.17)), so that this function is determined (up to translation-noninvariant discretization errors and nonlinearity effects) by the function $T^A_b(x)$ (see (3.27)). In the case when $\mathrm{MTF}(\lambda)$ is constructed using rectangular inclusions, it is more convenient from the theoretical point of view to use the *jump transfer* function, which we now define.

The jump transfer function characterizes the smoothing of a discontinuity of $\mu(\vec{r})$ on the tomogram. To construct this function we can consider a (phantom) object of the form

$$\mu(\vec{r}) = \mu_0(\vec{r}) + \mu_1(\vec{r}), \qquad \mu_1(\vec{r}) = \Delta\mu\chi_{\vec{a}}(\vec{r}), \tag{3.34}$$

where $\chi_{\vec{a}}(\vec{r})$ is the characteristic function of the disk with radius $b \gg \Delta q$ centered at the point $\vec{a}$, or of the square of size $b \gg \Delta q$ centered at the same point. The jump transfer function $P^A(x)$ is defined by the formula

$$\mu_1^A(\vec{r}) = \Delta\mu P^A(x), \tag{3.35}$$

where

$$\vec{r} = \vec{r}_0 + \vec{v}\cdot x, \tag{3.36}$$

$\vec{r}_0$ is a point on the smooth part of the inclusion boundary (square or disk), and $\vec{v}$ is the outward normal vector at $\vec{r}_0$. The function $P^A(x)$ is defined in the region

$$x \le C\Delta q. \tag{3.37}$$

In a BAM one can easily compute the asymptotic behavior of the function $P^A(x)$ in the region (3.37) using the expression (3.25) for $T^0_b(r)$. We obtain

$$P^A(x) \underset{\Omega}{\simeq} P^A_0(x), \tag{3.38}$$

$$P^A_0(x) = \frac{1}{2} - \frac{1}{\pi}\int_0^\infty \frac{\widehat{\Pi}(\lambda)R_A(\lambda)}{\lambda}\sin\lambda x\, d\lambda. \tag{3.39}$$

One can define the function $P^A_0(x)$ for $x < 0$ as well. We have

$$P^A_0(x) + P^A_0(-x) = 1. \tag{3.40}$$

If we rewrite $P^A_0(x)$ in the form

$$\begin{gathered} P^A_0(x) = (1-\theta(x)) - \frac{1}{\pi}\int_0^\infty \frac{\widehat{\Pi}(\lambda)R_A(\lambda)-1}{\lambda}\sin(\lambda x)\, d\lambda, \\ \theta(x) = \begin{cases} 1, & x > 0, \\ 0, & x < 0, \end{cases} \end{gathered} \tag{3.41}$$

then the second term in the sum describes the regularization error near the jump. We remark that even in a BMM the rigorous proof of (3.38) can be obtained only for algorithms without interpolation. Once again, the problem is to prove that the discretization error is small in the close zone (3.37).

Similarly to (2.97), one can give the following definition of spatial resolution:

$$h_A = -\left(\frac{dP^A}{dx}\bigg|_{x=0}\right)^{-1}. \tag{3.42}$$

The corresponding quantity for BAM,

$$h_A^0 = -\left(\frac{dP_0^A}{dx}\bigg|_{x=0}\right)^{-1}, \tag{3.43}$$

is given by

$$h_A^0 = \pi / \int_0^\infty R_A(\lambda)\, d\lambda, \tag{3.44}$$

in complete agreement with (2.98).

§3.3. Artifact level and discretization errors

Let us consider a (phantom) object of the form

$$\mu(\vec{r}) = \mu_0(\vec{r}) + \mu_1(\vec{r}), \qquad \mu_1(\vec{r}) = \Delta\mu\chi_{\mathscr{D}}(\vec{r}). \tag{3.45}$$

Again we assume that the inclusion $\mu_1(\vec{r})$ with contrast $\Delta\mu$ is located inside the disk $|\vec{r}| < R_0$ sufficiently far from its boundary. By *artifacts* one usually mean systematic reconstruction errors that are localized sufficiently far from the boundary of the region $\mathscr{D}$.

Unlike noise, artifacts possess a clear well-ordered geometric structure that depends on the nature of systematic errors. For example, the error in one direction in a BMM,

$$\Delta J^{\Pi}(\varphi_k, q_j) = C_J \delta_{jj_0} \cdot \delta_{kk_0}, \tag{3.46}$$

leads to artifacts $\delta\mu^A(\vec{r})$ (that do not depend on $\mu_1(\vec{r})$) of the form

$$\delta\mu^A(\vec{r}) = C_J H_A(\langle \vec{r}, \vec{\eta}_{k_0}\rangle - q_{j_0})\Delta\varphi\Delta q. \tag{3.47}$$

These artifacts are localized along the line (φ_{k_0}, q_{j_0}) and have the magnitude of order C_J.

The measurement error of the form

$$\Delta J^{\Pi}(\varphi_k, q_j) = C_J \delta_{jj_0} \tag{3.48}$$

leads to artifacts that look like concentric circles centered at the origin; such errors model the disruption of one of measurement channels in a third generation tomograph. The appearance of artifacts related to similar measurement errors indicates the wrong functioning of a tomograph, and will not be considered here.

On the other hand, there are artifacts that are inherent to all tomographic measurements, namely those related to discretization errors. The present section is devoted to these artifacts, while in the next section we will briefly discuss nonlinearity artifacts.

The criterion related to the level of artifacts is never used in practical tomography. This can be explained by several circumstances, the main being that the discretization artifacts are proportional to contrasts $\Delta\mu$ and in (medical) practice they are small and dominated by the noise or by other errors. Therefore, the analysis in this section pertains to a BMM more than to any practical tomograph. Estimates for the size of these artifacts are necessary for understanding the work of a tomograph, and also interesting from the theoretical point of view. These artifacts have a specific geometric structure, and the presence of this structure on a tomogram indicates that a tomograph is working properly. Furthermore, the analysis of the level of these artifacts allows us to evaluate the quality of the reconstruction algorithm. For example, a natural requirement for tomographs of the third and the fourth generations would be that the artifact level (in the framework of the corresponding mathematical model) would not be much larger that the artifact level for a BMM.

Discretization artifacts, their level, and their geometrical structure strongly depend on the geometry of the region $\mathscr{D}$ and its position with respect to the scanning center. The theory of these artifacts was briefly considered back in §2.3. Experiments show that to estimate the level of discretization artifacts at points $\vec{r}_0$ it suffices to take $\mathscr{D}$ in (3.45) to be the disk $\mathscr{D}(b, \vec{a})$, i.e., to take the phantom of the form (3.17) and to consider the case

$$\vec{a} = (-15\Delta q, 0) = (-A, 0), \qquad b = 5\Delta q. \tag{3.49}$$

If we are in the framework of a BMM and the condition (2.196) is satisfied, we use (2.198) to obtain theoretical estimates. The artifacts must be localized in the region $T(\partial\mathscr{D})$ where the conditions

$$0 < \xi_c^{\varepsilon_2} < 2 \quad \text{and} \quad m = 0 \tag{3.50}$$

are satisfied, and in our case (when $m = 0$) formula (2.194) implies

$$\xi_c^{\varepsilon_2} \equiv \xi_{c,n} = -\varepsilon_c l^{-1}(s_c) \cdot 2n \cdot \langle \vec{r}(s_c), \vec{\tau}(s_c) \rangle. \tag{3.51}$$

The points s_c correspond to two tangent lines from $\vec{r}_0$ to $\partial\mathscr{D}$. Since in all typical cases (see (2.178) and (2.179)) the function $f_n(\xi)$ (2.177) decreases as ξ and $\xi + 2n$ increase, the main contribution to $\Delta\mu_q^A$ (see (2.183)) comes from the term with $n = -1$ and the region of the largest artifacts can be defined from the condition

$$0 < \xi_{c,-1} < 2, \qquad m = 0. \tag{3.52}$$

Figure 7 (which has $\Delta q = 0.2$) shows the disk (3.49), and the curve Γ_- such that $r_0(s) \in \Gamma_-$ is defined from the condition

$$\xi_{c,-1} = 2. \tag{3.53}$$

This condition can be rewritten in the form

$$\langle l(s_c(\vec{r}_0)), \vec{r}_0 \rangle = 0. \tag{3.54}$$

The region of vectors $\vec{r}_0$ satisfying (3.52) (i.e., the region where the artifacts should be maximal) is shaded. To give a qualitative evaluation of these artifacts one can consider points where $\vec{r}_0 = (x_0, 0)$, $x_0 > 0$. Then (2.183) implies

$$\begin{aligned} \Delta\mu_q^A(x_0) &\simeq -8\pi \left(\frac{2\pi}{\Omega}\right)^{1/2} \frac{b^{1/2}}{l(s_c)} \sum_{n \geq 1} \frac{v(\xi_n) \sin\beta_n}{|\xi_n - 2n|^{1/2}}, \\ v(\xi) &= \frac{S_v(\xi) T(\xi) S_\Pi(\xi + 2n)}{4\pi^2(\xi - 2n)}. \end{aligned} \tag{3.55}$$

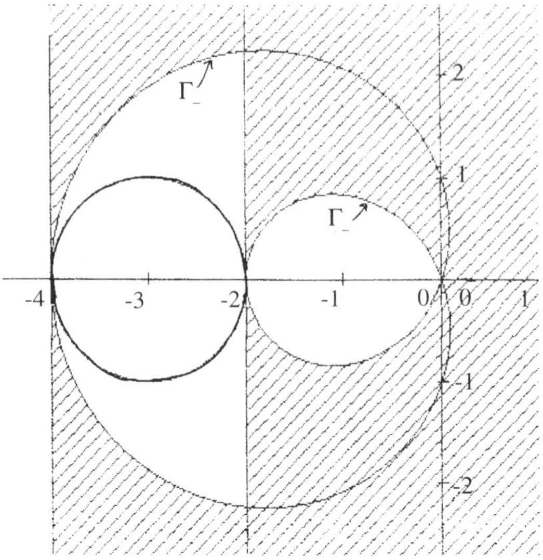

FIGURE 7

In (3.55) we denote

$$\xi_n = \frac{2nA}{x_0 + A}, \qquad \beta_n = \frac{2n\Omega x_0 b}{x_0 + A} - \frac{\pi}{4} \tag{3.56}$$

and assume that

$$x_0 + A > b. \tag{3.57}$$

Therefore we can separate the discretization artifacts by their geometry, which was described earlier (see Figure 7), and give a qualitative evaluation of these artifacts using the graph of the function $\mu_1^A(x_0)$ for the phantom described by (3.17) and (3.49). To compare the experimental results with the theory one must use the artifacts given by (3.55). This will be done in the next section.

§3.4. Results of the numerical experiment

In this section we present some results on the computation of reconstruction quality criteria. These results were obtained using a software package that provides a realization of all stages and algorithms for modeling of tomography systems given earlier in this paper. We will not describe that package here. Instead, we present several examples of computations and compare the results with the theoretical predictions, i.e., with the results that are given by BAM and artifact theory described in §3.3. We restrict ourselves to the analysis of several very simple models, more precisely, to BMM and to a third generation tomograph with the averaging described by (1.35). Therefore, we compare the results obtained by using BMM, BAM, and a third generation tomograph. The main conclusion we get from experiments is that BAM satisfactory describes all the properties of BMM, except, of course, the geometry of discretization artifacts. In its turn, BMM gives a satisfactory description (for an appropriate choice of $\Delta\varphi$ and Δq) of a third generation tomograph with the moderate opening angle (1.52). Below we mainly consider linear models. Nonlinearity effects are usually small (at realistic values of the contrast and with realistic apparatus functions); we will analyze them at the end of the section.

Everywhere below we assume that the analyzed object is the disk of radius $R_0 = 10\,\text{cm}$ with several inclusions. For BMM we take

$$\Delta q = 0.2\,\text{cm}, \qquad N_\varphi = 180, \tag{3.58}$$

and choose the apparatus function (1.6) with $d = \Delta\varphi$. This corresponds to the model (1.72) with S_Π (2.178). Therefore,

$$\Omega = 5\pi\,\text{cm}^{-1}, \qquad L = N_\varphi \Omega^{-1} \simeq 14.46 > R_0, \tag{3.59}$$

and the numerical experiment corresponds to the situation when we have a sufficiently large number of samples. Let us note here that for most of the results given below the value of Δq is not important, and all these results become universal if we measure the length in units Δq. To analyze a third generation model (1.85) we must specify Δ, R_M, R_D, $\Delta\alpha$, $\Delta\beta$ and choose the parameters $\Delta\varphi$, Δq in the beam straightening algorithm B. To be able to compare our results with BMM we will assume that for the third generation tomograph, $\Delta\varphi$ and Δq are also determined by (3.58). We choose $\Delta\alpha$ and $\Delta\beta$ from the conditions

$$\Delta\alpha = \Delta\varphi, \qquad R/\Delta q = \Delta/2\Delta\beta. \tag{3.60}$$

Let us recall that if we specify $R_H = R_0$ and Δ, we actually determine R_m also, while the value of R_D is not important (for a given $\Delta\beta$). Below we consider the cases when the opening angle Δ is small, $\Delta = \Delta_1$, and large, $\Delta = \Delta_2$. We take

$$\Delta_1 = 27.26^\circ, \qquad \Delta_2 = 72.5^\circ. \tag{3.61}$$

To pass to a parallel beam we use a version of the straightening algorithm $B = B^2$ (see (2.63)) that was described earlier. In the reconstruction we use the main algorithm $A_0 = A_1(R, V^1)$ with $\alpha = 1$ and with linear interpolation (2.110). As regularizers (windows) we use R_1 and R_3 (the R-L-window and the MS-L-window) with S_R defined by (2.166) and kernel samples H_j given by (2.135) and (2.137). The apparatus function $S_\Pi(\xi)$ is defined by (2.164).

Below we present several tomograms (Figures 12, 13, 17) that were obtained using pixel printing according to a certain visualization algorithm. In a realization of this algorithm we choose 16 numbers $B(1), \dots, B(16)$ that define the brightness window. The value $\mu^A(\alpha\Delta x, \beta\Delta y)$ is assigned to the entire rectangle (pixel) with sides Δx, Δy centered at the point $(\alpha\Delta x, \beta\Delta y)$. The brightness reconstruction is achieved by various fillings of these rectangles (pixels) by points according to a certain ordering that is apparent from the corresponding figure. If $\mu^A(\alpha\Delta x, \beta\Delta y) < B(1)$, then the corresponding pixel remains empty, and if $\mu^A(\alpha\Delta x, \beta\Delta y) > B(16)$ then the pixel is completely filled. If

$$B(j) < \mu^A(\alpha\Delta x, \beta\Delta y) < B(j+1), \tag{3.62}$$

then the pixel is filled according to the brightness scale shown in the corresponding figure. All these tomograms are reconstructed with the step

$$\Delta x = \Delta y = \Delta q. \tag{3.63}$$

After these preliminary remarks, we consider for each of our models the noise level, the jump transfer function, the disk image function, the geometry of artifacts, and the effects of nonlinearity.

1. The noise level. For algorithms we consider here the function $C_\sigma(A)$ can be computed precisely using (3.14):

$$C_\sigma(A) = \begin{cases} \frac{\pi}{6}\left(\frac{1}{3} - \frac{1}{\pi^2}\right) = 0.121481 & \text{(R-L window)}, \\ \frac{1}{12\pi} = 0.026528 & \text{(MS-L window)}. \end{cases} \tag{3.64}$$

In the numerical experiment we have considered a homogeneous phantom (the disk of radius 10 cm) with $\mu_0 = 0.2\,\text{cm}^{-2}$. The tomogram was reconstructed using a linear model. For BMM we took

$$\Delta I_{jk} = (\sigma_J^2(\varphi_k, q_j))^{-1/2}\varepsilon_{jk}, \tag{3.65}$$

where the ε_{jk} are independent Gaussian random variables with zero mean and variance 1. The random variables ε_{jk} were produced by a random number generator, and the $\sigma_J^2(\varphi_k, q_j)$ were computed by (3.8). The constant N_0 was obtained from the condition

$$N_0 e^{-0.2\cdot 20} = 10^4, \tag{3.66}$$

which corresponds to the case when the detector received 10^4 quanta during the measurement along the straight line passing through the center of the phantom. For a third generation tomograph we used similar conditions. The noise $\Sigma_{\mathscr{D}}^A$ on the tomogram was computed by formula (3.6), where $\mathscr{D}$ was taken to be the square with 5 cm side and centered at the origin. As we already noted, all tomograms were computed under the conditions (3.38). A sequence of experiments with different realizations of ε_{jk} gave, in the case of the BMM, the following average (over all realizations) value

$$\sum_{\mathscr{D}}^{A} = \begin{cases} 1.0\cdot 10^{-3}\,\text{cm}^{-1} & \text{(MS-L -window)}, \\ 2.2\cdot 10^{-3}\,\text{cm}^{-1} & \text{(R-L -window)}. \end{cases} \tag{3.67}$$

For a third generation tomograph, in the main algorithm we used the MS-L window only, and obtained the following results:

$$\sum_{\mathscr{D}}^{A} = \begin{cases} 8.7\cdot 10^{-4}\,\text{cm}^{-1}, & \Delta = \Delta_1, \\ 7.8\cdot 10^{-4}\,\text{cm}^{-1}, & \Delta = \Delta_2. \end{cases} \tag{3.68}$$

If we take a theoretical formula for $\sigma_J^2(\vec{r})$ and use a rough estimate $\sigma_J^2(\vec{r}) = 10^{-4}$ (i.e., ignore the dependence of σ_J^2 on $\vec{r}$) we obtain

$$\sqrt{\sigma_\mu^2} = \begin{cases} 1.08\cdot 10^{-3}\,\text{cm}^{-1} & \text{(MS-L -window)}, \\ 2.30\cdot 10^{-3}\,\text{cm}^{-1} & \text{(R-L -window)}, \end{cases} \tag{3.69}$$

which agrees quite well with (3.67). If we take into account the dependence of σ_J^2 on $(\vec{r})$, we can improve this agreement even further.

Comparing (3.67) with (3.68), we see that passing to a third generation tomograph decreases the noise. However, even in this case we can use the BMM estimate for $\Delta = \Delta_2$.

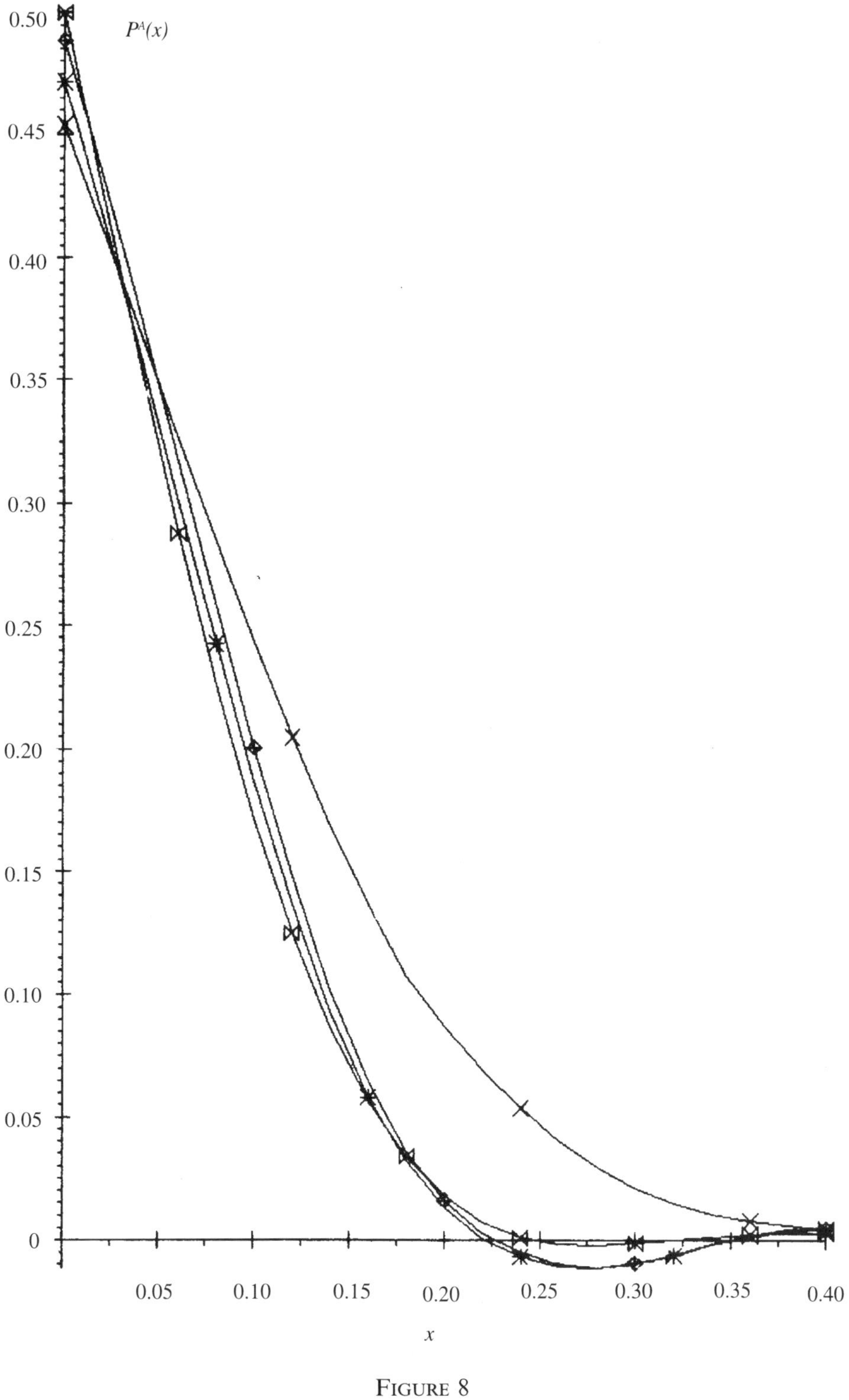
0.50
0.45
0.40
0.35
0.30
0.25
0.20
0.15
0.10
0.05
0
$P^A(x)$
0.05
0.10
0.15
0.20
0.25
0.30
0.35
0.40
x

FIGURE 8

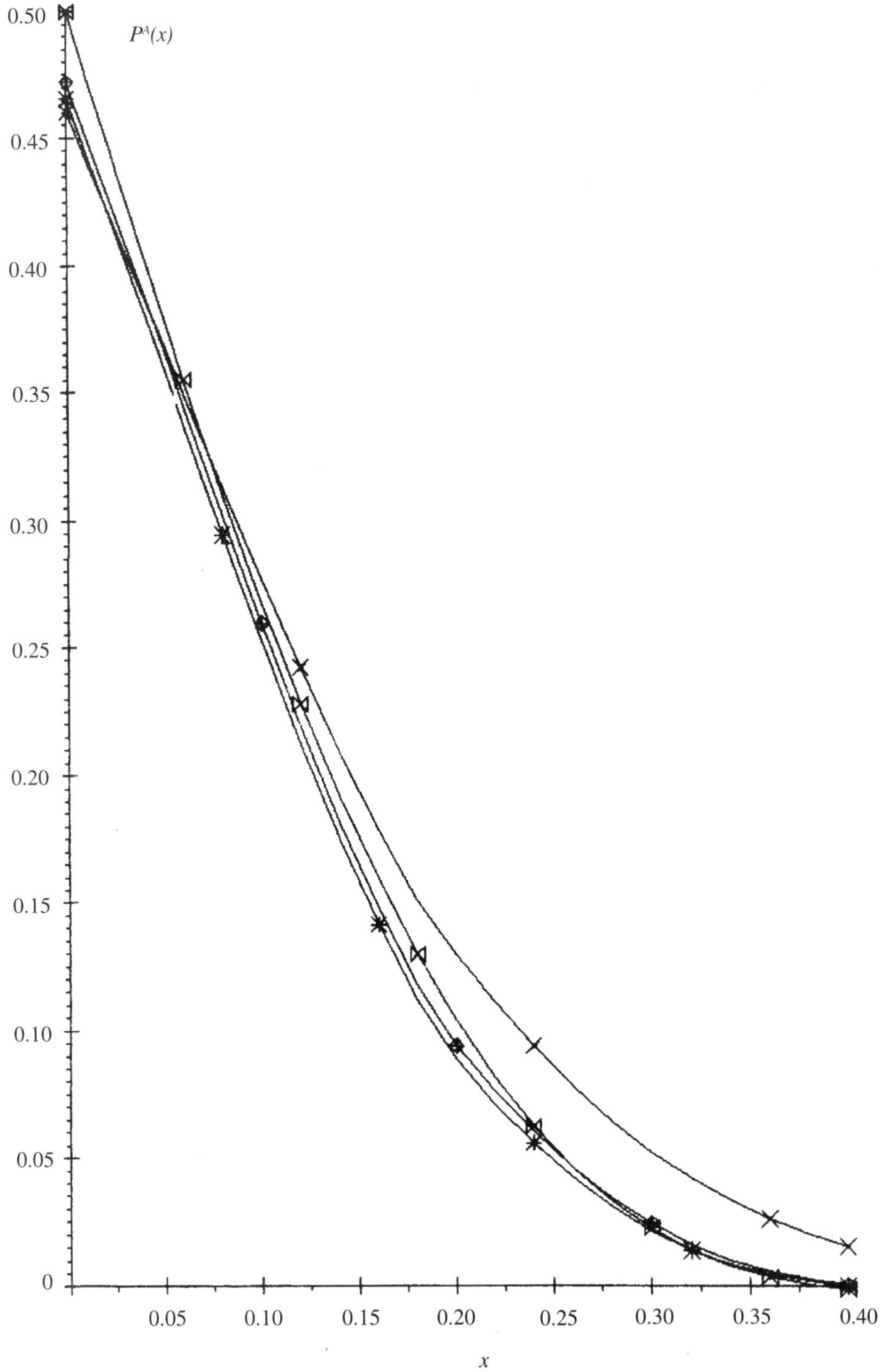
0.50
0.45
0.40
0.35
0.30
0.25
0.20
0.15
0.10
0.05
0
$P^A(x)$
0.05
0.10
0.15
0.20
0.25
0.30
0.35
0.40
x

FIGURE 9

2. Jump transfer function. Figures 8 and 9 show jump transfer functions corresponding to the R-L window (Figure 8) and to the MS-L window (Figure 9). The curves corresponding to BAM, BMM, a third generation tomograph with $\Delta = \Delta_1$, and a third generation tomograph with $\Delta = \Delta_2$ are marked by $\bowtie$, $*$, $\boxtimes$, $\times$ respectively. The x-variable is the distance from the jump (in centimeters). As we have already noted, the same curves will correspond to the general case if we recall that $\Delta q = 0.2\,\text{cm}$ and measure the distance in Δq units. The curve $\bowtie$ corresponds to $P_0^A(x)$ (see (3.39)). Three other curves corresponding to $P^A(x)$ (see (3.35)) are constructed from the tomogram of the phantom with one inclusion of contrast $\Delta\mu = 1\,\text{cm}^{-1}$ that has the form of the disk of radius $1\,\text{cm} = 5\Delta q$ centered at the point $(-3, 0)$. The reconstruction was performed with the step $\Delta x = 0.032\,\text{cm} = \Delta q/10$, so that the figures show the tomogram profiles corresponding to $y = 0$.

One can immediately see that the BAM ($P_0^A(x)$) gives a satisfactory reconstruction for moderate values of Δ. We also analyzed the dependence of the translation invariant part of the jump transfer function on the size and the form of the inclusion. The corresponding differences have about the same (or smaller) size as the differences inside the family of three curves $\bowtie$, $*$, $\boxtimes$. It is not clear whether or not we can describe the curves $\times$ corresponding to $\Delta = \Delta_2$ in the framework of the BMM. It could happen that to achieve that we must choose a different Δq with the corresponding change of the apparatus function.

3. Disk image function. Figures 10 and 11 show the disk image function. Figure 10 corresponds to the R-L window, and Figure 11 to the MS-L window. All graphs represent tomogram profiles (for $y = 0$) obtained in exactly the same way as the jump transfer functions, but with disks of different radii $b = \Delta q$, $b = \Delta q/2$, $b = \Delta q/4$ and with the x-variable representing the distance from the center of the disk (which is again the point $4(-3, 0)$. The curves $\bowtie$, $*$, $\boxtimes$ correspond to BMM, a third generation tomograph with $\Delta = \Delta_1$, and a third generation tomograph with $\Delta = \Delta_2$. Theoretical curves corresponding to BAM and constructed using (3.25) are not shown, since up to the graph precision they coincide with the curves $\bowtie$ corresponding to the BMM. As we might expect given the behavior of the jump transfer function, curves $\boxtimes$ corresponding to $\Delta = \Delta_2$ differ from the curves corresponding to BMM in a appropriate way, i.e., they have the smaller maximal value and decrease slower. Therefore, similarly to the case of the jump transfer function, BAM provides a reasonable description of the disk image function for BMM and for third generation tomographs with moderate values of Δ.

4. Discretization artifacts. As we have already pointed out, discretization artifacts are translation-noninvariant and depend strongly on the choice of a phantom. Experiments show that to analyze these artifacts it is convenient to choose a phantom in the form of the inclusion of radius $b = 5\delta q = 1\,\text{cm}$ centered at the point $(-A, 0)$, $A = 15\Delta q = 3\,\text{cm}$ (see (3.49)). It seems likely that artifacts corresponding to this phantom are close to the maximal ones (for a given inclusion radius).

Theoretical analysis of artifacts was carries out in §3.3. Here we compare results of this analysis with the numerical experiment. Figures 12 and 13 show tomograms for BMM and for a third generation tomograph with $\Delta = \Delta_2$ (in both cases we used the linear model and the R-L window). These figures immediately reveal that even for a very large opening angle ($\Delta = \Delta_2$) both the order of magnitude and the geometry of artifacts agree well with the theory. Comparing these figures with Figure 7, we see that the region where the artifacts are mainly located can be quite accurately described

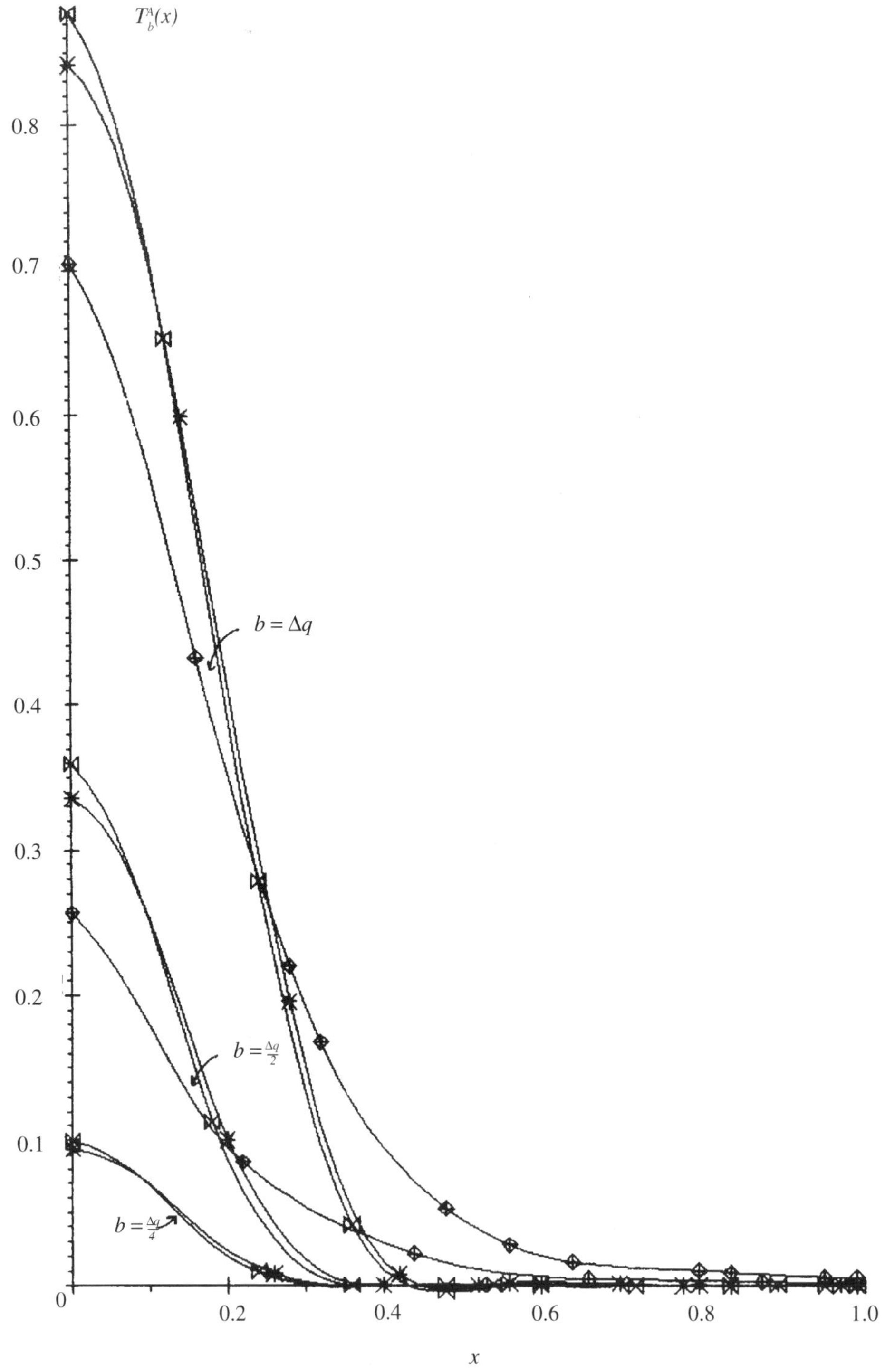
$T^{\Lambda}_{b}(x)$
0.8
0.7
0.6
0.5
0.4
0.3
0.2
0.1
0
0.2
0.4
0.6
0.8
1.0
x
$b = \Delta q$
$b = \frac{\Delta q}{2}$
$b = \frac{\Delta q}{4}$

FIGURE 10

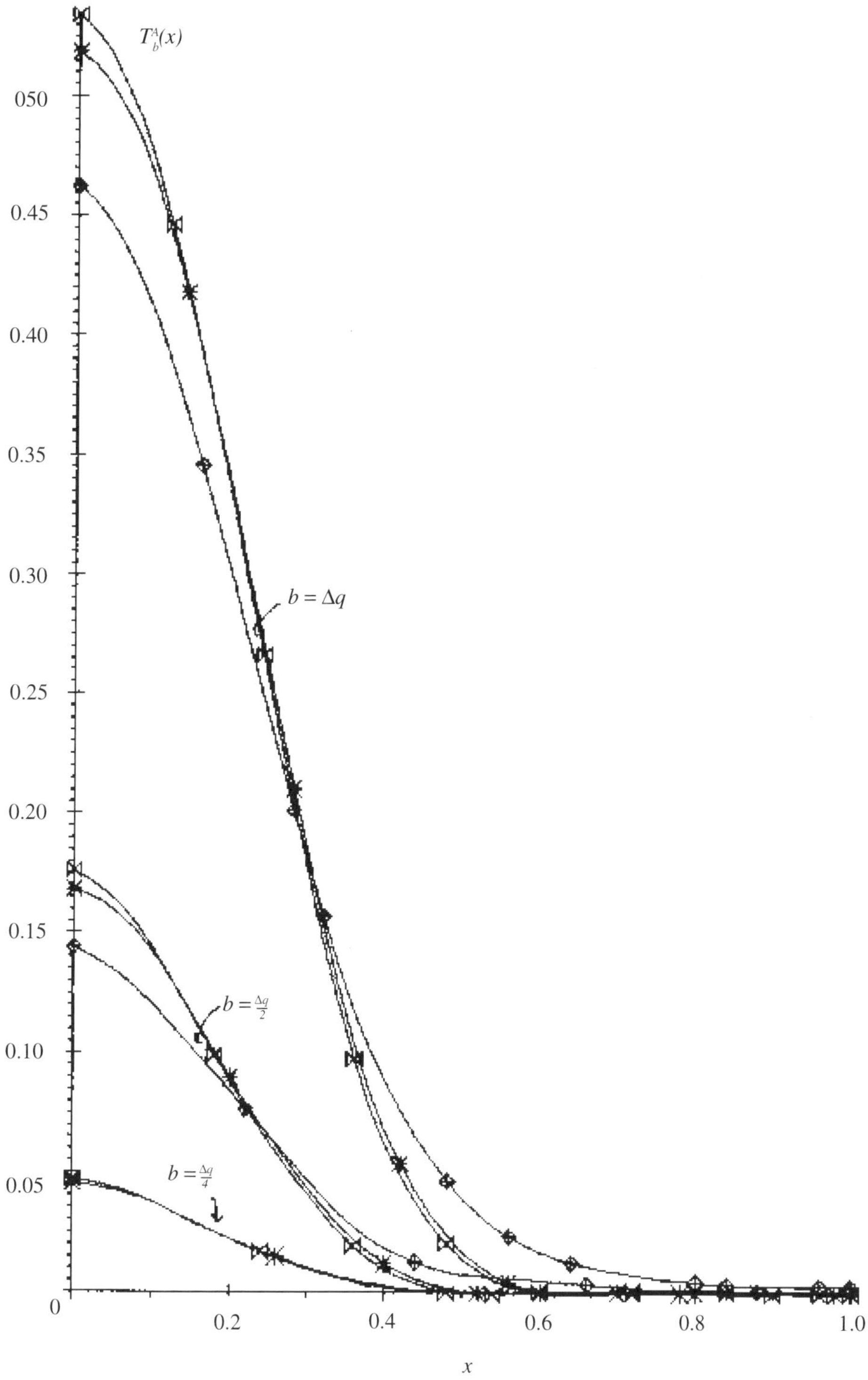
$T_b^A(x)$
050
0.45
0.40
0.35
0.30
0.25
0.20
0.15
0.10
0.05
0
0.2
0.4
0.6
0.8
1.0
$b = \Delta q$
$b = \frac{\Delta q}{2}$
$b = \frac{\Delta q}{4}$
x

FIGURE 11

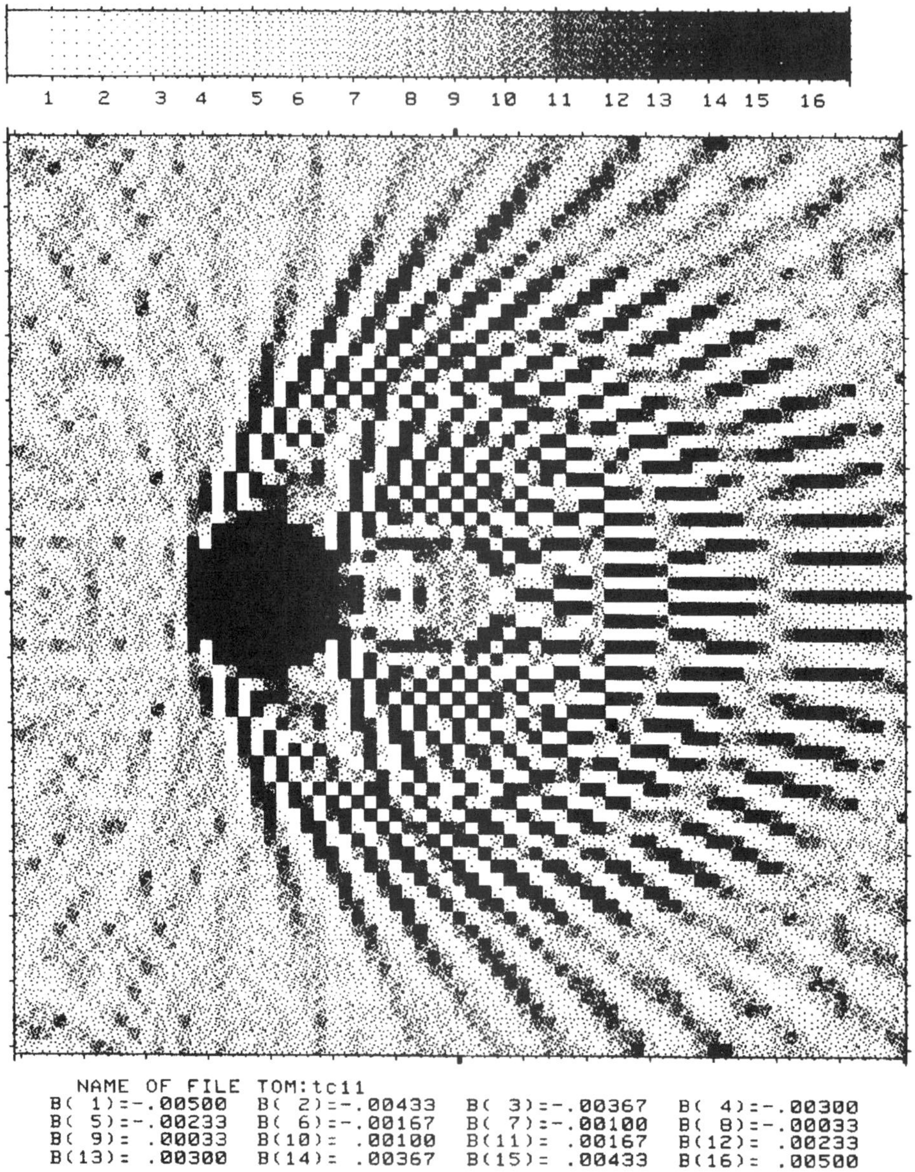
1 2 3 4 5 6 7 8 9 10 11 12 13 14 15 16
NAME OF FILE TOM:tc11
B(1)=-.00500 B(2)=-.00433 B(3)=-.00367 B(4)=-.00300
B(5)=-.00233 B(6)=-.00167 B(7)=-.00100 B(8)=-.00033
B(9)= .00033 B(10)= .00100 B(11)= .00167 B(12)= .00233
B(13)= .00300 B(14)= .00367 B(15)= .00433 B(16)= .00500

FIGURE 12

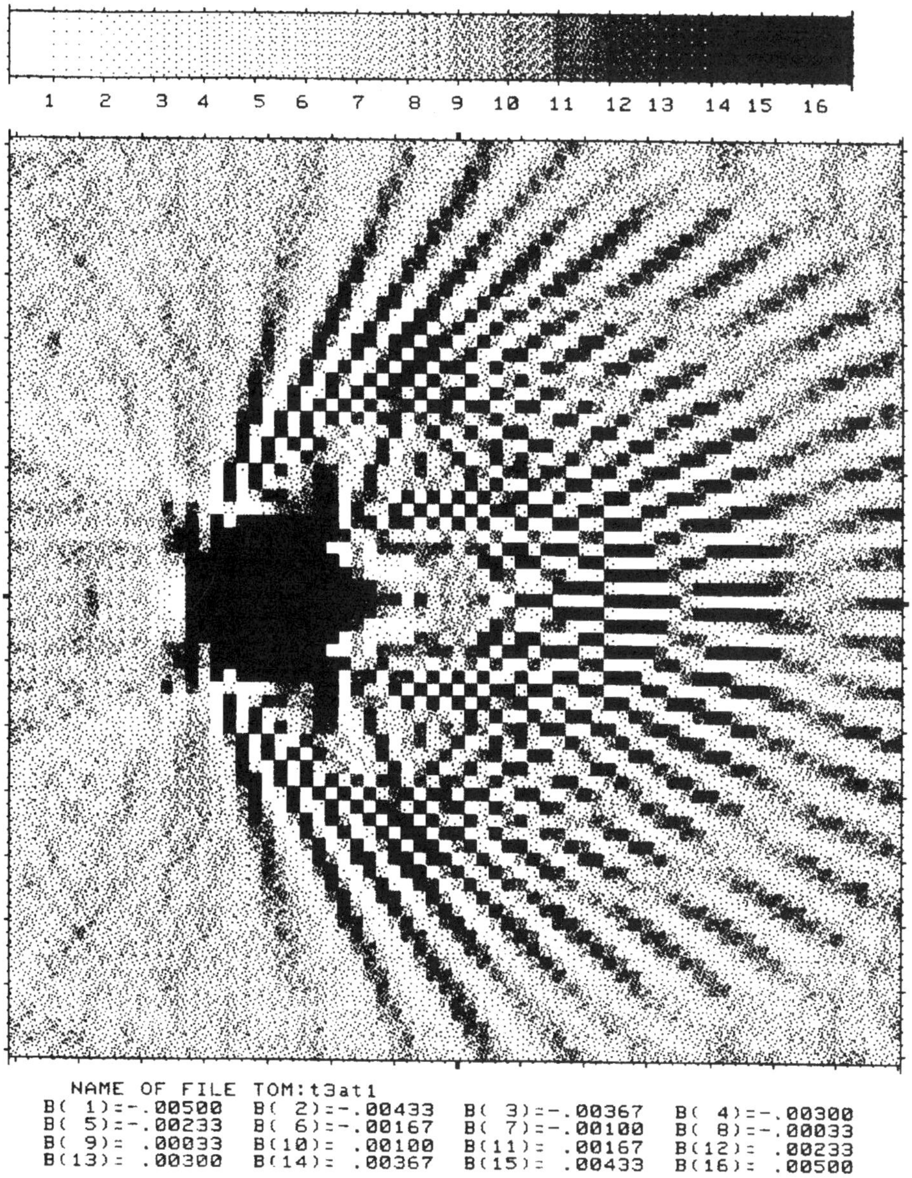
1 2 3 4 5 6 7 8 9 10 11 12 13 14 15 16
NAME OF FILE TOM:t3at1
B(1)=-.00500
B(2)=-.00433
B(3)=-.00367
B(4)=-.00300
B(5)=-.00233
B(6)=-.00167
B(7)=-.00100
B(8)=-.00033
B(9)= .00033
B(10)= .00100
B(11)= .00167
B(12)= .00233
B(13)= .00300
B(14)= .00367
B(15)= .00433
B(16)= .00500

FIGURE 13

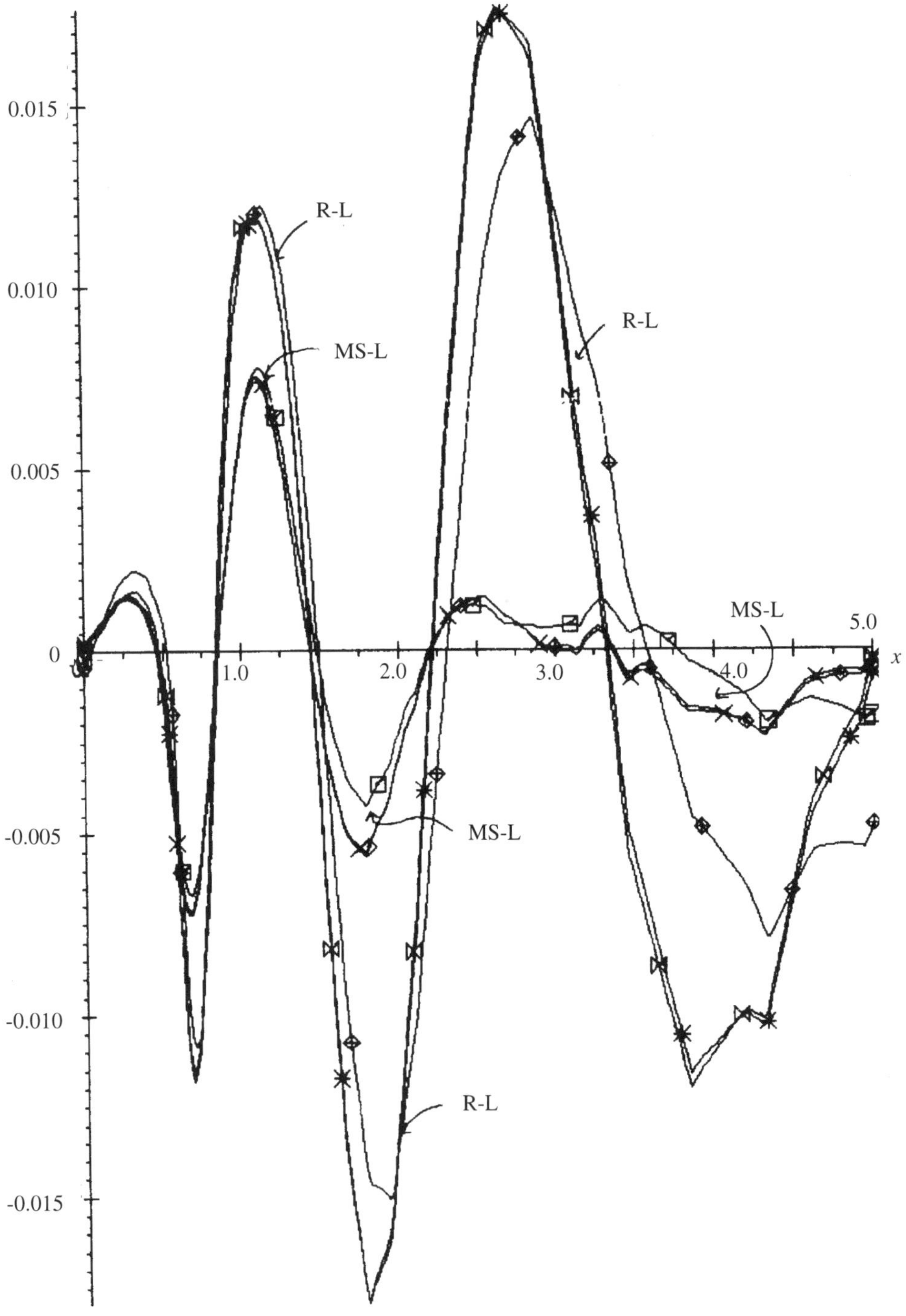
0.015
0.010
0.005
0
-0.005
-0.010
-0.015
1.0
2.0
3.0
4.0
5.0
x
R-L
R-L
R-L
MS-L
MS-L
MS-L

FIGURE 14

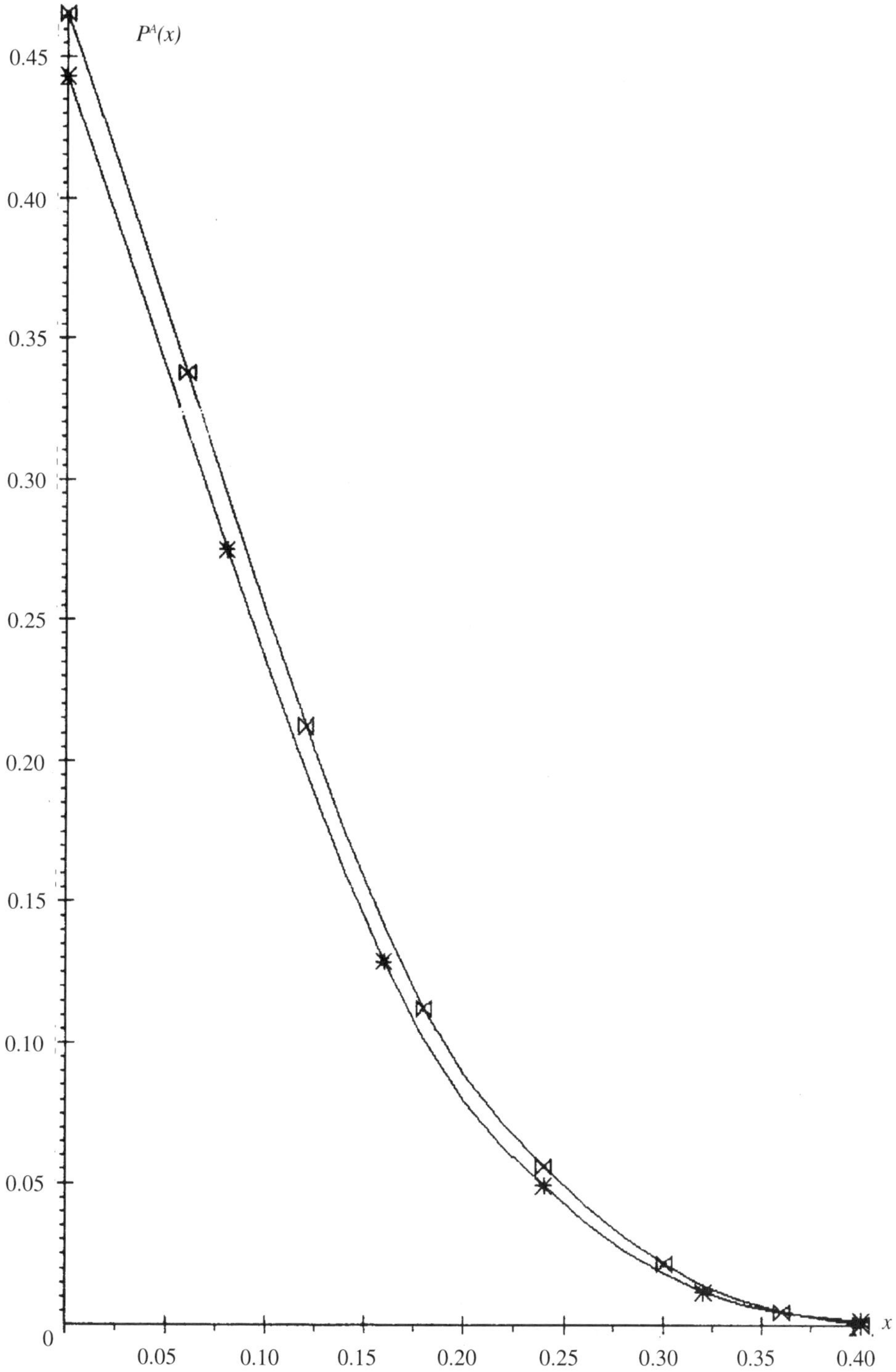
$P^A(x)$
0.45
0.40
0.35
0.30
0.25
0.20
0.15
0.10
0.05
0
0.05
0.10
0.15
0.20
0.25
0.30
0.35
0.40
x

FIGURE 15

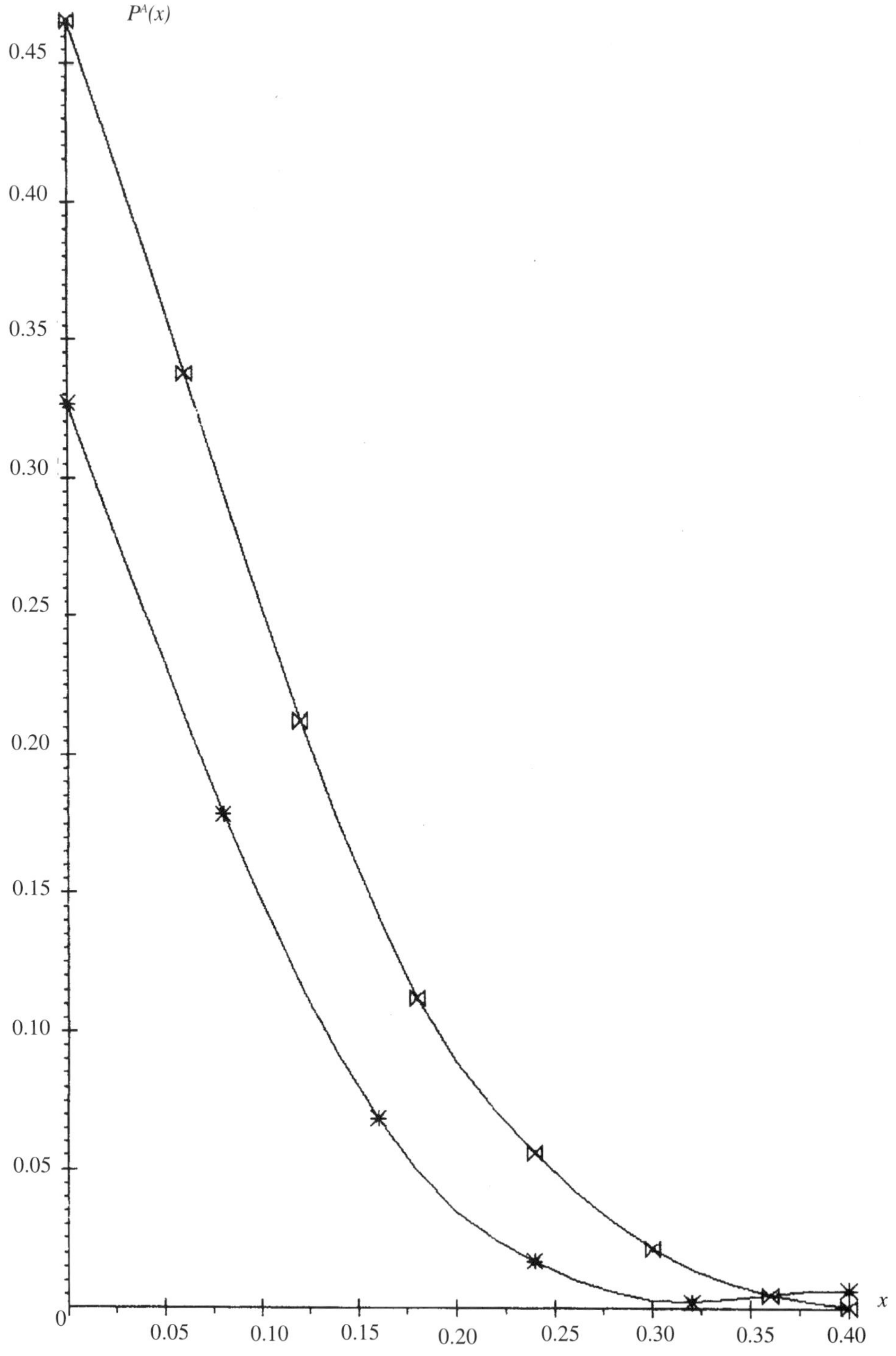
$P^A(x)$
0.45
0.40
0.35
0.30
0.25
0.20
0.15
0.10
0.05
0
0.05
0.10
0.15
0.20
0.25
0.30
0.35
0.40
x

FIGURE 16

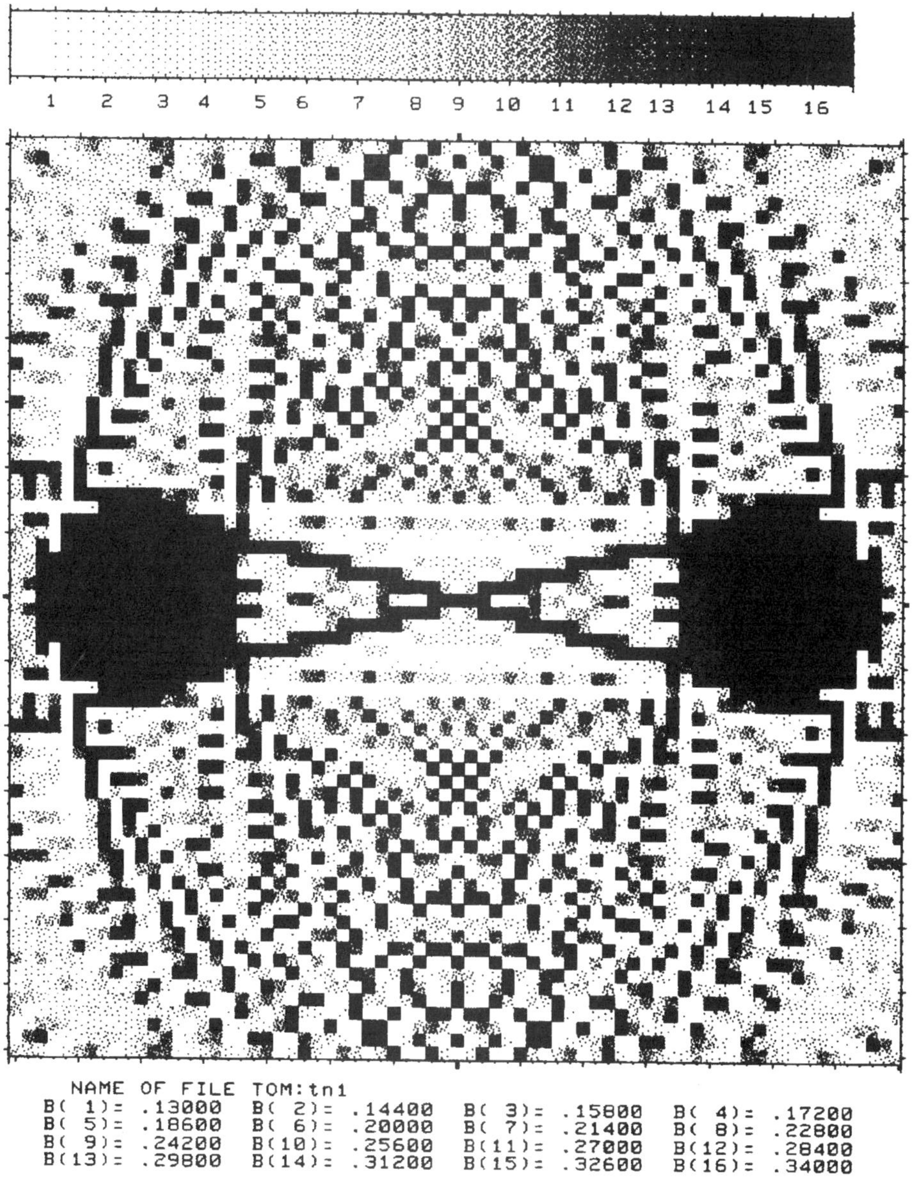
1 2 3 4 5 6 7 8 9 10 11 12 13 14 15 16
NAME OF FILE TOM:tn1
B(1)= .13000 B(2)= .14400 B(3)= .15800 B(4)= .17200
B(5)= .18600 B(6)= .20000 B(7)= .21400 B(8)= .22800
B(9)= .24200 B(10)= .25600 B(11)= .27000 B(12)= .28400
B(13)= .29800 B(14)= .31200 B(15)= .32600 B(16)= .34000

FIGURE 17

by the inequality (3.52). The detailed analysis of tomograms shows that artifacts are maximal (for the geometry we have chosen) on the axis $y = 0$. Figure 14 shows tomogram profiles along this axis for $0 \leq x \leq 4$ cm. These profiles were reconstructed with $\Delta x = \Delta q/10$ for the R-L window and for the MS-L window. The curves marked $\bowtie$, $*$, $\boxtimes$ correspond to the R-L window and to BMM, $\Delta = \Delta_1$, $\Delta = \Delta_1$ respectively, while the curves marked $\times$, $\diamondsuit$, $\boxdot$ correspond to the MS-L window and the same models.

Numerical comparison shows that for BMM and for $\Delta = \Delta_1$ experimental graphs practically coincide with those computed from (3.54). Figure 14 shows that for $\Delta = \Delta_2$ the artifact level somewhat decreases and remains close to the BMM case.

5. Nonlinearity effects. Analysis of nonlinearity effects was performed for the nonlinear version of BMM. The only difference of this version from the standard BMM is that instead of (1.72) we analyze the model (1.97) with $d = \Delta q$. In this case reasonable values of the contrast $\Delta\mu < 1$ cm lead to small nonlinearity effects, and the inclusion of nonlinearity essentially does not change the noise level or the disk image function. The change of the jump transfer function for the MS-L window is shown in Figures 15 and 16. The first figure corresponds to the contrast $\Delta\mu = 1$ cm, the second to the contrast $\Delta\mu = 10$ cm. The reconstruction was performed similarly to the linear case. The curves marked $\bowtie$ correspond to the linear BMM, and those marked $*$ to its nonlinear version. Let us note that the contrast $\Delta\mu = 1$ cm is already rather large (and almost never occurs in practice).

Figure 17 shows the appearance of nonlinear artifacts in the model we have described. The phantom consists of two round inclusions with radii 1.5 cm centered at the points $(\pm 5\,\text{cm}, 0)$. Roughly speaking, nonlinear artifacts are localized near four common tangent lines to these two disks, with greater contrast on "exterior" tangent lines and smaller constrast on the "inner" lines.

At present the authors do not have a reasonable theory of nonlinear effects (see **[17]**).

Conclusion

In conclusion let us consider some unsolved problems of two-dimensional Radon tomography. First of all, note that the results of this paper, together with the results of **[8]**, allow us to describe all principal properties of the linear BMM. Some unsolved problems remain here, but they are, presumably, of purely theoretical significance. These problems include the justification of the use of BAM in the computation of the jump transfer function for algorithms with interpolation, and possible generalizations of the results of **[8]** to the case of slowly decreasing functions $S_A(\xi)$. Let us recall that some algorithms used in practice belong to this class, and for these algorithms formulas (2.179) for the level of artifacts, which were obtained based on the results of **[8]**, lack a rigorous proof. The solution of these problems in the framework of **[8]** requires further analysis of the remainder in the stationary phase method. The complexity of this approach justifies attempts to find a different approach to the analysis of the convergence in BMM. In this connection we call the attention to certain results published in **[18]**. They were obtained without passing to the frequency domain. It is not clear whether the methods used in **[18]** yield sharper bounds.

On the other hand, there are no rigorous results about convergence even for the simplest models of third and fourth generation tomographs. Numerical experiments show that these models can be rather well described (at least in the case when the opening angle Δ is not too large) by BMM with the appropriately chosen apparatus function and parameters $\Delta\varphi$, Δq. These problems require further analysis. Let us recall that in the description of third and fourth generation tomographs we consider algorithms with beam straightening. Therefore, from a practical point of view the problems here consist in the optimal choice of the parameters $\Delta\varphi$ and Δq and in the choice of the apparatus function that allows us to describe the results in the framework of the BMM.

All these results were true for linear models. On the other hand, for the case when even a simplest nonlinearity of the type (1.97) is introduced into BMM, the authors do not know any rigorous convergence results. Numerical experiments show that the main characteristics of the linear and nonlinear BMM's practically coincide. Features that are special for nonlinear models are nonlinearity artifacts (see Figure 17). We do not have a qualitative description of these artifacts, and as far as geometry is concerned, let us mention the paper **[17]**. A majority of the problems that occur here can be reduced to the analysis of the stability of main parameters of the reconstruction quality with respect to variations of the initial data array. Earlier we have considered the example (3.46) of the variation of one of the parameters in the BMM. If we take $C_J \sim 1$ in (3.46), the reconstruction error will be of order 1 along some line. On the other hand, let us consider two apparatus functions Π_1 and Π_2, and let μ_1^A and μ_2^A be the corresponding reconstructions of the function $\mu = \chi_{\mathscr{D}}$ in the framework of BMM. Then $\Delta J^{\Pi}(\varphi_k, q_j) = J^{\Pi_2}(\varphi_k, q_j) - J^{\Pi_1}(\varphi_k, q_j)$ can be considered as the initial data error for $\Pi = \Pi_1$. Here we assume that $|\widehat{\Pi}_1 - \widehat{\Pi}_2| \sim 1$. Then $\Delta J^{\Pi}(\varphi_k, q_j) \sim 1$ if the line (φ_k, q_j) is tangential or almost tangential to the contour $\partial\mathscr{D}$. Results of **[8]** show that the "reconstruction error" $\mu_1^A - \mu_2^A$ is localized near $\partial\mathscr{D}$ (where it is of order 1) and is small far from $\partial\mathscr{D}$. This example shows that the stability properties of an algorithm depend strongly on how we vary the initial data array. It also leads to a conjecture about the stability of the algorithm with respect to a variation of initial data that is localized on a tangent line to $\partial\mathscr{D}$. We remark that passage from a linear model to a nonlinear one can be described by variations of exactly similar form. The following nonrigorous arguments support this conjecture. Let the lines $(\varphi, q^\alpha(\varphi))$ be tangent to $\partial\mathscr{D}$. Let us consider

$$\Delta J(\varphi_k, q_j) = \begin{cases} 1, & |q_j - q^\alpha(\varphi_k)| < C\Delta q, \\ 0, & |q_j - q^\alpha(\varphi_k)| > C\Delta q \end{cases} \tag{4.1}$$

(here $C \lesssim 1$), and try to estimate $\delta\mu^A = A_0(\Delta J^{\Pi}(\varphi_k, q_j))$ for $\mu = \chi_{\mathscr{D}}$. We have

$$\delta\mu^A(\vec{r}) \simeq \frac{1}{2}\sum_{k=0}^{2N_\varphi - 1}\sum_{\alpha}(\langle\vec{r}, \eta_k\rangle - q_{j(\alpha,k)})\Delta\varphi\Delta k, \tag{4.2}$$

where the $j(\alpha, k)$ are determined from the condition

$$|q_j - q^\alpha(\varphi_k)| < C\Delta q. \tag{4.3}$$

Replacing the sum by the integral, we obtain, instead of $\delta\mu^A$,

$$\widetilde{\delta\mu}^A(\vec{r}) = \frac{\Delta q}{2}\sum_{\alpha}\int_0^{2\pi} H_A(\langle\vec{r}, \eta\rangle - q^\alpha(\varphi))\, d\varphi. \tag{4.4}$$

In the case when $\mathscr{D}$ is the disk of radius b centered at the point $\vec{a}$, the last equality can be rewritten in the form

$$\widetilde{\delta\mu}^A(\vec{r}) = \Omega \int_0^\infty \xi S_R^A(\xi) J_0(\xi \cdot \Omega \cdot |\vec{r} - \vec{a}|) \cos(\xi \cdot b \cdot \Omega)\, d\xi. \tag{4.5}$$

Therefore,

$$\widetilde{\delta\mu}^A(\vec{r}) = \begin{cases} O(\Omega^{-1}), & d(\vec{r}, \partial\mathscr{D}) \cdot \Omega \gg 1; \\ O(\Omega^{1/2}), & \vec{r} \in \partial\mathscr{D}. \end{cases} \tag{4.6}$$

Now we come to the following problem: determine those variations of initial data for which the reconstruction error is localized near the boundary $\partial\mathscr{D}$, and determine whether we can consider the passage to a nonlinear model or to tomographs of third and fourth generations as one such variation.

Up to now, we have considered properties of a given model. In particular, when considering the BMM we assumed the functions SA_R, S_Π, S_V to be given. It seems that the most interesting, from both a theoretical and a practical point of view, is the *problem of optimal algorithms*. For example, for the BMM it means that we must find optimal (in some sense) functions S_R, S_V for a given S_Π. Below we will consider only the BMM. Let us note that the problem about optimal algorithms remains meaningful even if we ignore discretization errors and consider the BAM. Therefore it is reasonable to consider problems of this type. This approach agrees with the remark above that the discretization errors are usually unimportant. In particular, we can consider interpolation algorithms and assume that

$$S_R(\xi) = 0, \quad |\xi| > 1, \qquad S_\Pi(\xi) = 0, \quad |\xi| > 1, \tag{4.7}$$

or more general interpolation algorithms, and assume that

$$S_A(\xi) = 0, \quad |\xi| > 1, \qquad S_\Pi(\xi) = 0, \quad |\xi| > 1, \tag{4.8}$$

Let us note that in this case discretization errors are exponentially small for a sufficiently large number of angle samples **[5, 8]**, so they can ignored. The first condition in (4.8) can be written in the form

$$S_V(\xi) = 0, \quad |\xi| > 1. \tag{4.9}$$

This violates the locality of $V(s)$. However, even among local V's one can find functions for which (4.9) holds approximately. This is related to the existence of entire functions of exponential type that decrease sufficiently fast as $|s| \to \infty$ along the real axis.

The reconstruction quality is characterized in the BAM by the noise coefficient $C_\sigma(A)$ (see (3.13)), where

$$C_\sigma(A) = \frac{\pi}{4} \int_0^\infty \xi^2 (S_R^A(\xi))^2\, d\xi \tag{4.10}$$

and, depending on a parameter that evaluates the spatial resolution, either by the jump transfer function (see (3.39))

$$P_0^A(z) = \frac{1}{2} - \frac{1}{\pi} \int_0^\infty \frac{S_R^A(\xi) S_\Pi(\xi)}{\xi} \sin(\xi z)\, d\xi \qquad (z = \Omega x) \tag{4.11}$$

or by the normalized point image function $\delta^A(z)$ (see (2.89))

$$\delta^A(z) = 2\pi\Omega^{-2}\delta_A(r) \qquad (z = \Omega r), \tag{4.12}$$
$$\delta^A(z) = \int_0^\infty \xi S_R^A(\xi) S_\Pi(\xi) J_0(\xi z)\, d\xi.$$

The choice of one of these two parameters ($P_0^A(z)$ or $\delta^A(z)$) depends on the type of inclusion we want to be reconstructed better: large inclusions with smooth boundary or pointlike inclusions. Let us recall that

$$S_R^A(0) = S_\Pi(0) = 1. \tag{4.13}$$

Furthermore,

$$S_R^A(\xi) S_\Pi(\xi) = \int_0^\infty z\delta^A(z) J_0(\xi z)\, dz. \tag{4.14}$$

In particular,

$$\int_0^\infty z\delta^A(z)\, dz = 1 \tag{4.15}$$

and the Parseval identity for the Hankel transform gives

$$\int_0^\infty z(\delta^A(z))^2\, dz = \int_0^\infty \xi (S_R^A(\xi) S_\Pi(\xi))^2\, d\xi. \tag{4.16}$$

As a measure of spatial resolution one can take one of two constants

$$C_P(A) = -\left(\frac{dP_0^A}{dz}(0)\right)^{-1} = \pi\left(\int_0^\infty \xi S_R^A(\xi) S_\Pi(\xi)\, d\xi\right)^{-1}, \tag{4.17}$$
$$C_P(A) = \delta^A(0)^{-1} = \left(\int_0^\infty \xi S_R^A(\xi) S_\Pi(\xi)\, d\xi\right)^{-1}.$$

Let us take some $z_0 > 0$ and define artifact levels $B(z_0|A)$ for $z > z_0$ by the formulas

$$B_P(z_0|A) = \max_{z>z_0} |P_0^A(z)|, \qquad B_\delta(z_0|A) = \max_{z>z_0} |\delta^A(z)|, \tag{4.18}$$

We can also use the L^2-metric, defining

$$\widetilde{B_P}(z_0|A) = \int_{z_0}^\infty |P_0^A(z)|^2\, dz, \qquad \widetilde{B_\delta}(z_0|A) = \int_{z_0}^\infty z(\delta^A(z))^2\, dz. \tag{4.19}$$

If we choose an algorithm A, i.e., the functions S_R^A and S_Π, then its performance for some z_0 can be characterized by one of the triples

$$C_\sigma(A),\ C_P(A),\ B_P(z_0|A) \quad \text{or} \quad C_\sigma(A),\ C_\delta(A),\ B_\delta(z_0|A). \tag{4.20}$$

For a fixed S_Π these numbers depend on S_R^A. We say that an algorithm A_1 (for given S_Π, z_0) *performs better than* A_2 if

$$C_\sigma(A_1) \le C_\sigma(A_2), \quad C_P(A_1) \le C_P(A_2), \quad B_P(z_0|A_1) \le B_P(z_0|A_2), \tag{4.21}$$

and at least one of these inequalities is strict. We say that A_1 *is absolutely better that* A_2 if (4.21) holds for all z_0.

As an example, let us consider the simplest case (4.7) of algorithms without interpolation. For a given S_Π the algorithm is completely described by a choice of the function S_R (the window). We can ask whether or not there exist windows that are absolutely better than the R-L window or the S-L window, and if they exist, how much better they are (in terms of constants (4.20)). Numerical experiments suggest that there are no windows that are "significantly better" than the R-L (or the S-L) window. It would be interesting to prove this conjecture.

Let us give a possible formulation of the problem about optimal regularizers (windows) S_R. For given C_σ, C_P, S_Π, z_0 we can try to find an optimal window from either of the two similar conditions

$$B_P(z_0|S_R) = \min_{S_R} \equiv b_P(z_0), \tag{4.22}$$

$$B_\delta(z_0|S_R) = \min_{S_R} \equiv b_\delta(z_0) \tag{4.23}$$

(for given C_σ, C_δ, S_Π, z_0). This formulation needs refinements; in particular, we must describe the class of admissible function S_R. Another interesting problem is to describe the achievable regions in the space of parameters $C_\sigma, C_P, b_P(z_0)$. In the other words, we must determine when (for a given S_Π) there exists a function S_R for which the above parameters take prescribed values.

References

1. F. Natterer, *The mathematics of computerized tomography*, Teubner, Stuttgart, and Wiley, New York, 1986.
2. G. T. Herman, *Image reconstruction from projections. The fundamentals of computerized tomography*, Academic Press, New York, 1980.
3. S. Helgason, *The Radon transform*, Birkhäuser, Boston, MA, 1980.
4. A. Macovski, *Physical methods of computerized tomography*, Proc. IEEE **71** (1983), no. 3, 409–418.
5. A. K. Louis and F. Natterer, *Mathematical methods of computerized tomography*, Proc. IEEE **71** (1983), no. 3, 379–389.
6. R. W. Lewitt, *Reconstruction algorithms: Transform methods*, Proc. IEEE **71** (1983), no. 3, 390–408.
7. S. W. Rowland, *Computer implementation of image reconstruction formulas*, Image Reconstruction from Projections: Implementation and Application, Springer-Verlag, Heidelberg, 1979, pp. 9–80.
8. D. A. Popov, *On convergence of a class of algorithms for the inversion of the numerical Radon transform*, Mathematical Methods in Tomography, Transl. Math. Monographs, vol. 81, Amer. Math. Soc., Providence, RI, 1990, pp. 7–65.
9. G. T. Herman, *Correction for beam hardening in computed tomography*, Physics in Medicine & Biology **24** (1979), 81–106.
10. J. G. Verly, *Collimator effects in high resolution X-ray computed tomography*, IEEE Trans. Medical Imaging **MI-1** (1982), no. 2, 122–136.
11. W. K. Pratt, *Digital image processing*, Wiley, New York, 1978.
12. A. N. Tikhonov and V. Ya. Arsenin, *Methods for solving ill-posed problems*, 2nd ed., "Nauka", Moscow, 1979; English transl. of 1st ed., Wiley, New York, 1977.
13. D. A. Popov and D. V. Sushko, *On the convergence of algorithms for the numerical solution of convolution equations*, Dokl. Akad. Nauk SSSR **315** (1990), no. 2, 309–313; English transl. in Soviet Math. Dokl. **42** (1991).
14. ———, *Computation of singular convolutions*, this collection.
15. F. J. Harris, *Use of windows for harmonic analysis with the discrete Fourier transform*, Proc. IEEE **66** (1978), no. 1, 51–83.
16. N. I. Akhiezer, *Lectures on the therory of approximation*, 2nd ed., "Nauka", Moscow, 1965; English transl. of 1st ed., Ungar, New York, 1956.
17. V. P. Palamodov, *Nonlinear effects in tomography*, Dokl. Akad. Nauk SSSR **291** (1986), no. 2, 333–336; English transl. in Soviet Phys. Dokl. **31** (1986).
18. S. N. Gonchar, *On the convergence of numerical algorithms for reconstruction of discontinuous functions from Radon transforms*, Uspekhi Mat. Nauk **41** (1986), no. 3, 175–176; English transl. in Russian Math. Surveys **41** (1986).

Amer. Math. Soc. Transl.
(2) Vol. **162**, 1994

Mathematical Aspects of Polarization Tomography

V. A. Sharafutdinov

It is well known that the anisotropy of a characteristic of a medium—for example, dielectric permittivity, magnetic permeability, or conduction—leads to a polarization of a wave travelling in this medium. The same is true about elastic waves in solids. This makes it possible to detect and estimate anisotropy of a medium in a bounded volume by comparing the polarizations of incident and passing waves. In the framework of geometric optics, evolution of the polarization ellipse is usually described by a system of ordinary differential equations connecting components of electric field and the analyzed parameter of the medium along the light ray (for definiteness we consider electromagnetic waves, although similar phenomena can occur for elastic waves as well). Therefore, the polarization of the passing way for each ray is determined by the values of the analyzed parameter on this ray only. This means that our problem is of tomographic nature. Therefore, to solve this problem it is natural to use the tomographic scheme of information gathering, i.e., to perform polarization measurements along a sufficiently large family of rays. By polarization tomography we mean the collection of measurement schemes and methods used to solve corresponding inverse problems.

Up to now the polarization tomography has not received proper attention in the literature on tomography. To the best of the author's knowledge, such methods have been systematically analyzed only in the framework of photoelasticity problems [**1, 2**]. On the other hand, possible applications of polarization tomography are plentiful: fiber optics, plasma analysis, and earthquake prediction being examples.

Mathematical problems that arise in polarization tomography differ substantially from problems in classical tomography. There are two reasons for this. First, polarization effects are caused by the vector nature of waves. Therefore any reduction of polarization tomography problems to a search of scalar fields seems unnatural, and even impossible, so these problems essentially belong to vector tomography. The second difference is caused by the transverse nature of electromagnetic waves and can be explained as follows: the result of any measurement is the "integral along the line" of the analyzed parameter of the medium, and the contribution to this integral of any point of the line depends only on the component of this parameter orthogonal to the line.

The first section, which has a physical nature, is included in the paper only to convince the reader that our main object of study, the transverse ray transform of a vector field, is not a kind of weird author's invention, but reflects the above feature of polarization tomography problems. In §2 we give the definition of the transverse ray transform on a compact Riemannian scattering manifold and discuss some of its properties. In §3 we formulate Theorem 3.1, which is the main result of the paper. This theorem claims that in sufficiently simple cases the transverse ray transform is invertible, and also gives the corresponding stability estimates. The rest of the paper is devoted to the proof of this theorem.

§1. Evolution of the polarization ellipse along a ray

To begin with, we briefly recall the geometric optics method for the Maxwell equations. As a parameter of the medium, we consider the dielectric permittivity tensor. We start with the analysis of an isotropic medium, and after that we will consider our main subject: quasi-isotropic geometric optics approximation. After writing down the main system of differential equations describing the evolution of the polarization ellipse in a quasi-isotropic medium, we show that this system has a simple and clear interpretation from the point of view of the geometry of the corresponding Riemannian metric. After that we discuss briefly the nonlinear inverse problem of determining the dielectric permittivity tensor from polarization measurements, and show that the linearization of this problems leads to the inversion problem for the transverse ray transform of a degree 2 tensor field.

The relations presented at the beginning of this section, including equations (1.20), are well known and can be found in textbooks in optics (see, e.g., **[3]**). Equation (1.22) seems to be new.

1. Isotropic media. Let us consider a homogeneous (without charges and currents) system of Maxwell equations

$$\begin{aligned}&\operatorname{curl}\overline{\mathscr{H}}-\frac{1}{c}\frac{\partial}{\partial t}\overline{\mathscr{D}}=0, \qquad \operatorname{div}\overline{\mathscr{D}}=0\\ &\operatorname{curl}\overline{\mathscr{E}}-\frac{1}{c}\frac{\partial}{\partial t}\overline{\mathscr{B}}=0, \qquad \operatorname{div}\overline{\mathscr{B}}=0,\end{aligned} \tag{1.1}$$

which we supplement with the matter equations

$$\overline{\mathscr{D}}=\varepsilon\overline{\mathscr{E}}, \qquad \overline{\mathscr{B}}=\overline{\mathscr{H}}. \tag{1.2}$$

We assume the magnetic permeability to be equal to 1. Therefore, the only parameter of the medium is the dielectric permittivity $\varepsilon=\varepsilon(x)$ (or, equivalently, the refractive index $n=\sqrt{\varepsilon}$), which we first assume to be a scalar function of the argument $x\in\mathbb{R}^3$.

We restrict ourselves to fields that are harmonic in time, i.e., have the form

$$\overline{\mathscr{E}}(x,t)=\overline{E}(x)e^{-i\omega t}, \quad \overline{\mathscr{D}}(x,t)=\overline{D}(x)e^{-i\omega t}, \quad \overline{\mathscr{H}}(x,t)=\overline{H}(x)e^{-i\omega t}.$$

The system (1.1)–(1.2) becomes $(k=\omega/c)$

$$\operatorname{curl}\overline{H}+ik\overline{D}=0, \qquad \operatorname{curl}\overline{E}-ik\overline{H}=0, \tag{1.3}$$

$$\overline{D}=\varepsilon\overline{E}. \tag{1.4}$$

The geometric optics method consists in expanding each field $\overline{A}=\overline{E},\overline{D},\overline{H}$ in a power series of the form

$$\overline{A}(x)=\sum_{m=0}^{\infty}\frac{\overline{A}_m(x)}{(ik)^m}e^{ik\varphi(x)}. \tag{1.5}$$

After substituting these series in (1.3) and (1.4), and differentiating, we compare coefficients of equal powers of the wave number k in the left- and right-hand sides of the resulting equalities. In the physical literature this is usually done formally, without any discussion of the conversion of the series. Here we will follows this example.

As the first consequence of this procedure we see that the phase φ satisfies the eikonal equation

$$|\nabla\varphi|^2 = n^2. \tag{1.6}$$

Characteristics of this equation are geodesics of the Riemannian metric

$$d\tau^2 = n^2|dx|^2 = n^2((dx^1)^2 + (dx^2)^2 + (dx^3)^2). \tag{1.7}$$

The amplitudes $\overline{E}_m$ and $\overline{H}_m$ satisfy an infinite chain of equations. The first term of this chain is

$$[\nabla\varphi, \overline{H}_0] + \varepsilon\overline{E}_0 = 0, \qquad [\nabla\varphi, \overline{E}_0] - \overline{H}_0 = 0, \tag{1.8}$$

and the higher order approximations are

$$[\nabla\varphi, \overline{H}_m] + \varepsilon\overline{E}_m = -\operatorname{curl}\overline{H}_{m-1}, \qquad [\nabla\varphi, \overline{E}_0] - \overline{H}_0 = -\operatorname{curl}\overline{E}_{m-1}, \tag{1.9}$$

$m = 1, 2, \ldots$. Here $[\cdot,\cdot]$ denotes the vector product.

From the formal point of view, the eikonal equation (1.6) means that the determinant of the linear system (1.8) vanishes. It is important to note that in this case the corank of the linear system (1.8) becomes 2.

Let γ be a ray, i.e., a geodesics of the metric (1.7), and let $\overline{l}, \overline{\nu}, \overline{\beta}$ be the Frenet frame along γ. A general solution of the system (1.8) is of the form

$$\overline{E}_0 = \Phi_\nu\overline{\nu} + \Phi_\beta\overline{\beta}, \qquad \overline{H}_0 = n(-\Phi_\beta\overline{\nu} + \Phi_\nu\overline{\beta}), \tag{1.10}$$

where Φ_ν, Φ_β are arbitrary functions on the ray. The first order approximation, i.e., the system (1.9) for $m = 1$, gives differential equations for these functions. Indeed, the corank of the left-hand side of this system equals 2, so its compatibility requires two linear relations of the right-hand side. These compatibility conditions can be easily written down:

$$\begin{aligned} &\langle 2n\nabla\Phi_\nu + \Phi_\nu\nabla n, \overline{l}\rangle + \Phi_\nu n \operatorname{div}\overline{l} + 2n\kappa\Phi_\beta = 0, \\ &\langle 2n\nabla\Phi_\beta + \Phi_\beta\nabla n, \overline{l}\rangle + \Phi_\beta n \operatorname{div}\overline{l} + 2n\kappa\Phi_\nu = 0. \end{aligned} \tag{1.11}$$

Here κ is the torsion of the ray γ, and $\langle\cdot,\cdot\rangle$ denotes the inner product.

The system (1.11) is a system of ordinary differential equations along the ray γ. It has a simple family of first integrals, which allows us to give a simple qualitative interpretation of (1.11). Define the real and the complex amplitudes as follows:

$$A^2 = |\Phi_\nu|^2 + |\Phi_\beta|^2, \qquad \Phi^2 = \Phi_\nu^2 + \Phi_\beta^2. \tag{1.12}$$

From (1.11) we obtain the following equations:

$$\operatorname{div}(A^2\overline{l}) = 0, \qquad \operatorname{div}(\Phi^2\overline{l}) = 0. \tag{1.13}$$

These equations can easily be integrated, and give

$$A = A_0/\sqrt{J}, \qquad \Phi = \Phi_0/\sqrt{J}, \tag{1.14}$$

where J is the so-called geometric divergence. In particular, $\Phi/A = \text{const}$ along the ray.

Let us fix a point $x \in \gamma$. The end of the electric vector $\overline{E}(t) = \mathrm{Re}(\overline{E}(x)e^{i\omega t}$ runs over an ellipse in the plane spanned by vectors $\overline{\nu}, \overline{\beta}$. The eccentricity of this ellipse is a function of Φ/A, hence is constant along the ray. By (1.14), the size of the ellipse is proportional to $1/\sqrt{J}$. The last parameter that characterizes the position of the polarization ellipse in the $(\overline{\nu}, \overline{\beta})$-plane, namely the angle θ between its major axis and the vector ν, satisfies the Rytov law

$$d\theta/ds = \kappa, \tag{1.15}$$

where s is the arc length on γ. Relation (1.15) follows from (1.11). These three rules—shape conservation, proportionality of the size to $1/\sqrt{J}$, and the Rytov law—completely describe the evolution of the polarization ellipse for isotropic media.

2. Quasi-isotropic media. There are several methods for generalizing the above scheme to the case when (1.4) is replaced by

$$D_\alpha = \varepsilon - \alpha\beta E_\beta. \tag{1.16}$$

We consider one of these methods, which is known as the *quasi-isotropic generalization* of geometric optics. It is based on the representation of the permittability tensor in the form

$$\varepsilon_{\alpha\beta} = \varepsilon\delta_{\alpha\beta} + \chi_{\alpha\beta}, \qquad \chi_{\alpha\beta} \sim 1/k, \tag{1.17}$$

where $\varepsilon\delta_{\alpha\beta}$ is the isotropic part of the tensor $\varepsilon_{\alpha\beta}$, and the tensor $\chi_{\alpha\beta}$ is of the same order as the parameter $1/k$ of the asymptotic expansion (1.5). The formal procedure for deriving the quasi-isotropic approximation equations is similar to the previous scheme with the following additional rule: terms $\chi\overline{A}/k^m$ should be attributed to the $(m+1)$th term of the asymptotic expansion. For example, the decomposition of the electric induction vector takes the form

$$\overline{D} = \sum_{m=0}^{\infty} \frac{\varepsilon\overline{E}_m + \chi\overline{E}_{m-1}}{(ik)^m} e^{ik\varphi}.$$

The eikonal equation (1.6), as well as the zero approximation equations (1.8), do not change. In particular, on the zero approximation level the field still have the transverse character (1.10). Higher approximation equations (1.9) are replaced by the following equations:

$$\begin{aligned} [\nabla\varphi, \overline{H}_m] + \varepsilon\overline{E}_m &= -\operatorname{curl}\overline{H}_{m-1} + ik\chi\overline{E}_{m-1}, \\ [\nabla\varphi, \overline{E}_0] - \overline{H}_0 &= -\operatorname{curl}\overline{E}_{m-1}. \end{aligned} \tag{1.18}$$

The compatibility conditions (1.18) of the first order approximation equations take the form

$$\begin{aligned} &\langle 2n\nabla\Phi_\nu + \Phi_\nu\nabla n, \overline{l}\rangle + \Phi_\nu n \operatorname{div}\overline{l} + 2n\kappa\Phi_\beta - ik(\chi_{\nu\nu}\Phi_\nu + \chi_{\nu\beta}\Phi_\beta) = 0, \\ &\langle 2n\nabla\Phi_\beta + \Phi_\beta\nabla n, \overline{l}\rangle + \Phi_\beta n \operatorname{div}\overline{l} + 2n\kappa\Phi_\nu - ik(\chi_{\beta\nu}\Phi_\beta + \chi_{\beta\beta}\Phi_\beta) = 0. \end{aligned} \tag{1.19}$$

where

$$\begin{pmatrix} \chi_{ll} & \chi_{l\nu} & \chi_{l\beta} \\ \chi_{\nu l} & \chi_{\nu\nu} & \chi_{\nu\beta} \\ \chi_{\beta l} & \chi_{\beta\nu} & \chi_{\beta\beta} \end{pmatrix}$$

are the components of the tensor χ in the basis $\overline{l}, \overline{\nu}, \overline{\beta}$. Let us note that, as we mentioned in the Introduction, system (1.19) contains only the components of χ that are transverse to the ray.

If the tensor $\varepsilon_{\alpha\beta}$ is Hermitian: $\varepsilon_{\alpha\beta} = \overline{\varepsilon}_{\beta\alpha}$, then the real amplitude A defined by the first equality in (1.12) satisfies the relations (1.13)–(1.14), whereas the corresponding equalities for the complex amplitude Φ do not hold. Using the first relation in (1.13), we can simplify (1.19) by setting $F_\nu = A\Phi_\nu$, $F_\beta = A\Phi_\beta$. We obtain

$$\begin{aligned} \frac{dF_\nu}{ds} &= \frac{ik}{2n}(\chi_{\nu\nu}F_\nu + \chi_{\nu\beta}F_\beta) - \kappa F_\beta, \\ \frac{dF_\beta}{ds} &= \frac{ik}{2n}(\chi_{\beta\nu}F_\nu + \chi_{\beta\beta}F_\beta) + \kappa F_\nu, \end{aligned} \tag{1.20}$$

which is equivalent to (1.19).

Further simplification of the system (1.20) is possible from the point of view of the geometry associated to the metric (1.7). To this end, let us make in (1.20) the following change of variables:

$$f = \frac{ik}{2n}\chi, \qquad \eta = \frac{1}{n}\overline{F}, \qquad \dot{\gamma} = \frac{1}{n}\overline{l}. \tag{1.21}$$

From now on we adopt a mathematical approach and notation; in particular, we stop denoting vectors by overbars. The meaning of the last two equalities in (1.21) is that the vectors η and $\dot{\gamma}$ have unit length in the metric (1.27), whereas the vectors $\overline{F}$ and $\overline{l}$ have unit length in the Euclidean metric. One can show that the changes (1.21) transform the system (1.20) into the equation

$$D\eta/d\tau = P_{\dot{\gamma}} f \eta. \tag{1.22}$$

Here τ is the length function along the geodesics γ in the metric (1.7), $D/d\tau = \nabla_{\dot{\gamma}} = \dot{\gamma}^i \nabla_i$ is the covariant derivative operator along γ, and $P_{\dot{\gamma}}$ is the orthogonal projection onto the plane orthogonal to the vector $\dot{\gamma} = d\gamma/d\tau$. The right-hand side of (1.22) is understood as follows: the tensor f considered as a linear operator is applied to the vector η, and then the operator $P_{\dot{\gamma}}$ is applied to the resulting vector.

The equivalence of (1.20) and (1.22) is verified as follows. We write down the Christoffel symbols of the metric (1.7), express d/ds in terms of $D/d\tau$, use the relations

$$\frac{D\overline{\nu}}{d\tau} = n^{-2}\langle\nabla n, \overline{l}\rangle\overline{\nu} - n^{-1}\kappa\overline{\beta}, \qquad \frac{D\overline{\beta}}{d\tau} = n^{-1}\kappa\overline{\nu} n^{-2}\langle\nabla n, \overline{l}\rangle\overline{\beta},$$

resulting from the Frenet formulas, and substitute these relations in (1.20). The torsion κ cancels, and we come to the equation (1.22).

The realization of this scheme is a sequence of purely technical and rather cumbersome computations, and we do not present it here.

In the case when the medium is isotropic, i.e., $f = 0$, (1.22) implies that the vector field η is parallel to itself along γ in the metric (1.7). It is known that this fact is equivalent to the Rytov law (1.15). Therefore, equation (1.22) can be considered as a generalization of the Rytov law to the case of a quasi-isotropic medium.

3. Inverse problem. Let the analyzed medium fill a bounded region $D \subset \mathbb{R}^3$, and let the quasi-isotropic approximation hold. Let us assume that somehow we know the isotropic part $\varepsilon(x)\delta_{ij}$ of the tensor (1.17), i.e., we know the metric (1.7) and its geodesics. Our problem is to determine the anisotropic part χ_{ij} of the dielectric permittibility tensor. We assume that we can perform tomographic measurements of the following type: we test the region D along any geodesic of the metric (1.7) (say, using a laser if they are in the visible light range), choosing polarization parameters arbitrarily at the input to the region D and measuring them at the output.

The mathematical formulation of this problem is as follows. The metric (1.7) in the region D is assumed to be known. For any geodesics $\gamma: [0,1] \to D$ with ends at the boundary of D we know the value $\eta(1)$ of a solution of the system (1.22) as a function on the initial value $\eta(0)$ and the geodesics γ:

$$\eta(1) = U(\gamma)\eta(0). \tag{1.23}$$

In other words, we know the fundamental matrix $U(\gamma)$ of (1.22). We want to determine $f(x)$ from $U(\gamma)$.

Now we can forget the initial physical setup, considering the above problem for a region $D \subset \mathbb{R}^n$, $n \geq 2$, and for a general Riemannian metric

$$d\tau^2 = g_{ij}\,dx^i\,dx^j \tag{1.24}$$

in D. Of course, the factor $P_{\dot\gamma}$ in (1.22) is now the orthogonal projection in the sense of the metric (1.24).

Let us note that from the mathematical (and, possibly, also from the applied) point of view it makes sense to consider an analog of this problem without a factor $P_{\dot\gamma}$ in (1.22), i.e., with (1.22) replaced by

$$D\eta/d\tau = f\eta.$$

This vector tomography problem is considered in **[4]**, where under some additional smallness conditions on the region D and the function f the uniqueness of the solution is proved and the stability estimate is obtained. At present, we cannot extend the methods of **[4]** to the equation (1.22).

The inverse problem we have formulated is nonlinear. Let us linearize it. To this end we fix a geodesic $\gamma: [0,1] \to D$ with ends on the boundary of the region D and consider an orthonormal basis $e_1(\tau), \dots, e_{n-1}(\tau), e_n(\tau) = c\dot\gamma(\tau)$ parallel along γ. In this basis the system (1.22) takes the form

$$\dot\eta^j = \sum_{j=1}^{n-1} f_{ij}\eta^j, \qquad 1 \leq i \leq n-1.$$

Represent a solution of this Cauchy problem as a Neumann series

$$\eta(1) = \left[I + \int_0^1 F(\tau)\,d\tau + \int_0^1 F(\tau)\,d\tau \int_0^\tau F(\tau_1)\,d\tau_1 + \cdots\right]\eta(0), \tag{1.25}$$

where $F = (f_{ij})_{i,j=1}^{n-1}$, I is the identity matrix. Disregarding in (1.25) terms that are nonlinear in f, we get

$$\eta^i(1) - \eta^i(0) = \int_0^1 \sum_{j=1}^{n-1} f_{ij}(\tau)\eta^i(0)\,d\tau, \qquad 1 \leq i \leq n-1. \tag{1.26}$$

Multiplying each equality by ξ^i and summing, we obtain the relation

$$Jf(\gamma;\xi,\eta) = \int_0^1 \sum_{j=1}^{n-1} f_{ij}(\tau)\xi^i\eta^i(0)\,d\tau, \tag{1.27}$$

where $Jf(\gamma;\xi,\eta) = \sum_{i=1}^{n-1} \xi^i(\eta^i(1) - \eta^i(0))$ is a known function. To transform the equation (1.27) into an invariant form we put $\xi^n = \eta^n(0) = 0$ and change the upper summation limit in (1.27) to n. Noting that the vector fields $\xi(\tau) = \xi^i e_i(\tau)$ and $\eta(\tau) = \eta^i(0)e_i(\tau)$ are parallel along γ and orthogonal to the vector $\dot{\gamma}$, we see that the equation (1.27) takes the form

$$Jf(\gamma;\xi,\eta) = \int_0^1 f_{ij}(\gamma(\tau))\xi^i(\tau)\eta^i(\tau)\,d\tau. \tag{1.28}$$

In this formula, and everywhere in this paper, we assume summation from 1 to n over any pair of repeated upper and lower indices. Evidently, the integrand in (1.28) does not depend on the choice of a local coordinate system in a neighborhood of the point $\gamma(\tau)$. Hence, we arrive at the following linear problem.

Suppose that in a region $D \subset \mathbb{R}^n$ we are given the Riemannian metric (1.24). We must find a tensor field $f = (f_{ij})$ on D provided that for any geodesic $\gamma\colon [0,1] \to D$ with ends at the boundary of D we know the bilinear form (1.28) for all $\xi, \eta \in \gamma^\perp$, where $\gamma^\perp$ is the space of vector fields that are parallel along γ and perpendicular to $\dot{\gamma}$.

Below we restrict ourselves to the analysis of symmetric tensor fields, $f_{ij} = f_{ji}$. In this case the bilinear form (1.28) can be replaced by the quadratic form

$$Jf(\gamma,\eta) = \int_0^1 f_{ij}(\gamma(t))\eta^i(t)\eta^j(t)\,dt, \qquad \eta \in \gamma^\perp. \tag{1.29}$$

The function $Jf(\gamma,\eta)$ defined by this formula is called the *transverse ray transform* of the field f.

Like any tomographic problem, the inversion problem for the transverse ray transform is dimensionally overdetermined in the case $n > 2$. Indeed, the field f depends on the n-dimensional variable $x \in D$, whereas the known function $Jf(\gamma,\eta)$ depends on the $2(n-1)$-parameter family of geodesics γ. This remark suggests that we restrict measurements to an n-dimensional family of geodesics. Such a reduction of dimensionality was performed in **[2]** for a very specific problem. On the other hand, the problem is underdetermined with respect to the number of required functions: we are looking for $n(n+1)/2$ components of the field f, while knowing only $n(n-1)/2$ coefficients a_{ij} of the quadratic form $Jf(\gamma,\eta) = a_{ij}(f,\gamma)\eta^i\eta^j$ (since $\dim \gamma^\perp = n-1$).

To conclude this section, we show that if the metric (1.24) is Euclidean (i.e., $\varepsilon = \text{const}$ in (1.17)), the inversion problem for the transverse ray transform of a tensor field is reduced to the classical tomography problem of inverting the ray transform of a scalar function **[5]** (to the Radon inversion problem, when $n = 3$). Indeed, in this case geodesics are straight lines that can be parametrized by a point $x \in \mathbb{R}^n$ and a director $0 \neq \xi \in \mathbb{R}^n$. Extending f by zero outside D, we can rewrite (1.28) as follows:

$$Jf(x,\xi;\eta) = \int_{-\infty}^{\infty} f_{ij}(x + t\xi)\eta^i\eta^j\,dt, \tag{1.30}$$
$$x,\eta \in \mathbb{R}^n, \quad 0 \neq \xi \in \mathbb{R}^n, \quad \xi \perp \eta.$$

Let us fix $0 \neq \eta \in \mathbb{R}^n$ and consider the function $\varphi(y) = f_{ij}(y)\eta^i\eta^j$ on the hyperplane $\mathbb{R}^{n-1}_{\eta,p} = \{y \in \mathbb{R}^n \mid \langle y,\eta\rangle = p\}$. By (1.30), we know the integrals of φ over all lines in $\mathbb{R}^{n-1}_{\eta,p}$. Therefore we can determine the values of $f_{ij}(y)\eta^i\eta^j$ on any hyperplane $\mathbb{R}^{n-1}_{\eta,p}$, hence the field f on $\mathbb{R}^n$.

§2. Transverse ray transform

For a manifold M (by a manifold we mean a smooth locally compact finite-dimensional manifold; "smooth" means "infinitely differentiable") we denote by $\tau_M = (TM, p, M)$ and $\tau'_M = (T'M, p', M)$ the tangent and the cotangent bundle respectively. Points of TM are pairs (x, ξ), where $x \in M$, $\xi \in T_xM$. Let $S^m\tau'_M = (S^mT'_M, p'_m, M)$ be the mth symmetric power of the bundle τ'_M. Sections $f \in C^\infty(S^m\tau'_M)$ are covariant symmetric tensor fields of order μ on M. We restrict ourself to the analysis of real tensor fields, although all notions and results can be transferred to complex fields almost word for word. For $u \in S^kT'_xM$, $v \in S^lT'_xM$ we define their product as $uv = \sigma(u \otimes v)$, where σ is the symmetrization. This makes $S^*\tau'_M = \bigoplus_{m=1}^{\infty} S^m\tau'_M$ a bundle of commutative graded algebras.

For a Riemannian manifold (M, g) the metric g establishes a canonical isomorphism of bundles τ_M and τ'_M; sometimes we will use the identification $\tau_M = \tau'_M = S^1\tau'_M$. We will often use the coordinate representation of tensors. If $x^1, \dots, x^n$ is a local coordinate system in a region $U \subset M$, then a field $u \in C^\infty(S^m\tau'_M; U)$ can be uniquely represented in the form

$$u = u_{i_1 \cdots i_m} dx^{i_1} \otimes \cdots \otimes dx^{i_m}, \tag{2.1}$$

where $u_{i_1 \cdots i_m} \in C^\infty(U)$ are called *covariant components* (or coordinates) of the field u in the given coordinate system. Assuming that the choice of the coordinate system is clear from the context (or can be arbitrary), we will usually shorten (2.1) to $u = (u_{i_1 \cdots i_m})$. It is convenient to consider also *contravariant coordinates*

$$u^{i_1 \cdots i_m} = g^{i_1 j_1} \cdots g^{i_m j_m} u_{j_1 \cdots j_m},$$

where $(g^{ij}) = (g_{ij})^{-1}$. The inner product $\langle \xi, \eta \rangle = g_{ij}(x)\xi^i\eta^j = \xi_i\eta^i$ $(\xi, \eta \in T_xM)$ can be extended to $S^mT'_xM$ by the formula $\langle u, v \rangle = u_{i_1 \cdots i_m} v^{i_1 \cdots i_m}$. Let us note that for $\xi \in T_xM$, $u \in S^mT'_xM$ we have the equality $u_{i_1 \cdots i_m}\xi^{i_1} \cdots \xi^{i_m} = \langle u, \xi^m \rangle$. Below we will use this equality to shorten certain formulas. For $\xi \in T_xM$ by $i_\xi \colon S^mT'_xM \to S^{m+1}T'_xM$ we denote the operator of symmetric multiplication by ξ, i.e., $i_\xi u = \xi u$, and by $j_\xi \colon S^{m+1}T'_xM \to S^mT'_xM$ we denote the adjoint operator. In coordinates, the operator j_ξ is given by $(j_\xi u)_{i_1 \cdots i_m} = \xi^p u_{p i_1 \cdots i_m}$. We have the following orthogonal decomposition:

$$S^mT'_xM = \ker j_\xi \oplus \operatorname{im} i_\xi. \tag{2.2}$$

Denote by $P_\xi \colon S^mT'_xM \to S^mT'_xM$ the orthogonal projection to the first term of the decomposition (2.2). For $\xi \neq 0$, the operator P_ξ is given in coordinates by the following formula:

$$(P_\xi u)_{i_1 \cdots i_m} = \left(\delta^{j_1}_{i_1} - \frac{1}{|\xi|^2}\xi_{i_1}\xi^{j_1}\right) \cdots \left(\delta^{j_m}_{i_m} - \frac{1}{|\xi|^2}\xi_{i_m}\xi^{j_m}\right) u_{j_1 \cdots j_m}, \tag{2.3}$$

where (δ^j_i) is the Kronecker tensor.

Let (M, g) be a Riemannian manifold with boundary ∂M. For $x \in \partial M$ denote by $\nu(x)$ the unit outward normal vector to ∂M at x. Let $\Omega M = \{(x, \xi) \in TM \mid |\xi|^2 = \langle \xi, \xi \rangle = 1\}$ be the manifold of unit tangent vectors to M. The boundary $\partial\Omega M$ of this manifold can be decomposed into the union of two submanifolds

$$\partial_\pm \Omega M = \{(x, \xi) \in \Omega M \mid x \in \partial M, \pm\langle \xi, \nu(x) \rangle \geq 0\}$$

with the common boundary $\partial_0\Omega M = \partial_+\Omega M \cap \partial_-\Omega M$. We use the notation $S^m\pi_M =$

$(S^m\Pi M, q_m, \partial_+\Omega M)$ for the bundle on $\partial_+\Omega M$ induced from $S^m\tau'_M$ by the restriction $p\colon \partial_+\Omega M \to M$ of the projection of the tangent bundle, i.e., $S^m\pi_M = p^*S^m\tau'_M$. Hence, sections $\varphi \in C^\infty(S^m\pi_M)$ of this bundle are functions that associate to a point $(x,\xi) \in \partial_+\Omega M$ a tensor $\varphi(x,\xi) \in S^m T'_x M$.

A compact Riemannian manifold with boundary (M, g) is called a *compact scattering Riemannian manifold* (CSRM for short) if

(1) the boundary ∂M is strictly convex, i.e., for any $x \in \partial M$ the second quadratic form $\mathbf{I}(x,\xi) = \langle \nabla_\xi \nu, \xi\rangle$ on $T_x(\partial M)$ is positive definite;

(2) for any $(x,\xi) \in TM$, $\xi \neq 0$, the maximal geodesic $\gamma_{x\xi}$ satisfying the initial conditions $\gamma_{x\xi}(0) = x$ and $\dot\gamma_{x\xi}(0) = \xi$ is defined on a finite interval $[\tau_-(x,\xi), \tau_+(x,\xi)]$.

The *transverse ray transform* on a CSRM (M, g) is a linear operator

$$J\colon C^\infty(S^m\tau'_M) \to C^\infty(S^m\pi_M) \tag{2.4}$$

defined by the formula

$$Jf(x,\xi) = \int_{\tau_-(x,\xi)}^0 I_\gamma^{t,0}(P_{\dot\gamma(t)} f(\gamma(t)))\,dt, \qquad (x,\xi) \in \partial_+\Omega M, \tag{2.5}$$

where $\gamma = \gamma_{x\xi}\colon [\tau_-(x,\xi), 0] \to M$ is the geodesic determined by the conditions $\gamma(0) = x$, $\dot\gamma(0) = \xi$, and $I_\gamma^{t,0}$ is the parallel transport along γ from $\gamma(t)$ to $x = \gamma(0)$.

Let us comment on the relation of this definition to the definition (1.29) in §1. Note that for $\xi, \eta \in T_x M$ we have a formula

$$P_\xi \eta^m = (P_\xi)^m, \tag{2.6}$$

which easily follows from (2.3). Let $(x,\xi) \in \partial_+\Omega M$, $\eta \in T_x M$, $\langle \xi, \eta\rangle = 0$. Denote by $\eta(t)$ the vector field that is parallel along $\gamma = \gamma_{x\xi}$ and satisfies $\eta(0) = \eta$. Taking the inner product of (2.5) with $(\eta + a\xi)^m$, $a \in \mathbb{R}$, and using (2.6), we can transform the integrand in the resulting formula as follows:

$$\begin{aligned}
&\langle I_\gamma^{t,0}(P_{\dot\gamma(t)} f(\gamma(t))), (\eta + a\xi)^m\rangle \\
&\quad = \langle (P_{\dot\gamma(t)} f(\gamma(t))), I_\gamma^{t,0}(\eta + a\xi)^m\rangle = \langle (P_{\dot\gamma(t)} f(\gamma(t))), (\eta(t) + a\dot\gamma(t))^m\rangle \\
&\quad = \langle (f(\gamma(t))), P_{\dot\gamma(t)}(\eta(t) + a\dot\gamma(t))^m\rangle = \langle (f(\gamma(t))), (P_{\dot\gamma(t)}(\eta(t) + a\dot\gamma(t)))^m\rangle \\
&\quad = \langle f(\gamma(t)), (\eta(t))^m\rangle.
\end{aligned}$$

Therefore,

$$\begin{aligned}
\langle Jf(x,\xi), (\eta + a\xi)^m\rangle &= \langle Jf(x,\xi), \eta^m\rangle \\
&= \int_{\tau_-(x,\xi)}^0 f_{i_1\cdots i_m}(\gamma(t))\eta^{i_1}(t)\cdots\eta^{i_m}(t)\,dt,
\end{aligned} \tag{2.7}$$

which for $m = 2$ coincides with (1.27) up to a constant factor.

It is interesting to compare (2.7) with the operator

$$If(x,\xi) = \int_{\tau_-(x,\xi)}^0 f_{i_1\cdots i_m}(\gamma(t))\dot\gamma^{i_1}(t)\cdots\dot\gamma^{i_m}(t)\,dt, \qquad (x,\xi) \in \partial_+\Omega M, \tag{2.8}$$

which is studied in **[6, 7]**. In our setup this operator can be naturally called the *longitudal ray transform* (in **[6, 7]** it is called the ray transform). First, for $m = 0$ these operators coincide. Second, for $n = \dim M = 2$ these operators can be reduced to each other by the diffeomorphism $TM \to TM$ that maps (x,ξ) to (x,ξ'), where ξ' is obtained from ξ by rotation through the angle $\pi/2$ in the positive direction (for simplicity we assume M to be oriented). For other values of m,n these transform are, presumably, unrelated. It might be quite interesting to consider these two transforms together, but we will not do this in the present paper.

Let us recall **[8]** that for a smooth vector bundle α over a compact manifold and for an integer $s \geq 0$ we can define the topological Hilbert space $H^s(\alpha)$ of sections whose components in a local coordinate system have locally square integrable derivatives of order up to s. Denote by $\|\cdot\|_s$ one of equivalent norms in this space. Similarly to Theorem 2.1 from **[6]**, one can prove the following result.

THEOREM 2.1. *Let (M,g) be a compact scattering Riemannian manifold. For any integer $s \geq 0$ the transverse ray transform* (2.5) *can be extended to a bounded operator*

$$J\colon H^s(S^m\tau'_M) \to H^s(S^m\pi_M). \tag{2.9}$$

§3. The main result

Let (M,g) be a Riemannian manifold. For $x \in M$ and a two-dimensional subspace $\sigma \subset T_xM$ we denote by $K(x,\sigma) = R_{ijkl}\xi^i\xi^k\eta^j\eta^l/|\xi\wedge\eta|$ the sectional curvature at x in the direction s; here ξ,η is a basis in σ and (R_{ijkl}) is the curvature tensor. For $x \in M$ denote

$$K(x) = \sup_\sigma |K(x,\sigma)|. \tag{3.1}$$

For a CSRM (M,g) we introduce the following parameter:

$$k(M,g) = \sup_{(x,\xi)\in\partial_-\Omega M} \int_0^{\tau_+(x,\xi)} tK(\gamma_{x\xi}(t))\,dt, \tag{3.2}$$

where $\gamma_{x\xi}\colon [0,\tau_+(x,\xi)] \to M$ is the geodesic determined by $\gamma_{x,\xi}(0) = x$, $\dot\gamma_{x\xi}(0) = \xi$.

Now we can formulate the main result of this paper.

THEOREM 3.1. *For any integers n,m satisfying the conditions $n \geq 3$, $n > m \geq 0$ there exists $\varepsilon(m,n) > 0$ such that for any compact scattering Riemannian manifold (M,g) of dimension n satisfying the condition*

$$k(M,g) < \varepsilon(m,n) \tag{3.3}$$

the transverse ray transform

$$J\colon H^1(S^m\tau'_M) \to H^1(S^m\pi_M)$$

is injective. Furthermore, for $f \in H^1(S^m\pi_M)$ the following stability estimate holds:

$$\|f\|_0 \leq C\|Jf\|_1, \tag{3.4}$$

with a constant C independent of f.

The condition $n \geq 3$ in the statement of the theorem is essential, since, as we have seen, for $n = 2$ the operator J can be reduced to the operator I, which has a nontrivial kernel. The second condition $n > m$ is, presumably, nonessential and is required only by the method of the proof we use.

Below we assume that $m \geq 1$, since, as we have seen, for $m = 0$ the operator J coincides with I and Theorem 3.1 follows from Theorem 1.1 in **[7]**.

The remaining part of the paper is devoted to the proof of Theorem 3.1. Here we only remark that Theorem 2.1 easily implies that it suffices to prove Theorem 3.1 for $f \in C^\infty(S^m\tau'_M)$.

§4. Pestov's differential identity

The main technique used in the proof of Theorem 3.1 is the technique of semibasic tensor fields on the total space TM of the tangent bundle to the Riemannian manifold (M, g); this technique is expounded in §3 of **[6]**. We assume that the reader is somewhat familiar with this technique. By $\beta^r_s M = (B^r_s M, p^r_s, TM)$ we denote the bundle of semibasic tensors of degree (r, s). Let $\overset{v}{\nabla}, \overset{h}{\nabla}\colon C^\infty(\beta^r_s M) \to C^\infty(\beta^r_{s+1} M)$ be the vertical and horizontal covariant derivative respectively. The operator $H\colon C^\infty(\beta^r_s M) \to C^\infty \beta^r_s M)$ is defined by the formula $H = \xi^i \overset{h}{\nabla}_i$. The metric g defines canonical isomorphisms of bundles $\beta^r_s M \sim \beta^{s+r}_0 M \sim \beta^0_{s+r} M$; in coordinates these isomorphisms are expressed by well-known operations of lowering and lifting of tensor indices, which we will constantly use. A similar convention will be used for differentiation operators: $\overset{v}{\nabla}{}^i = g^{ij}\overset{v}{\nabla}_j$, $\overset{h}{\nabla}{}^i = g^{ij}\overset{h}{\nabla}_j$. The inner product in $\beta^0_m M$ is defined by the formula

$$\langle u(x,\xi), v(x,\xi)\rangle - u_{i_1\cdots i_m}(x,\xi)v^{i_1\cdots i_m}(x,\xi), \qquad (x,\xi) \in TM.$$

We denote also $|u(x,\xi)|^2 = \langle u(x,\xi), u(x,\xi)\rangle$.

The next result is a generalization of Lemma 4.1 from **[6]** to semibasic tensor fields of arbitrary degree.

LEMMA 4.1. *For a field* $u = (u_{i_1\cdots i_m}(x,\xi)) \in C^\infty(\beta^0_m M)$ *on* TM *the following equality holds*:

$$\begin{aligned}(4.1)\qquad 2\langle \overset{h}{\nabla} u, \overset{v}{\nabla}(Hu)\rangle &= |\overset{h}{\nabla} u|^2 + \overset{h}{\nabla}_i v^i + \overset{v}{\nabla}_i w^i \\ &\quad - R_{ijkl}\xi^i\xi^k \overset{v}{\nabla}{}^j u^{i_1\cdots i_m}\overset{v}{\nabla}{}^l u_{i_1\cdots i_m} - \sum_{k=1}^{m} R^{i_k}{}_{jpl}\xi^p u^{i_1\cdots i_{k-1} j i_{k+1}\cdots i_m}\overset{v}{\nabla}{}^l u_{i_1\cdots i_m},\end{aligned}$$

where (R_{ijkl}) *is the curvature tensor and the semibasic vector fields* v, w *are defined by the formulas*

$$(4.2)\qquad v^i = \xi^i \overset{h}{\nabla}{}^j u^{i_1\cdots i_m}\overset{v}{\nabla}_j u_{i_1\cdots i_m} - \xi^j \overset{v}{\nabla}{}^i u^{i_1\cdots i_m}\overset{h}{\nabla}_j u_{i_1\cdots i_m},$$

$$(4.3)\qquad w^i = \xi^j \overset{h}{\nabla}{}^i u^{i_1\cdots i_m}\overset{h}{\nabla}_j u_{i_1\cdots i_m}.$$

PROOF. We have

$$\begin{aligned}2\langle \overset{h}{\nabla} u, \overset{v}{\nabla}(Hu)\rangle &= 2\overset{h}{\nabla}{}^j u^{i_1\cdots i_m}\overset{v}{\nabla}_j (Hu)_{i_1\cdots i_m} = 2\overset{h}{\nabla}{}^j u^{i_1\cdots i_m}\overset{v}{\nabla}_j(\xi^p \overset{h}{\nabla}_p u_{i_1\cdots i_m}) \\ &= 2\overset{h}{\nabla}{}^j u^{i_1\cdots i_m}\overset{h}{\nabla}_j u_{i_1\cdots i_m} + 2\xi^p \overset{h}{\nabla}{}^j u^{i_1\cdots i_m}\overset{v}{\nabla}_j \overset{h}{\nabla}_p u_{i_1\cdots i_m},\end{aligned}$$

which can be rewritten in the form

$$(4.4)\qquad 2\langle \overset{h}{\nabla} u, \overset{v}{\nabla}(Hu)\rangle = 2|\overset{h}{\nabla} u|^2 + 2\xi^p \overset{h}{\nabla}{}^j u^{i_1\cdots i_m}\overset{v}{\nabla}_j \overset{h}{\nabla}_p u_{i_1\cdots i_m}.$$

Represent the second term in the right-hand side of (4.4) as follows:

$$
\begin{aligned}
&2\xi^p \overset{h}{\nabla}{}^j u^{i_1\cdots i_m} \overset{v}{\nabla}_j \overset{h}{\nabla}_p u_{i_1\cdots i_m} \\
(4.5)\qquad &\quad = \overset{v}{\nabla}_j(\xi^p \overset{h}{\nabla}{}^j u^{i_1\cdots i_m} \overset{h}{\nabla}_p u_{i_1\cdots i_m}) + \overset{h}{\nabla}_p(\xi^p \overset{h}{\nabla}{}^j u^{i_1\cdots i_m} \overset{v}{\nabla}_j u_{i_1\cdots i_m}) \\
&\quad - \overset{h}{\nabla}{}^j(\xi^p \overset{v}{\nabla}_j u^{i_1\cdots i_m} \overset{h}{\nabla}_p u_{i_1\cdots i_m}) - \varphi,
\end{aligned}
$$

where φ is a function on TM defined by this equality. Let us show that φ does not depend on second derivatives of the field u. Indeed, expressing derivatives of products in (4.5) in terms of derivatives of factors, we obtain

$$
\begin{aligned}
\varphi = 2|\overset{h}{\nabla}u|^2 &+ \xi^p \overset{v}{\nabla}{}^j u_{i_1\cdots i_m}(\overset{h}{\nabla}_p \overset{h}{\nabla}_j - \overset{h}{\nabla}_j \overset{h}{\nabla}_p) u^{i_1\cdots i_m} \\
&+ \xi^p \overset{h}{\nabla}_p u_{i_1\cdots i_m}(\overset{v}{\nabla}_j \overset{h}{\nabla}{}^j - \overset{h}{\nabla}{}^j \overset{v}{\nabla}_j) u^{i_1\cdots i_m} \xi^p \overset{h}{\nabla}{}^j u_{i_1\cdots i_m}(\overset{v}{\nabla}_j \overset{h}{\nabla}_p - \overset{h}{\nabla}_p \overset{v}{\nabla}_j) u^{i_1\cdots i_m}.
\end{aligned}
$$

Using commutation rules from **[6]** for the operators $\overset{v}{\nabla}$ and $\overset{h}{\nabla}$, from the last equality we get

$$
\varphi = 2|\overset{h}{\nabla}u|^2 + R_{ijkl}\xi^i\xi^k \overset{h}{\nabla}{}^j u^{i_1\cdots i_m} \overset{v}{\nabla}{}^l u_{i_1\cdots i_m} + \sum_{k=1}^{m} R_{i_k pqj}\xi^q u^{i_1\cdots i_{k-1} p i_{k+1}\cdots i_m} \overset{v}{\nabla}{}^j u_{i_1\cdots i_m}.
$$

Substituting this expression for φ into (4.5) and then substituting (4.5) into the right-hand of (4.4). we complete the proof of the lemma. □

§5. Reduction of Theorem 3.1 to the inverse problem for the kinetic equation

Let (M, g) be a CSRM, $f \in C^\infty(S^m\tau'_M)$. Denote $T^0M = \{(x,\xi) \in TM \mid \xi \neq 0\}$ and define a semibasic tensor field $u = (u_{i_1\cdots i_m}(x,\xi))$ on T^0M by the formula

$$
(5.1)\qquad u(x,\xi) = \int_{\tau_-(x,\xi)}^{0} I_\gamma^{t,0}(P_{\dot\gamma(t)} f(\gamma(t)))\,dt, \qquad (x,\xi) \in T^0M,
$$

where we use the same notation as in the definition (2.6) of the transverse ray transform. The only difference between (2.5) and (5.1) is that (2.5) is considered only for $(x,\xi) \in \partial_+\Omega M$, whereas (5.1) is defined for all $(x,\xi) \in T^0M$. In particular, for u we have the boundary condition

$$
(5.2)\qquad u|_{\partial_+\Omega M} = Jf.
$$

Since $\tau_-(x,\xi) = 0$ for $(x,\xi) \in \partial_-\Omega M$, we get the second boundary condition

$$
(5.3)\qquad u|_{\partial_-\Omega M} = 0.
$$

The field u depends smoothly on $(x,\xi) \in T^0M$ everywhere except at points of $T^0(\partial M)$, where some partial derivatives of the field u can become infinite. Therefore some of the integrals below are improper, and their convergence must be verified. This verification is performed in exactly the same way as in **[6]**, since singularities of the field u are caused by singularities of the lower integration limit in (5.1). Therefore we will skip this verification.

The field $u(x,\xi)$ is homogeneous with respect to the second argument:

$$u(x,t\xi) = t^{-1}u(x,\xi), \qquad t>0, \tag{5.4}$$

and satisfies on $T^0M \setminus T^0(\partial M)$ the differential equation

$$Hu(x,\xi) = P_\xi f(x). \tag{5.5}$$

Relations (5.4) and (5.5) are derived from (5.1) by almost literal repetition of the corresponding arguments in **[6]**, which we skip.

Finally, let us note that the field $u = (u_{i_1\cdots i_m}(x,\xi))$ is symmetric with respect to all indices and satisfies the relation

$$j_\xi u(x,\xi) = 0, \tag{5.6}$$

which immediately follows from the corresponding properties of the integrand in (5.1).

Let us indicate some properties of the right-hand side of (5.5). Roughly speaking, it is the product of two factors depending on different variables. This property turns out to be crucial in further arguments.

Equation (5.5) (with an arbitrary function of (x,ξ) in the right-hand side) is called *the kinetic equation of the metric* g. Written in coordinates, it is a *system* of differential equations for components of the field u. This fact express the fundamental difference between our situation and the situation in **[6, 7]**, where a *single* equation was considered.

Hence, we come to the following inverse problem for the kinetic equation: to compute the factor $f(x)$ in the right-hand side of (5.6) given the boundary value (5.3) of the solution of the kinetic equation.

§6. Integral identity for the kinetic equation

Let (M,g) be a CSRM. Fix $\rho>1$ and denote $T^\rho M = \{(x,\xi)\in TM \mid 1\le|\xi|\le\rho\}$. For the solution $u(x,\xi)$ of the boundary value problem (5.2)–(5.5) we write down the identity in Lemma 4.1 multiplied by the symplectic volume form

$$dV^{2n} = \det(g_{ij})\,d\xi\wedge dx = \det(g_{ij})\,d\xi^1\wedge\cdots\wedge d\xi^n\wedge dx^1\wedge\cdots\wedge dx^n \tag{6.1}$$

and integrate over $T^\rho M$. Transforming summands of the resulting equality containing $\overset{h}{\nabla}_i v^i$, $\overset{v}{\nabla}_i w^i$ using the Gauss-Ostrogradskiĭ formulas for the horizontal and the vertical divergence **[6]**, we get the relation

$$\begin{aligned}
&\int_{T^\rho M} |\overset{h}{\nabla} u|^2\,dV^{2n} + \frac{1}{\rho}\int_{\Omega^\rho M}\langle w,\xi\rangle\,d\Sigma^{2n-1} - \int_{\Omega M}\langle w,\xi\rangle\,d\Sigma^{2n-1}\\
&\quad = 2\int_{T^\rho M}\langle \overset{h}{\nabla} u, \overset{v}{\nabla}(Hu)\rangle\,dV^{2n} - \int_{T^\rho(\partial M)}\langle v,\nu\rangle\,dV^{2n-1}\\
&\qquad + \int_{T^\rho M}\Big(R_{ijkl}\xi^i\xi^k\overset{v}{\nabla}{}^j u^{i_1\cdots i_m}\overset{v}{\nabla}{}^l u_{i_1\cdots i_m}\\
&\qquad\qquad + \sum_{k=1}^m R^{i_k}{}_{pql}\xi^q u^{i_1\cdots i_{k-1}pi_{k+1}\cdots i_m}\overset{v}{\nabla}{}^j u_{i_1\cdots i_m}\Big)\,dV^{2n-1},
\end{aligned} \tag{6.2}$$

where ν is the outward normal vector to ∂M,

$$\Omega^\rho = \{(x,\xi)\mid |\xi|=\rho\}, \qquad T^\rho(\partial M) = \{(x,\xi)\mid x\in\partial M, 1\le|\xi|\le\rho\},$$

and $d\Sigma^{2n-1}$ and dV^{2n-1} are the corresponding volume forms on these manifolds. For details see [6].

By (5.4), all expressions under the integral sign in (6.2) are homogeneous in ξ. Using this fact, we can combine the two last integrals in the left-hand side of (6.2) and decrease the dimensionality of all other integrals by 1. Details of this procedure, which is quite similar to the corresponding arguments in [6], are omitted. Noting also that $\langle w, \xi\rangle = |Hu|^2$ by (4.3), we finally obtain

$$\begin{aligned}\int_{\Omega M} [|\overset{h}{\nabla} u|^2 + (n-2)]\, d\Sigma^{2n-1} \\ = 2\int_{\Omega M} \langle \overset{h}{\nabla} u, \overset{v}{\nabla}(Hu)\rangle\, d\Sigma^{2n-1} - \int_{\partial\Omega M} \langle v, \nu\rangle\, d\Sigma^{2n-2} + \int_{\Omega M} \mathscr{R}_1[u]\, d\Sigma^{2n-1},\end{aligned} \tag{6.3}$$

where we use the abbreviated notation

$$\mathscr{R}_1[u] = R_{ijkl}\xi^i\xi^k \overset{v}{\nabla}{}^j u^{i_1\cdots i_m} \overset{v}{\nabla}{}^l u_{i_1\cdots i_m} + \sum_{k=1}^{m} R^{i_k}{}_{pql}\xi^q u^{i_1\cdots i_{k-1} p i_{k+1}\cdots i_m} \overset{v}{\nabla}{}^j u_{i_1\cdots i_m}. \tag{6.4}$$

The volume forms $d\Sigma^{2n-1}$ and $d\Sigma^{2n-2}$ in (6.3) have a simple geometric meaning. Namely, definitions in [6] easily imply that

$$d\Sigma^{2n-1}(x,\xi) = d\omega_x(\xi)\wedge dV^n(x), \qquad d\Sigma^{2n-2}(x,\xi) = d\omega_x(\xi)\wedge dV^{n-1}(x), \tag{6.5}$$

where $d\omega_x(\xi)$ is the angular measure on the sphere $\Omega_x M = \Omega M \cap T_x M$ induced by the metric g and dV^n, dV^{n-1} are the Riemannian volumes on M, ∂M respectively.

§7. Estimation of the summand related to the right-hand side of the kinetic equation

Most troublesome is the first summand in the right-hand side of (6.3). In the similar identity in [6, 7] the corresponding term was a divergence, whereas in our case it is not so.

According to the definition of the operator P_ξ, the right-hand side of (5.5) can be represented in the form

$$P_\xi f(x) = f(x) - i_\xi y(x,\xi) \tag{7.1}$$

with some symmetric semibasic tensor field y of order $m-1$. In its turn, by (2.2) this field can be represented in the form

$$y(x,\xi) = \widetilde{y}(x,\xi) + i_\xi h(x,\xi), \qquad j_\xi \widetilde{y}(x,\xi) = 0. \tag{7.2}$$

From (5.5) and (7.12) we get

$$\overset{v}{\nabla}(Hu) = \overset{v}{\nabla}(P_\xi f) = \overset{v}{\nabla}(f - i_\xi y) = -\overset{v}{\nabla}(i_\xi y).$$

Written in coordinates, this relation gives

$$\begin{aligned}\overset{v}{\nabla}_i (Hu)_{i_1\cdots i_m} &= -\overset{v}{\nabla}_i (i_\xi y)_{i_1\cdots i_m} = -\sigma(i_1\cdots i_m)\overset{v}{\nabla}_i(\xi_{i_1} y_{i_2\cdots i_m} \\ &= -\sigma(i_1\cdots i_m)(g_{ii_1} y_{i_2\cdots i_m} + \xi_{i_1}\overset{v}{\nabla}_i(\xi_{i_1} y_{i_2\cdots i_m}),\end{aligned}$$

where $\sigma(i_1\cdots i_m)$ is the symmetrization with respect to $i_1,\dots,i_m$. Therefore,

$$\begin{aligned}\langle \overset{v}{\nabla} u, \overset{v}{\nabla}(Hu)\rangle &= \overset{h}{\nabla}{}^i u^{i_1\cdots i_m}\overset{v}{\nabla}_i (Hu)_{i_1\cdots i_m} = \overset{h}{\nabla}{}^i u^{i_1\cdots i_m}(g_{ii_1} y_{i_2\cdots i_m} + \xi_{i_1}\overset{v}{\nabla}_i(\xi_{i_1} y_{i_2\cdots i_m})) \\ &= -\overset{h}{\nabla}_i u^{ii_2\cdots i_m} y_{i_2\cdots i_m} - \overset{h}{\nabla}{}^i(\xi_{i_1} u^{i_1\cdots i_m})\overset{v}{\nabla}_i y_{i_2\cdots i_m} = -\overset{h}{\nabla}_i u^{ii_2\cdots i_m} y_{i_2\cdots i_m};\end{aligned}$$

in deriving the last equality we used the condition (5.6). Substituting the expression (7.2) for y and using (5.6) once again, we get

$$
\begin{aligned}
\langle \overset{v}{\nabla} u, \overset{v}{\nabla}(Hu)\rangle &= -\overset{h}{\nabla}_i u^{ii_2\cdots i_m}(\widetilde{y}_{i_2\cdots i_m} + \xi_{i_2} h_{i_3\cdots i_m}) \\
&= -\overset{h}{\nabla}_i u^{ii_2\cdots i_m}\widetilde{y}_{i_2\cdots i_m} - \overset{h}{\nabla}_i(\xi_{i_2} u^{ii_2\cdots i_m}) h_{i_3\cdots i_m} = -\overset{h}{\nabla}_i u^{ii_2\cdots i_m}\widetilde{y}_{i_2\cdots i_m}.
\end{aligned} \tag{7.3}
$$

Defining the semibasic $\overset{h}{\delta} u$ by the formula

$$
(\overset{h}{\delta} u)_{i_1\cdots i_{m-1}} = \overset{h}{\nabla}{}^p u_{pi_1\cdots i_{m-1}}, \tag{7.4}
$$

we can rewrite (7.3) in the coordinate-free form:

$$
\langle \overset{h}{\nabla} u, \overset{v}{\nabla}(Hu)\rangle = -\langle \overset{h}{\delta} u, \widetilde{y}\rangle. \tag{7.5}
$$

Using the inequality for arithmetic and geometric means, we obtain from (7.5) that

$$
2|\langle \overset{h}{\nabla} u, \overset{v}{\nabla}(Hu)\rangle| \le b|\overset{h}{\delta} u|^2 + (1/b)|\widetilde{y}|^2, \tag{7.6}
$$

where b is an arbitrary positive number. We transform the first summand in the right-hand side of this inequality, separating out the part that has the divergence form. We get

$$
\begin{aligned}
|\overset{h}{\delta} u|^2 &= (\overset{h}{\delta} u)^{i_2\cdots i_m}(\overset{h}{\delta} u)_{i_2\cdots i_m} = \overset{h}{\nabla}_p u^{pi_2\cdots i_m}\overset{h}{\nabla}{}^q u_{qi_2\cdots i_m} \\
&= \overset{h}{\nabla}_p(u^{pi_2\cdots i_m}\overset{h}{\nabla}{}^q u_{qi_2\cdots i_m}) - u^{pi_2\cdots i_m}\overset{h}{\nabla}_p\overset{h}{\nabla}{}^q u_{qi_2\cdots i_m} \\
&= \overset{h}{\nabla}_p(u^{pi_2\cdots i_m}\overset{h}{\nabla}{}^q u_{qi_2\cdots i_m}) - u^p_{\cdot i_2\cdots i_m}\overset{h}{\nabla}_p\overset{h}{\nabla}_q u^{qi_2\cdots i_m}.
\end{aligned} \tag{7.7}
$$

Commutation formulas for the operator $\overset{h}{\nabla}$ (see [**6**]) give

$$
\begin{aligned}
\overset{h}{\nabla}_p\overset{h}{\nabla}_q u^{qi_2\cdots i_m} &= \overset{h}{\nabla}_q\overset{h}{\nabla}_p u^{qi_2\cdots i_m} - R^i{}_{jpq}\xi^j\overset{v}{\nabla}_i u^{qi_2\cdots i_m} \\
&\quad + R^q{}_{ipq}u^{ji_2\cdots i_m} + \sum_{s=2}^m R^{i_s}{}_{jpq}u^{qi_2\cdots i_{s-1}ji_{s+1}\cdots i_m}.
\end{aligned}
$$

Substituting this into the second summand on the right-hand side of (7.7), we obtain

$$
|\overset{h}{\delta}|^2 = -u^p_{\cdot i_2\cdots i_m}\overset{h}{\nabla}_q\overset{h}{\nabla}_p u^{qi_2\cdots i_m} + \overset{h}{\nabla}_p(u^{pi_2\cdots i_m}\overset{h}{\nabla}_q u_{qi_2\cdots i_m}) + \mathscr{R}_2[u], \tag{7.8}
$$

where

$$
\begin{aligned}
\mathscr{R}_2[u] &= R_{ijkl}\xi^i u^k_{\cdot i_2\cdots i_m} - R^k{}_{ijk} - u^j_{\cdot i_2\cdots i_m}u^{ii_2\cdots i_m} \\
&\quad + \sum_{s=2}^m R^{i_s}{}_{jkl}u^k_{\cdot i_2\cdots i_m}u^{li_2\cdots i_{s-1}ji_{s+1}\cdots i_m}
\end{aligned} \tag{7.9}
$$

Now we transform the first summand in the right-hand side of (7.8) in the order inverse to the one used in (7.7). We get

(7.10)
$$\begin{aligned}|\overset{h}{\delta}|^2 &= \overset{h}{\nabla}_q(u^p_{\cdot i_2\cdots i_m}\overset{h}{\nabla}_p u^{qi_2\cdots i_m}) + \overset{h}{\nabla}_q u^p_{\cdot i_2\cdots i_m}\overset{h}{\nabla}_p u^{qi_2\cdots i_m}\\ &\quad + \overset{h}{\nabla}_p(u^{pi_2\cdots i_m}\overset{h}{\nabla}{}^q u_{qi_2\cdots i_m}) + \mathscr{R}_2[u]\\ &= \overset{h}{\nabla}{}^p u^{qi_2\cdots i_m}\overset{h}{\nabla}_q u_{pi_2\cdots i_m} + \overset{h}{\nabla}_i(u^{ii_2\cdots i_m}\overset{h}{\nabla}{}^j u_{ji_2\cdots i_m} - u_{ji_2\cdots i_m}\overset{h}{\nabla}{}^j u^{ii_2\cdots i_m}) + \mathscr{R}_2[u].\end{aligned}$$

Introducing a semibasic vector field $\widetilde{v}$ by the formula

$$\widetilde{v}^i = u^{ii_2\cdots i_m}\overset{h}{\nabla}{}^j u_{ji_2\cdots i_m} - u_{ji_2\cdots i_m}\overset{h}{\nabla}{}^j u^{ii_2\cdots i_m}, \tag{7.11}$$

we can rewrite (7.10) in the form

$$|\overset{h}{\delta}u|^2 = \overset{h}{\nabla}{}^i u^{ji_2\cdots i_m}\overset{h}{\nabla}_j u_{ii_2\cdots i_m} + \overset{h}{\nabla}_i\widetilde{v}^i + \mathscr{R}_2[u]. \tag{7.12}$$

Introduce one more (the last one!) semibasic tensor field z on T^0M by the formula

$$\overset{h}{\nabla}u_{i_1\cdots i_m} = (1/|\xi|)\xi_i(Hu)_{i_1\cdots i_m} + z_{ii_1\cdots i_m}. \tag{7.13}$$

The meaning of this new tensor z is that it is orthogonal to the vector ξ with respect to all indices, i.e.,

$$\xi^i z_{ii_1\cdots i_m} = \xi^{i_1} z_{ii_1\cdots i_m} = 0, \tag{7.14}$$

whereas the tensor $\overset{h}{\nabla}u = (\overset{h}{\nabla}u_{i_1\cdots i_m})$ is orthogonal to ξ only with respect to the last m indices. Indeed, the last equality in (7.14) follows from (5.6), and the first one follows immediately from (7.13) and the definition of the operator H.

Formula (7.14) implies that two summands in the right-hand side of (7.13) are orthogonal to each other, so that

$$|\overset{h}{\nabla}u|^2 = |Hu|^2 + |z|^2. \tag{7.15}$$

The first summand in the right-hand side can be expressed in terms of z. Indeed,

$$\begin{aligned}&\overset{h}{\nabla}{}^i u^{ji_2\cdots i_m}\overset{h}{\nabla}_j uii_2\cdots i_m\\ &\quad = \left(z^{iji_2\cdots i_m} + \frac{1}{|\xi|^2}\xi^i(Hu)^{ji_2\cdots i_m}\right)\left(z_{jii_2\cdots i_m} + \frac{1}{|\xi|^2}\xi^j(Hu)_{ii_2\cdots i_m}\right)\\ &\quad = z^{iji_2\cdots i_m}z_{jii_2\cdots i_m} + \frac{1}{|\xi|^2}\xi_j z^{iji_2\cdots i_m}(Hu)_{ii_2\cdots i_m}\\ &\quad\quad + \frac{1}{|\xi|^2}\xi^i z_{jii_2\cdots i_m}(Hu)^{ji_2\cdots i_m} + \frac{1}{|\xi|^4}\xi^i\xi_j(Hu)^{ji_2\cdots i_m}(Hu)_{ii_2\cdots i_m}.\end{aligned}$$

The last three terms in the right-hand side of this formula vanish due to (7.14) and a similar property of the tensor Hu (which follows from (5.5)), so we get

$$\overset{h}{\nabla}{}^i u^{ji_2\cdots i_m}\overset{h}{\nabla}_j u_{ii_2\cdots i_m} = z^{iji_2\cdots i_m}z_{jii_2\cdots i_m}.$$

Using this and (7.12), we get the inequality

$$|\overset{h}{\delta} u|^2 \le |z|^2 \overset{h}{\nabla}_i \widetilde{v}^i + \mathscr{R}_2[u]. \tag{7.16}$$

From (7.6) and (7.16) we conclude that

$$2|\langle \overset{h}{\nabla} u, \overset{v}{\nabla}(Hu)\rangle| \le b|z|^2 + (1/b)|\widetilde{y}|^2 + b\overset{h}{\nabla}_i \widetilde{v}^i + b\mathscr{R}_2[u]. \tag{7.17}$$

Now we express $\widetilde{y}$ in terms of f. Recalling relations (7.1) and (7.2), we get

$$f = P_\xi f + i_\xi \widetilde{y} + i_\xi^2 h, \qquad j_\xi \widetilde{y} = 0. \tag{7.18}$$

Applying the operator j_ξ to the first of these identities, we get

$$j_\xi f = j_\xi i_\xi \widetilde{y} + j_\xi i_\xi^2 h. \tag{7.19}$$

Now we use the following result.

LEMMA 7.1. *For an integer $k \ge 1$, the following formula holds in the space of semibasic tensor fields of order m:*

$$j_\xi i_\xi^k = \frac{k}{m-k}|\xi|^2 i_\xi^{k-1} + \frac{m}{m+k} i_\xi^k j_\xi.$$

We give the proof of this lemma at the end of this section, and now we continue with the main arguments.

Transforming each term on the right-hand side of (7.19) using the above lemma and taking the second equality (7.18) into account, we get

$$j_\xi f = \frac{1}{m}|\xi|^2 \widetilde{y} + i_\xi \left(\frac{2}{m} + \frac{m-2}{m} i_\xi j_\xi\right) h.$$

Since the second summand in the right-hand side of this equality belongs to the kernel of P_ξ, we have

$$\widetilde{y} = \frac{m}{|\xi|^2} P_\xi j_\xi f.$$

Substituting this into (7.17), we get

$$2|\langle \overset{h}{\nabla} u, \overset{v}{\nabla}(Hu)\rangle| \le b|z|^2 + \frac{m^2}{b|\xi|^4}|P_\xi i_\xi f|^2 + b\overset{h}{\nabla}_i \widetilde{v}^i + b\mathscr{R}_2[u]. \tag{7.20}$$

Integrating (7.20) and using the Gauss-Ostrogradskiĭ formula for the horizontal divergence to transform the third summand in the right-hand side, we obtain the estimate

$$\begin{aligned} 2\int_{\Omega M} |\langle \overset{h}{\nabla} u, \overset{v}{\nabla}(Hu)\rangle|\, d\Sigma^{2n-1} &\le \int_{\Omega M} \left(b|z|^2 + \frac{m^2}{b}|P_\xi i_\xi f|^2\right) d\Sigma^{2n-1} \\ &+ b\int_{\partial\Omega M} \langle \widetilde{v}, \nu\rangle\, d\Sigma^{2n-2} + b\int_{\Omega M} \mathscr{R}_2[u]\, d\Sigma^{2n-1}. \end{aligned} \tag{7.21}$$

Combining (6.3) and (7.21), we get

$$\begin{aligned} \int_{\Omega M} [|\overset{h}{\nabla} u|^2 + (n-2)|Hu|^2]\, d\Sigma^{2n-1} &\le \int_{\Omega M} \left(b|z|^2 + \frac{m^2}{b}|P_\xi i_\xi f|^2\right) d\Sigma^{2n-1} \\ &+ \int_{\partial\Omega M} \langle b\widetilde{v} - v, \nu\rangle\, d\Sigma^{2n-2} + \int_{\Omega M} \mathscr{R}[u]\, d\Sigma^{2n-1}, \end{aligned} \tag{7.22}$$

where

$$\mathscr{R}[u] = \mathscr{R}_1[u] + b\mathscr{R}_2[u]. \tag{7.23}$$

Replacing the summands on the left-hand side of (7.22) by their representations (5.5) and (7.15) and using formula (6.5) for the form $d\Sigma^{2n-1}$, we can rewrite (7.22) as follows:

(7.24)
$$\int_M \left\{ \int_{\Omega_x M} \left[(1-b)|z|^2 + (n-1)|P_\xi f|^2 - (m^2/b)|P_\xi j_\xi f|^2\right] d\omega_x(\xi) \right\} dV^2(x)$$
$$\leq \int_{\partial\Omega M} \langle b\widetilde{v} - v, v\rangle \, d\Sigma^{2n-2} + \int_{\Omega M} \mathscr{R}[u] \, d\Sigma^{2n-1}.$$

At this intermediate step we can draw the following conclusion. For the solution u of equation (5.5) satisfying the conditions (5.4) and (5.6) we have obtained the estimate (7.24), in which b is an arbitrary positive number, semibasic vector fields v and $\widetilde{v}$ are determined by formulas (4.2) and (7.11), and the function $\mathscr{R}[u]$ is defined by formulas (6.34), (7.9), and (7.13). The only property of the field z that will be used later is the equality

$$|\overset{h}{\nabla} u|^2 = |z|^2 + |P_\xi f|^2, \tag{7.25}$$

which follows from (5.5) and (7.15). Let us remark that so far we have not used the boundary conditions (5.2) and (5.3).

Proof of Lemma 7.1. It suffices to consider the case $k = 1$, since the general case follows immediately by induction on k. For a symmetric semibasic tensor field x of order m we have

$$(j_\xi i_\xi x)_{i_1\cdots i_m} = \xi^{i_{m+1}} \sigma(i_1 \cdots i_{m+1})(x_{i_1\cdots i_m} \xi_{m+1}),$$

where $\sigma(i_1 \cdots i_{m+1})$ is the symmetrization with respect to indices $i_1, \dots, i_{m+1}$. Using the decomposition of the symmetrization described in Lemma 4.1 of **[9]**, we transform the right-hand side of the last equality as follows:

$$\begin{aligned}
(j_\xi i_\xi x)_{i_1\cdots i_m} &= \frac{1}{m+1} \xi^{i_{m+1}} \sigma(i_1 \cdots i_m) \left(x_{i_1\cdots i_m} \xi_{i_{m+1}} + m x_{i_2\cdots i_{m+1}} \xi_{i_1}\right) \\
&= \frac{1}{m+1} \xi^{i_{m+1}} \sigma(i_1 \cdots i_m) \left(x_{i_1\cdots i_m} \xi_{i_{m+1}} \xi^{i_{m+1}} + m \xi_{i_1} x_{i_2\cdots i_{m+1}} \xi^{i_{m+1}}\right) \\
&= \left(\frac{1}{m+1} |\xi|^2 x + \frac{m}{m+1} i_\xi j_\xi x\right)_{i_1\cdots i_m}.
\end{aligned}$$

The lemma is proved. □

§8. Estimate of terms containing the curvature

In this section we estimate the last integral on the right-hand side of (7.24) in terms of $\int_{\Omega M} |\overset{h}{\nabla} u|^2 \, d\Sigma^{2n-1}$.

By the letter C we denote various constants that depend only on n and m.

For a Riemannian manifold (M, g), a point $x \in M$, and vectors $\xi, \eta, \lambda, \mu \in T_x M$ we have the inequality

$$|R_{ijkl}(x)\xi^i \eta^j \mu^k \lambda^l| \le CK(x)|\xi|\,|\eta|\,|\lambda|\,|\mu|, \tag{8.1}$$

where $K(x)$ is defined by (3.1). The proof follows, for example, from formulas in **[10]** that express components of the curvature tensor in terms of sectional curvature.

Using (6.4), (7.9), and (7.23), we conclude from (8.1) that the following inequality holds on ΩM:

$$|\mathscr{R}[u](x,\xi)| \le CK(x)\left(|u(x,\xi)|^2 + |\overset{v}{\nabla} u(x,\xi)|^2\right). \tag{8.2}$$

Here we assume that the number b in (7.23) satisfies the condition $0 < b \le 1$.

The proof of the following statement can be found in **[7]**.

Lemma 8.1. *For a smooth semibasic tensor field φ on a CSRM (M, g) satisfying the boundary condition $\varphi\big|_{\partial_-\Omega M} = 0$ and a continuous nonnegative function $K(x,\xi)$ in ΩM the following inequality holds*:

$$\int_{\Omega M} K(x,\xi)|\varphi(x,\xi)|^2\, d\Sigma^{2n-1} \le k \int_{\Omega M} |H\varphi(x,\xi)|^2\, d\Sigma^{2n-1},$$

where

$$k = \sup_{(x,\xi)\in\partial_-\Omega M} \int_0^{\tau_+(x,\xi)} tK(\gamma_{x\xi}(t), \dot\gamma_{x,\xi}(t))\, dt$$

and $\gamma_{x,\xi}\colon [0, \tau_+(x,\xi)] \to M$ is the geodesic determined by the boundary conditions $\gamma_{x\xi}(0) = x$, $\dot\gamma_{x,\xi}(0) = \xi$.

The boundary condition (5.3) implies that both fields u and $\overset{v}{\nabla} u$ vanish on $\partial_-\Omega M$. Integrating (8.2) and using Lemma 8.1, we obtain the inequality

$$\int_{\Omega M} |\mathscr{R}[u]|\, d\Sigma^{2n-1} \le Ck \int_{\Omega M} \left(|Hu|^2 + |H\overset{v}{\nabla} u|^2\right) d\Sigma^{2n-1}, \tag{8.3}$$

where $k = k(M, g)$ is defined by (3.2).

Let us estimate $\int |H\overset{v}{\nabla} u|^2\, d\Sigma$ in terms of $\int |\overset{v}{\nabla} u|^2\, d\Sigma$. To do this, we note that the definition of H immediately implies that $\overset{v}{\nabla} H - H\overset{v}{\nabla} = \overset{h}{\nabla}$, so that

$$|H\overset{v}{\nabla} u|^2 \le 2(|\overset{h}{\nabla} u|^2 + |\overset{v}{\nabla} Hu|^2). \tag{8.4}$$

Furthermore, the following inequality holds on ΩM:

$$|Hu|^2 = |\langle \xi, \overset{h}{\nabla}\rangle u|^2 \le |\overset{h}{\nabla} u|^2. \tag{8.5}$$

Using (8.4) and (8.5), we transform (8.3) to the form

$$\begin{aligned} &\int_{\Omega M} |\mathscr{R}[u]|\, d\Sigma^{2n-1} \\ &\qquad \le Ck\left[\int_{\Omega M} |\overset{h}{\nabla} u|^2\, d\Sigma^{2n-1} + \int_M \int_{\Omega_x M} |H\overset{v}{\nabla} Hu|^2\, d\omega_x(\xi)\, dV^n(x)\right]. \end{aligned} \tag{8.6}$$

Fix a point $x \in M$ and choose coordinates in a neighborhood of this point in such a way that $g_{ij}(x) = \delta_{ij}$. Applying the operator $\overset{v}{\nabla}_i = \partial/\partial\xi^i$ to the equality

$$(Hu)_{i_1\cdots i_m} = \left(\delta_{i_1}^{j_1} - (1/|\xi|^2)\xi_{i_1}\xi^{j_1}\right)\cdots\left(\delta_{i_m}^{j_m} - (1/|\xi|^2)\xi_{i_m}\xi^{j_m}\right) f_{j_1\cdots j_m},$$

which follows from (5.5) and (2.3), we get the following representation:

$$(\overset{v}{\nabla} Hu)_{i_1\cdots i_{m+1}} = |\xi|^{-2m-2} P_{i_1\cdots i_{m+1}}^{j_1\cdots j_m}(\xi) f_{j_1\cdots j_m}(x)$$

with some polynomials $P_{i_1\cdots i_{m+1}}^{j_1\cdots j_m}(\xi)$ independent of x. This representation implies the estimate

$$\int_{\Omega_x M} |\overset{v}{\nabla} Hu|^2\, d\omega_x(\xi) \le C|f(x)|^2. \tag{8.7}$$

Lemma 10.1 below shows that the quadratic form $\int_{\Omega_x M} |P_\xi f|^2 \omega_x(\xi)$ is positive definite on $S^m T'_x M$ and can be estimated as follows:

$$|f|^2 \le C \int_{\Omega_x M} |P_\xi f|^2\, d\omega_x(\xi), \tag{8.8}$$

where C is a constant independent of x.

Combining (8.7) and (8.8), we see that a solution of (5.5) satisfies the inequality

$$\int_{\Omega_x M} |\overset{v}{\nabla} Hu|^2\, d\omega_x(\xi) \le C \int_{\Omega_x M} |Hu|^2\, d\omega_x(\xi). \tag{8.9}$$

Inequalities (8.9) and (8.5) allow us to present the estimate (8.6) in the following final form:

$$\int_{\Omega M} |\mathscr{R}[u]|\, d\Sigma^{2n-1} \le Ck \int_{\Omega M} |\overset{h}{\nabla} u|^2\, d\Sigma^{2n-1}. \tag{8.10}$$

Using (8.10), we rewrite our main inequality (7.24) as follows:

(8.11)
$$\int_M \left\{ \int_{\Omega_x M} \left[(1-b)|z|^2 + (n-1)|P_\xi f|^2 - (m^2/b)|P_\xi j_\xi f|^2\right] d\omega_x(\xi) \right\} dV^2(x)$$
$$- Ck \int_{\Omega M} |\overset{h}{\nabla} u|^2\, d\Sigma^{2n-1} \le \int_{\partial\Omega M} \langle b\widetilde{v} - v, \nu\rangle\, d\Sigma^{2n-2}.$$

Let us remark that in deriving this inequality we used the boundary condition (5.3), but did not use (5.2).

§9. Estimation of boundary terms

In this section we estimate the right-hand side of (8.11) in terms of Jf. By (4.2) and (7.11), we have on $\partial\Omega M$

$$\begin{aligned} \langle b\widetilde{v} - v, \nu\rangle = {} & b\left(\nu_i u^{ii_2\cdots i_m} \overset{h}{\nabla}{}^j u_{ji_2\cdots i_m} - \nu^i u^{ji_2\cdots i_m} \overset{h}{\nabla}_j u_{ii_2\cdots i_m}\right) \\ & + \nu_i \xi^j \overset{v}{\nabla}{}^i u^{i_1\cdots i_m} \overset{h}{\nabla}_j u_{i_1\cdots i_m} - \nu_i \xi^i \overset{h}{\nabla}{}^j u^{i_1\cdots i_m} \overset{v}{\nabla}_j u_{i_1\cdots i_m}. \end{aligned} \tag{9.1}$$

Let us prove that the right-hand side of (9.1) depends only on values of u on $\partial\Omega M$. To do this we choose a coordinate system $x^1, \dots, x^m$ in a neighborhood of a point $x_0 \in \partial M$ in such a way that the boundary ∂M is given by the equation $x^n = 0$, and $g_{in} = \delta_{in}$. Then the vector v has coordinates $(0, 0, \dots, 1)$, and (9.1) can be written as follows:

$$\begin{aligned}\langle b\widetilde{v} - v, v\rangle = Lu \equiv b(u^{ni_2\dots i_m}\overset{h}{\nabla}{}^{\alpha} u_{\alpha i_2\dots i_m} - u^{\alpha i_2\dots i_m}\overset{h}{\nabla}_{\alpha} u_{ni_2\dots i_m})\\ + \xi^{\alpha}\overset{v}{\nabla}{}^{n} u^{i_1\dots i_m}\overset{h}{\nabla}_{\alpha} u_{i_1\dots i_m} - v_n\xi^{i}\overset{h}{\nabla}{}^{\alpha} u^{i_1\dots i_m}\overset{v}{\nabla}_{\alpha} u_{i_1\dots i_m}.\end{aligned} \tag{9.2}$$

with the summation over α from 1 to $n-1$.

It is essential that Lu does not include the derivatives $\overset{h}{\nabla}_n$. Therefore, if we choose a local coordinate system $y_1, \dots, y^{2n-1}$ on $\partial\Omega M$, then Lu becomes a quadratic form in components of the fields u, $\partial u/\partial y^i$, and $\partial u/\partial|\xi|$. Since (5.4) is homogeneous, $\partial u/\partial|\xi| = -u$; hence L is a quadratic differential operator on the bundle $p^*(S^m\tau'_M)$, where $p\colon \partial\Omega M \to M$ is the restriction of the projection of the tangent bundle. Therefore, (9.2) implies the estimate

$$\left|\int_{\partial\Omega M} d\Sigma^{2n-2}\langle b\widetilde{v} - v, v\rangle\right| \le D \parallel u|_{\partial\Omega M} \parallel_1^2, \tag{9.3}$$

where the constant D depends on m and on (M, g), in contrast to the constant C from (8.11). Dependence of D on b can be excluded assuming that $0 < b \le 1$.

Recalling boundary conditions (5.2) and (5.3), we can rewrite the estimate (9.3) as follows:

$$\left|\int_{\partial\Omega M} d\Sigma^{2n-2}\langle b\widetilde{v} - v, v\rangle\right| \le D\|u\|Jf_1^2. \tag{9.4}$$

With the help of (9.4), our main inequality (8.11) can be rewritten in the form

(9.5)
$$\int_M \left\{\int_{\Omega_x M} \left[(1-b)|z|^2 + (n-1)|P_\xi f|^2 - (m^2/b)|P_\xi j_\xi f|^2\right] d\omega_x(\xi)\right\} dV^2(x)$$
$$- Ck\int_{\Omega M} |\overset{h}{\nabla} u|^2\, d\Sigma^{2n-1} \le D\|u\|Jf_1^2.$$

§10. Proof of Theorem 3.1

The next statement collects the main algebraic difficulties of our problem.

LEMMA 10.1. *Let m, n be integers satisfying the conditions $n \ge 3$, $n > m \ge 1$. For a Riemannian manifold (M, g) of dimension n and a point $x \in M$ the quadratic form*

$$\langle Bf, f\rangle = \int_{\Omega_x} \left[(n-1)|P_\xi f|^2 - m^2|P_\xi j_\xi f|^2\right] d\omega_x(\xi) \tag{10.1}$$

is positive definite on $S^m T'_x M$ and satisfies the estimate

$$\int_{\Omega_x} \left[(n-1)|P_\xi f|^2 - m^2|P_\xi j_\xi f|^2\right] d\omega_x(\xi) \ge \delta|f|^2 \tag{10.2}$$

with a positive coefficient δ depending only on m and n.

Postponing the proof of this lemma for a moment, we use it to complete the proof of Theorem 3.1.

In proving Lemma 10.1 we will obtain the estimate

$$\int_{\Omega_x} |P_\xi f|^2 - m^2|\, d\omega_x(\xi) \tag{10.3}$$

with a constant C depending only on m and n. Formulas (10.2) and (10.3) imply the inequality

$$\int_{\Omega_x} \left[(n-1)|P_\xi f|^2 - m^2|P_\xi j_\xi f|^2\right] d\omega_x(\xi) \ge \delta \int_{\Omega_x} |P_\xi f|^2\, d\omega_x(\xi) \tag{10.4}$$

with a factor δ that differs from the one in (10.2), but still is positive and depends only on m and n.

Formula (10.2) implies, in particular, the estimate

$$\int_{\Omega_x} |P_\xi j_\xi f|^2 - m^2|\, d\omega_x(\xi) \le C_1 \int_{\Omega_x} |P_\xi f|^2\, d\omega_x(\xi) \tag{10.5}$$

with a constant C_1 depending only on m and n.

Assuming that $0 < b \le 1$, we obtain from (10.2), (10.3), and (10.5) that

$$\begin{aligned} &\int_{\Omega_x} \left[(n-1)|P_\xi f|^2 - (m^2/b)|P_\xi j_\xi f|^2\right] d\omega_x(\xi) \\ &\quad = \int_{\Omega_x} \left[(n-1)|P_\xi f|^2 - m^2|P_\xi j_\xi f|^2\right] d\omega_x(\xi) \\ &\qquad - m^2\left(\frac{1}{b}-1\right)\int_{\Omega_x} |P_\xi j_\xi f|^2\, d\omega_x(\xi) \\ &\quad \ge \left(\delta - C_1 m^2\left(\frac{1}{b}-1\right)\right)\int_{\Omega_x} |P_\xi f|^2\, d\omega_x(\xi). \end{aligned}$$

Using this inequality, we obtain from (9.5) that

(10.6)
$$\int_{\Omega M} \left[(1-b)|z|^2 + \left(\delta - C_1 m^2\left(\frac{1}{b}-1\right)\right)|P_\xi|^2 - Ck|\overset{h}{\nabla} u|^2\right] d\Sigma^{2n-1} \le D\|Jf\|_1^2.$$

Up to now the only condition the number b must satisfy is $0 < b \le 1$. Now we choose β in such a way that

$$\delta - C_1 m^2\left(\frac{1}{b}-1\right) = \frac{\delta}{2}$$

and denote by δ_1 the smaller of two numbers $1-b$ and $\delta/2$. Then (10.6) implies

$$\int_{\Omega M} \left[\delta_1\left(|z|^2 + |P_\xi|^2\right) - Ck|\overset{h}{\nabla} u|^2\right] d\Sigma^{2n-1} \le D\|Jf\|_1^2.$$

Recalling the definition (7.25), we rewrite this inequality as follows:

$$(\delta_1 - Ck)\int_{\Omega M} |\overset{h}{\nabla} u|^2\, d\Sigma^{2n-1} \le D\|Jf\|_1^2. \tag{10.7}$$

In (10.7) the constants δ_1 and C_1 depend on m and n only, and the number $k = k(M, g)$ satisfies the condition (3.3) of Theorem 3.1. Choosing $\varepsilon(m, n)$ in the formulation of this theorem in such a way that $\delta_1 - C\varepsilon(m,n) = \delta_1/2$, we obtain from (10.7)

$$\int_{\Omega M} |\overset{h}{\nabla} u|^2 \, d\Sigma^{2n-1} \le D_1 \|Jf\|_1^2, \tag{10.8}$$

where $D_1 = 2D/\delta_1$.

Using the inequality

$$|f(x)|^2 \le \int_{\Omega_x M} |P_\xi f(x)|^2 \, d\omega_x(\xi),$$

which follows from Lemma 10.1, and also equation (5.5), we obtain the following estimate:

$$\begin{aligned}\|f\|_0^2 &= \int_M |f(x)|^2 \, dV^n(x) \\ &\le C \int_M \left[\int_{\Omega_x M} |P_\xi f(x)|^2 \, d\omega_x(\xi)\right] dV^n(x) = \int_{\Omega M} |Hu|^2 \, d\Omega^{2n-1}(\xi).\end{aligned}$$

With the help of (8.5), we can transform this estimate to the form

$$\|f\|_0^2 \le C \int_{\Omega M} |\overset{h}{\nabla} u|^2 \, d\Omega^{2n-1}(\xi). \tag{10.9}$$

Estimates (10.8) and (10.9) imply the estimate (3.4), completing the proof of Theorem 3.1.

§11. Decomposition of operators A_0 and A_1

The rest of the paper is devoted to the proof of Lemma 10.1. Under the conditions of the lemma, we choose an orthonormal basis in $T_x M$ and use it to identify $T_x M$ with the space $\mathbb{R}^n$ endowed with the standard inner product $\langle \cdot, \cdot \rangle$. Under this identification, $S^m T_x' M$ is identified with the mth symmetric power $S^m = S^m \mathbb{R}^n$ of $\mathbb{R}^n$, the sphere $\Omega_x M$ with $\Omega = \{x \in \mathbb{R}^n \mid |\xi| = 1\}$, and the measure $d\omega_x$ with the standard angular measure $d\omega$ on Ω. Let $\omega = 2\pi^{n/2}/\Gamma(n/2)$ be the volume of Ω.

Define operators A_0 and A_1 by the formulas

$$A_0 = \frac{1}{\omega} \int_\Omega P_\xi \, d\omega(\xi), \qquad A_1 = \frac{1}{\omega} \int_\Omega i_\xi P_\xi j_\xi \, d\omega(\xi) \tag{11.1}$$

and set

$$B = (n-1)A_0 - m^2 A_1. \tag{11.2}$$

Then we have

$$\langle Bf, f \rangle = \frac{1}{\omega} \int_\Omega \left[(n-1)|P_\xi f|^2 - m^2 |P_\xi j_\xi f|^2\right] d\omega(\xi).$$

Therefore, Lemma 10.1 is equivalent to the fact that the operator B is positive definite.

Let $\delta = (\delta_{ij}) \in S^2$ be the Kronecker tensor. Denote by $i\colon S^m \to S^{m+2}$ the operator of symmetric multiplication by δ and by $j\colon S^{m+2} \to S^m$ the operator of convolution with δ. The operators i and j are conjugate to each other.

LEMMA 11.1. *The following equalities hold on* S^m, $m \geq 1$:

$$A_\alpha = (m-\alpha)!\Gamma(n/2)\sum_{p=0}^{[m/2]} a_\alpha(p,m,m) i^p j^q, \qquad \alpha = 0,1, \tag{11.3}$$

where $[m/2]$ *is the integral part of* $\mu/2$ *and*

$$a_\alpha(p,m,m) = \frac{(-1)^\alpha}{2^{2p}(p!)^2}\sum_{k=2p}^{m}(-1)^k \frac{(1+\alpha k-\alpha)k!}{2^k(m-k)!(k-2p)!\Gamma(k+n/2)}. \tag{11.4}$$

PROOF. First, let us note that vectors $\{\eta^m \mid \eta \in \mathbb{R}^n\}$ generate the linear space S^m, due to the formula

$$\frac{\partial^m}{\partial t^\beta}\bigg|_{t=0}\left(\sum_i t_i e_i\right)^m = m! e^\beta,$$

which holds for a basis $(e_1, \dots, e_n)$ of the space $\mathbb{R}^n$ and a multi-index β with $|\beta| = m$. Therefore, to prove (11.3) it suffices to establish, for any $\eta, \zeta \in \Omega$, the formula

$$\langle A_\alpha, \eta^m, \zeta^m\rangle = (m-\alpha)!\Gamma(n/2)\sum_{p=0}^{[m/2]} a_\alpha(p,m,m)\langle i^p j^p \eta^m, \zeta^m\rangle. \tag{11.5}$$

Let us note that for $|\eta| = |\zeta| = 1$ we have

$$\langle i^p j^p \eta^m, \zeta^m\rangle = \langle j^p\eta^m, j^p\zeta^m\rangle = \langle \eta^{m-2p}, \zeta^{m-2p}\rangle = \langle \eta, \zeta\rangle^{m-2p}.$$

Therefore, the required equalities (11.5) can be rewritten in the form

$$\langle A_\alpha, \eta^m, \zeta^m\rangle = (m-\alpha)!\Gamma(n/2)\sum_{p=0}^{[m/2]} a_\alpha(p,m,m)\langle \eta, \zeta\rangle^{m-2p}. \tag{11.6}$$

By the definition (11.1) of the operators A_α we have

$$\langle A_\alpha \eta^m, \zeta^m\rangle = \frac{1}{\omega}\int_\Omega \langle P_\xi j_\xi^\alpha \eta^m, j_\xi^\alpha \zeta^m\rangle \, d\omega(\xi). \tag{11.7}$$

Let us note now that for $|\xi| = |\eta| = 1$ we have

$$j_\xi \eta^m = \langle \eta, \xi\rangle \eta^{m-1}, \tag{11.8}$$

and, as one can easily see from (2.3),

$$P_\xi \eta^m = (P_\xi \eta)^m (\eta - \langle \eta, \xi\rangle \xi)^m. \tag{11.9}$$

By (11.8) and (11.9) the integral in (11.7) can be transformed as follows:

$$\begin{aligned}\langle P_\xi j_\xi^\alpha \eta^m, j_\xi^\alpha \zeta^m\rangle &= (\langle \eta, \xi\rangle\langle \zeta, \xi\rangle)^\alpha \langle P_\xi \eta^{m-\alpha}, \zeta^{m-\alpha}\rangle \\ &= (\langle \eta, \xi\rangle\langle \zeta, \xi\rangle)^\alpha (\langle \eta, \zeta\rangle - \langle \eta, \xi\rangle\langle \zeta, \xi\rangle)^{m-\alpha}.\end{aligned}$$

Substituting this expression into (11.7) and denoting for simplicity $x = \langle \eta, \zeta\rangle$, we obtain

$$\langle A_\alpha \eta^m, \zeta^m\rangle = (-1)^\alpha \sum_{l=0}^{m}(-1)^l \binom{m-\alpha}{l-\alpha} x^{m-l}\frac{1}{\omega}\int_\Omega (\langle \eta, \xi\rangle\langle \zeta, \xi\rangle)^l \, d\omega(\xi). \tag{11.10}$$

with the convention $\binom{p}{q} = 0$ for $q < 0$.

Let us calculate the integral in the right-hand side of (11.10). Choose an orthonormal basis in $\mathbb{R}^n$ in such a way that $\eta = e_1$, $\zeta = xe_1 + (1-x^2)^{1/2}e_2$. Then

$$\langle \eta, \xi \rangle = \xi_1, \quad \langle \zeta, \xi \rangle = x\xi_1 + (1-x^2)^{1/2}\xi_2.$$

Therefore,

$$\begin{aligned}\frac{1}{\omega}\int_\Omega (\langle \eta, \xi \rangle \langle \zeta, \xi \rangle)^l \, d\omega(\xi) &= \frac{1}{\omega}\int_\Omega \xi_1^l \left[x\xi_1 + (1-x^2)^{1/2}\xi_2\right]^l d\omega(\xi) \\ &= \sum_{r=0}^{[l/2]} \binom{l}{2r} x^{l-2r}(1-x^2)^r \frac{1}{\omega}\int_\Omega \xi_1^{2l-2r}\xi_2^{2r}\, d\omega(\xi).\end{aligned} \tag{11.11}$$

It is known (see **[11]**) that

$$\frac{1}{\omega}\int_\Omega \xi_1^{2l-2r}\xi_2^{2r}\, d\omega(\xi) = \frac{\Gamma(n/2)}{\pi\Gamma(l+n/2)}\Gamma(l-r+1/2)\Gamma(r+1/2).$$

Substituting this into (11.11), we obtain

$$\begin{aligned}&\frac{1}{\omega}\int_\Omega (\langle \eta, \xi \rangle \langle \zeta, \xi \rangle)^l \, d\omega(\xi) \\ &\quad = \frac{\Gamma(n/2)}{\pi\Gamma(l+n/2)} \sum_{r=0}^{[l/2]} \binom{l}{2r} \Gamma(l-r+1/2)\Gamma(r+1/2) x^{l-2r}(1-x^2)^r.\end{aligned}$$

Replacing the integral in (11.10) by its expression from the last formula, changing the order of summation in the resulting double sum, and introducing the notation

$$c_\alpha(r,m,n) = \Gamma(r+1/2)\sum_{l=2r}^{m} (-1)^l \binom{m-\alpha}{l-\alpha}\binom{l}{2r}\frac{\Gamma(l-r+1/2)}{\Gamma(l+n/2)}, \tag{11.12}$$

we come to the formula

$$\langle A_\alpha \eta^m, \zeta^m \rangle = (-1)^\alpha \frac{\Gamma(n/2)}{\pi} \sum_{r=0}^{[m/2]} c_\alpha(r,m,n) x^{m-2r}(1-x^2)^r.$$

Expanding the factor $(1-x^2)^r$ in the right-hand side of this formula in powers of x and changing the summation order in the resulting double sum, we obtain

$$\langle A_\alpha \eta^m, \zeta^m \rangle = (-1)^\alpha \frac{\Gamma(n/2)}{\pi} \sum_{p=0}^{[m/2]} (-1)^p \left[\sum_{r=p}^{[m/2]} (-1)^r \binom{r}{p} c_\alpha(r,m,n)\right] x^{m-2p}. \tag{11.13}$$

Recalling that $x = \langle \eta, \zeta \rangle$ and comparing the resulting formula (11.13) with the formula (11.5) that we want to prove, we see that (11.5) is valid with

$$a_\alpha(p,m,n) = \frac{(-1)^{p+\alpha}}{\pi(m-\alpha)!} \sum_{r=p}^{[m/2]} (-1)^r \binom{r}{p} c_\alpha(r,m,n). \tag{11.14}$$

To complete the proof it remain to verify that formula (11.14) is equivalent to (11.4).

Substituting into (11.14) the expression (11.12) for $c_\alpha(r,m,n)$, changing the summation order in the resulting double sum, and introducing the notation

$$\gamma(p,l) = \sum_{r=p}^{[l/2]} (-1)^r \binom{r}{p}\binom{l}{2r}\Gamma(r+1/2)\Gamma(l-r+1/2), \tag{11.15}$$

we come to the formula

$$a_\alpha(p,m,n) = \frac{(-1)^{p+\alpha}}{\pi(m-\alpha)!}\sum_{l=2p}^{[m/2]}(-1)^l\binom{m-\alpha}{l-\alpha}\frac{\gamma(p,l)}{\Gamma(l+n/2)}. \tag{11.16}$$

It turns out that the sum (11.15) can be simplified. To do this, we use the well-known formulas

$$\Gamma(r+1/2) = \frac{(2r-1)!!}{2^r}\sqrt{\pi}, \qquad \Gamma(l-r+1/2) = \frac{(2l-2r-1)!!}{2^{l-r}}\sqrt{\pi}.$$

Substituting into (11.15), we get

$$\gamma(p,l) = \frac{\pi}{2^l}\sum_{r=p}^{[l/2]}(-1)^r\binom{r}{p}\binom{l}{2r}(2r-1)!!(2l-2r-1)!!.$$

Using simple transformations, this equality can be rewritten in the form

$$\gamma(p,l) = \frac{\pi(l!)^2}{2^{2l}p!(l-p)!}\sum_{r=p}^{[l/2]}(-1)^r\binom{r}{p}\binom{2l-2r}{l}.$$

Changing the summation variable $k = r - p$ in the last sum, we get

$$\gamma(p,l) = (-1)^p\frac{\pi(l!)^2}{2^{2l}p!(l-p)!}\sum_{k=0}^{[l/2]-p}(-1)^k\binom{l-p}{k}\binom{2l-2p-2k}{l}. \tag{11.17}$$

Now we use the following relation **[12,** Russian p.620, formula (62)]:

$$\sum_{k=0}^{[n/2]}(-1)^k\binom{n}{k}\binom{2n-2k}{n+m} = 2^{n-m}\binom{n}{m}.$$

Taking $n = l - p$ and $m = p$ in this formula, we obtain

$$\sum_{k=0}^{[(l-p)/2]}(-1)^k\binom{l-p}{k}\binom{2l-2p-2k}{l} = 2^{l-2p}\binom{l-p}{p}. \tag{11.18}$$

Let us note that in this formula the upper summation limit can be decreased up to $[l/2]-p$, since $\binom{2l-2p-2k}{l} = 0$ for $k > [l/2]-p$. Substituting (11.18) into (11.17) we obtain

$$\gamma(p,l) = (-1)^p\frac{\pi(l!)^2}{2^{l+2p}(p!)^2(l-2p)!}.$$

Finally, substituting this value for $\gamma(p,l)$ into (11.16), we come to (11.14). Lemma 11.1 is proved. □

§12. Proof of Lemma 10.1

First we show that Lemma 10.1 follows from the following result.

LEMMA 12.1. *For $n \geq 3$, $m \geq 1$, $0 \leq p \leq [m/2]$ the numbers $a_0(p,m,n)$ defined by* (11.14) *are positive. The numbers $\widetilde{a}(p,m,n)$ defined by*

$$\widetilde{a}(p,m,n) = \frac{1}{2^{2p}(p!)^2}\sum_{k=2p}^{m}(-1)^k\frac{(k+1)!}{2^k(m-k)!(k-2p)!\Gamma(k+(n/2))} \tag{12.1}$$

are positive in each of the following two cases:
1) $n = 3$, $1 \leq m \leq 2$, $0 \leq p \leq [m/2]$, *and*
2) $n \geq 4$, $m \geq 1$, $0 \leq p \leq [m/2]$.

Indeed, Lemma 11.1 gives the following representation for the operator $B = (n-1)A_0 - m^2A_1$:

$$B = m!\Gamma(n/2)\sum_{p=0}^{[m/2]} b(p,m,n)i^p j^p, \tag{12.2}$$

where

$$b(p,m,n) = (n-1)a_0(p,m,n) - ma_1(p,m,n). \tag{12.3}$$

For $n > m \geq 1$ we use the positivity of $a_0(p,m,n)$ to obtain from (12.3) that

$$b(p,m,n) \geq m[a_0(p,m,n) - a_1(p,m,n)]. \tag{12.4}$$

Comparing (11.4) and (12.1), we see that

$$a_0(p,m,n) - a_1(p,m,n) = \widetilde{a}(p,m,n) \tag{12.6}$$

Relations (12.3) and (12.5) show that the positivity of $b(p,m,n)$ follows from the positivity of $\widetilde{a}(p,m,n)$.

So, for $n > m \geq 1$, $n \geq 3$ all coefficient of the sum (12.2) are positive. Therefore for $0 \neq f \in S^m$ we have

$$\langle Bf, f\rangle = m!\Gamma(n/2)\sum_{p=0}^{[m/2]} b(p,m,n)\langle j^p f, i^p f\rangle \geq m!\Gamma(n/2)b(0,m,n)|f|^2 > 0,$$

proving Lemma 10.1

PROOF OF LEMMA 12.1. Consider the integral

$$I_\alpha(p,m,n) = \int_0^1 x^{2p+\alpha}(1-x)^{(n/2)-p-\alpha}(1-x/2)^{m-2p}\,dx. \tag{12.6}$$

This integral converges under the following restrictions on parameters:

$$0 \leq p \leq [m/2], \qquad 0 \leq \alpha < (n/2) - 1, \tag{12.7}$$

and is, evidently, positive.

We transform (12.6), expanding the last factor in the integrand in powers of x:

$$I_\alpha(p,m,n) = (m-2p)! \sum_{r=0}^{m-2p} \frac{(-1)^r}{2^r r!(m-2p-r)!} \int_0^1 x^{r+2p+\alpha}(1-x)^{(n/2)-2-\alpha}\,dx.$$

Expressing the integral in the right-hand side of this formula in terms of the function Γ, we get

$$\begin{aligned} I_\alpha(p,m,n) \\ = \Gamma((n/2)-1-\alpha)(m-2p)! \sum_{r=0}^{m-2p} (-1)^r \frac{\Gamma(r+2p+\alpha+1)}{2^r r!(m-2p-r)!\Gamma(r+2p+(n/2))}. \end{aligned}$$

Changing the summation variable by the formula $k = r+2p$, we obtain

$$\begin{aligned} & I_\alpha(p,m,n) \\ \text{(12.8)} \quad & = \frac{\Gamma((n/2)-1-\alpha)(m-2p)!}{2^{2p}} \sum_{k=2p}^{m} (-1)^k \frac{\Gamma(k+1+\alpha)}{2^k (m-k)!(k-2p)!\Gamma(k+(n/2))}. \end{aligned}$$

In (12.8), set $\alpha = 0$. Conditions (12.7) become $n \ge 3$, $0 \le p \le [m/2]$. As a result, we get

$$I_0(p,m,n) = \frac{\Gamma((n/2)-1)(m-2p)!}{2^{2p}} \sum_{k=2p}^{m-2p} (-1)^k \frac{k!}{2^k (m-k)!(k-2p)!\Gamma(k+n/2)}.$$

The right-hand side of this formula differs from the right-hand side of (11.4) with $\alpha = 0$ by a positive factor. Therefore, positivity of $I_0(p,m,n)$ implies positivity of $a_0(p,m,n)$. The first statement of Lemma 12.1 is proved.

Now we set $\alpha = 1$ in (12.8). Conditions (12.7) become $n \ge 5$, $0 \le p \le [m/2]$. As a result, we get

$$I_1(p,m,n) = \frac{\Gamma((n/2)-2)(m-2p)!}{2^{2p}} \sum_{k=2p}^{m} (-1)^k \frac{(k+1)!}{2^k (m-k)!(k-2p)!\Gamma(k+n/2)}.$$

The right-hand side of this formula differs from the right-hand side of (12.1) by a positive factor. Therefore, positivity of $I_1(p,m,n)$ implies positivity of $\widetilde{a}_0(p,m,n)$. Therefore, the second statement of Lemma 12.1 is proved for $n \ge 5$.

For $n = 4$, formula (12.1) takes the form

$$\widetilde{a}(p,m,4) = \frac{1}{2^{2p}(p!)^2} \sum_{k=2p}^{m} \frac{(-1)^k}{2^k (m-k)!(k-2p)!}.$$

Changing the variable by the formula $k = 2p + r$, we get

$$\widetilde{a}(p,m,4) = \frac{1}{2^{4p}(p!)^2(m-2p)!} \sum_{r=0}^{m-2p} (-1/2)^r \binom{m-2p}{r} = \frac{1-1/2)^{m-2p}}{2^{4p}(p!)^2(m-2p)!} > 0.$$

Finally, for $n = 3$ the second statement is verified by direct computation using formula (12.1). □

§13. Concluding remarks

As we have already noted, the restriction $n > m$ is presumably not crucial for the validity of Theorem 3.1, and is required only by the approach we used. However, even in the framework of this approach this restriction does not exhaust its capacity. Indeed, we have used this restriction only in the proof of Lemma 10.1, which is equivalent to the positive definiteness of the operator B. Therefore we come to the following problem.

PROBLEM. For which m and n is the operator

$$B = (n-1)A_0 - m^2 A_1 = \frac{1}{\omega}\int_\Omega \left[(n-1)P_\xi - m^2 i_\xi P_\xi j_\xi\right] d\omega(\xi)$$

positive definite on the space $S^m\mathbb{R}^n$?

Theorem 3.1 is valid for those pairs m, n for which the answer to this question is positive.

Lemma 10.1 gives a partial answer to this problem, but the author could not get a complete solution.

If we change the condition $n > m$ to $n - 1 \geq \beta m$ with some $\beta < 1$, the inequality (12.4) becomes

$$b(p,m,n) \geq n[\beta a_0(p,m,n) - a_1(p,m,n)] = m\widetilde{a}_\beta(p,m,n),$$

where

$$\widetilde{a}_\beta(p,m,n) = \frac{1}{2^{2p}(p!)^2}\sum_{k=2p}^{m}(-1)^k \frac{(k+\beta)k!}{2^k(m-k)!(k-2p)!\Gamma(k+(n/2))}.$$

Therefore, the above problem is reduced to the following question: for which β are the numbers $\widetilde{a}_\beta(p,m,n)$ positive for $n-1 \geq \beta m$, $0 \leq p \leq [m/2]$?

Another possible approach to the solution of this problem can consist in the description of eigenvalues of the operator B and the verification that they are positive. One can easily see that each of the operators A_α, $\alpha = 0, 1$, has $[m/2]+1$ proper eigenspaces $S^m_k \subset S^m$ with S^m_k, $0 \leq k \leq [m/2]$, consisting of tensors of the form $i^k f$, where $f \in S^{m-2k}$ satisfy the condition $jf = 0$. The space S^m_k corresponds to the eigenvalue $\lambda_0(m-2k,m,n)$ of the operator A_0, which is related to the corresponding coefficient $\mu(m-2k,m,n)$ in the expansion

$$\frac{t^m|t|^{n-2}}{(1-t^2)^{(n-2)/n}} = \sum_{k=-\infty}^{[m/2]} \mu(m-2k,m,n)C_{m-2k}^{((n/2)-1)}(t) \tag{13.1}$$

with respect to Gegenbauer polynomials by the formula

$$\lambda_0(m-2k,m,n) = \frac{n-2}{n+2m-4k-2}\mu(m-2k,m,n).$$

At the same time, S^m_k corresponds to the eigenvalue $\lambda_1(m-2k,m,n)$ of the operator A_1, which is related to coefficients of the expansion (13.1) by the formula

$$\lambda_1(m-2k,m,n) = \frac{n-2}{m(n+2m-4k-2)} \times [(m+n-2) - \mu(m-2k,m,n)(m+n-3)\mu(m-2k,m-2,n)].$$

For $m-2k=0$, the corresponding eigenvalue of the operator A_1 equals zero. Therefore, our problem reduces to verifying the positivity of certain linear combinations of coefficients of the expansion (13.1), and this runs into serious algebraic difficulties.

Becoming desperate in attempts to find a theoretical solution, the author turned to an experiment and computed the eigenvalues of the operator B for $1 \le m \le 50$. Results of these computations allow him to conjecture that the answer to the problem is positive for $\nu \ge (8m+23)/13$.

References

1. H. K. Aben, *Integral photoelastisity*, "Valgus", Tallinn, 1975. (Russian)
2. V. A. Sharafutdinov, *On the method of integral photoelastisity in the weak optical anisotropy case*, Eesti NSV Tead. Akad. Toimetised Füüs.-Mat. **38** (1989), no. 4, 379–389. (Russian)
3. Yu. A. Kravtsov and Yu. I. Orlov, *Geometrical optics of nonhomogeneous media*, "Nauka", Moscow, 1980. (Russian)
4. L. B. Vertgeim, *Integral geometry with a matrix weight and a nonlinear problem of matrix reconstruction*, Dokl. Akad. Nauk SSSR **319** (1991), no. 3, 531–534; English transl. in Soviet Math. Dokl. **44** (1992).
5. S. Helgason, *The Radon transform*, Birkhäuser, Boston, MA, 1980.
6. L. N. Pestov and V. A. Sharafutdinov, *Integral geometry of tensor fields on manifolds of negative curvature*, Sibirsk. Mat. Zh. **29** (1988), no. 3, 114–130; English transl. in Siberian Math. J. **29** (1988).
7. V. A. Sharafutdinov, *Integral geometry of a tensor field on manifolds of bounded curvature*, Sibirsk. Mat. Zh. **33** (1992), no. 3, 192–204; English transl. in Siberian Math. J. **33** (1992).
8. R. Palais, *Seminar on the Atiyah-Singer index theorem*, Princeton Univ. Press, Princeton, NJ, 1965.
9. V. A. Sharafutdinov, *An integral geometry problem for tensor fields and the Saint-Venant equation*, Sibirsk. Mat. Zh. **24** (1983), no. 3, 176–187; English transl. in Siberian Math. J. **24** (1983).
10. D. Gromoll, W. Klingenberg, and W. Meyer, *Riemannsche Geometrie im Grossen*, Lecture Notes in Math., vol. 55, Springer-Verlag, Berlin, 1968.
11. L. Schwartz, *Méthodes mathématiques pour les sciences physiques*, Hermann, Paris, 1961.
12. A. P. Prudnikov, Yu. A. Brychkov, and O. I. Marichev, *Integrals and series*, "Nauka", Moscow, 1984; English transl., Gordon and Breach, New York, 1986.

Institute of Mathematics, Siberian Branch of the Russian Academy of Sciences, 4, Universitetskiĭ pr., Novosibirsk, 630090, Russia

Amer. Math. Soc. Transl.
(2) Vol. **162**, 1994

Exponential Radon Transform

I. Ya. Shneĭberg

§1. Introduction

In emission tomography, the Radon transform with the weight

$$g(w,p) = (R_\gamma f)(w,p) = \int_{x\cdot w=p} f(x)\gamma(w,x)\,dl \tag{1}$$

is sometimes used (see [1]); here $f:\mathbb{R}^2\to\mathbb{R}^1$, $w\in S^1$, $x\cdot w$ is the inner product of x and w, dl in the linear measure on the line $x\cdot w=p$,

$$\gamma(x,w) = \exp\left(\int_0^\infty \rho(x+tw^\perp)\,dt\right),$$

and $\rho(x)$ is the absorption coefficient of the medium at the point x. The mathematical theory of operators of the form (1) is related to problems of integral geometry [16] and to inverse problems for the kinetic equation (see [2]). Necessary conditions for the solvability of the equation (2) are obtained in [3]. In [4], the semi-Fredholm property of the operator R_γ in Sobolev spaces is established and a numerical algorithm for solving the equation (1) is suggested. More complete results are known for weights γ of a special form. If $\gamma(w,x)=e^{\nu(w)\cdot x}$, then the corresponding transformation is called the *exponential Radon transform*,

$$(R_\nu f)(w,p) = \int_{x\cdot w=p} f(x)e^{\nu(w)\cdot x}\,ds; \tag{2}$$

here $f:\mathbb{R}^n\to\mathbb{R}^1$ $(n\ge 2)$, $\nu: S^{n-1}\to\mathbb{R}^n$, and ds is the Lebesgue measure on the hyperplane $x\cdot w=p$. For $n=2$, the operator (2) occurs in the emission tomography of media with absorption coefficient independent of x, but depending on the direction of the radiation. For $n>2$ one can naturally introduce the so-called *ray exponential transform*

$$(\mathscr{P}_\mu f)(\theta,x) = \int_{-\infty}^{\infty} f(x+\theta t)e^{\mu(\theta)t}\,dt, \tag{3}$$

where $\mu: S^{n-1}\to\mathbb{R}^1$ and $x\cdot\theta=0$. The function $(\mathscr{P}_\mu f)(\theta,x)$ is defined on the set $T=\{(\theta,x): \theta\in S^{n-1},\ x\in\mathbb{R}^n,\ \theta\cdot x=0\}$. In the case $n=2$ the operators R_ν and $\mathscr{P}_\mu$ essentially coincide (in the first case w is the normal vector to the line, and in the second case w is the director vector). The inversion formula for a constant μ is obtained in this case in [5]. In [5, 6] for $n=2$ a formula is proved that expresses the function $g_0 = R_0 f$ $(\nu = 0)$ in terms of the function $g = R_\nu f$. This enabled the authors to write down certain relations for the function g that are important for the construction of algorithms for numerical solution of the equation (1) suggested in **[6]**. In **[7, 15]** it is proved that these relations provide a set of necessary and sufficient conditions for a function g to belong to the image of the operator R_ν. A number of interesting properties of the operators R_ν and $\mathscr{P}_\mu$ was established in **[5, 6]**.

Using the multidimensional Cauchy theorem for holomorphic functions, several formulas for the operator R_ν in the case of $n = 2$ and a constant function ν were established in **[10]**. An ingenious method for selecting the integration region suggested by Kuchment in **[11]** allowed him to obtain some new explicit inversion formulas. In this paper we prove inversion formulas for the operators R_ν and $\mathscr{P}_\mu$ for any $n \geq 2$ and for arbitrary smooth functions ν and μ. In §4 we present another inversion formula (see (28) and (32)) for the operator R_ν in the case when $n = 2$ and $\nu = \text{const}$. The numerical realization of this formula leads to significantly smaller artifacts than all algorithms known before.

§2. Auxiliary formulas for holomorphic functions

In this section we assume that $\nu\colon S^{n-1} \to \mathbb{R}^n$ and $\mu\colon S^{n-1} \to \mathbb{R}^1$ are smooth functions, with $\nu(w) \cdot w = 0$ for all $w \in S^{n-1}$.

In the space $\mathbb{C}^n$, let us consider the $(n+1)$-dimensional submanifold $\Omega_\nu = \{\xi + i\tau\varphi(w)\}$, where $\xi \in \mathbb{R}^n \setminus \{0\}$, $w = \xi/|\xi|$, $0 \leq \tau \leq \min(\xi/|\varphi(w)|, 1)$. The boundary of Ω_ν consists of three parts: $\Gamma_0 = \{\xi : \xi \in \mathbb{R}^n\}$, $\Gamma_1\{\xi + i|\xi|(\nu(w)/|\nu(w)|),\ |\xi| \leq \nu(w)|\}$, $\Gamma_2 = \{\xi + i\nu(w),\ |\xi| \geq |\nu(w)|\}$.

Set $z_j = \xi_j + i\eta_j$, $j = 1, \dots, n$, $\xi_j, \eta_j \in \mathbb{R}^1$. The restriction of the differential form $dz_1 \wedge \dots \wedge dz_n$ to Γ_0 coincides with the form $d\xi_1 \wedge \dots \wedge d\xi_n$, and its restriction to Γ_1 vanishes. Indeed, $\Gamma_1 = \{z = (z_1, \dots, z_n) : z_j = \xi_j + i|\xi|(\nu_j(w)/|\nu(w)|),\ j = 1, \dots, n\}$. We have

$$\sum_{j=1}^n z_j^2 = \sum_{j=1}^n \left(\xi_j + i|\xi|\frac{\nu_j(w)}{|\nu(w)|}\right)^2 = \sum_{j=1}^n \xi_j^2 - |\xi|^2 = 0.$$

The indicated choice of the set Ω_ν, when the form $dz_1 \wedge \dots \wedge dz_n$ vanishes on a piece of the boundary of Ω_ν that is not contained in the union of $\mathbb{R}^n$ and the manifold $\{\xi + i\nu(w)\}$, was suggested by Kuchment (see **[11]**).

The restriction of $dz_1 \wedge \dots \wedge dz_n$ to Γ_2, written in the coordinates ξ, has the form $V(\xi)d\xi_1 \wedge \dots \wedge d\xi_n$, where $V(\xi)$ is a function that can be computed from the mapping ν. Let us assume now that a function $F : \mathbb{R}^n \to \mathbb{R}^1$ can be analytically extended to Ω_ν and that $|F(z)| \leq c(1 + |\operatorname{Re} z|)^{-\alpha}$ for some $\alpha > n$ and for an arbitrary $z \in \Omega$. Denote

$$\varkappa(t) = \begin{cases} 1, & t > 0, \\ 0, & t < 0. \end{cases}$$

Cauchy's theorem, together with the above remarks, implies

LEMMA 1. *We have*

$$\begin{aligned} &\int_{\mathbb{R}^n} F(\xi) d\xi_1 \wedge \dots \wedge d\xi_n \\ &\quad = \int_{\mathbb{R}^n} F(\xi + i\nu(\xi/|\xi|)) V(\xi) \varkappa(|\xi| - |\nu(\xi)|) d\xi_1 \wedge \dots \wedge d\xi_n. \end{aligned} \tag{4}$$

Now we consider formula (4) in the case $\nu = 2$. Since $\nu(w)\cdot w = 0$, in this case we have $\nu(w) = \mu(w^\perp)w^\perp$, where $w = (\cos\varphi, \sin\varphi)$, $w^\perp = (-\sin\varphi, \cos\varphi)$, $\mu\colon S^1 \to \mathbb{R}^1$. In Γ_2, introduce polar coordinates $\xi_1 = \sigma\cos\varphi$, $\xi_2 = \sigma\sin\varphi$. Then

$$
\begin{aligned}
dz_1 \wedge dz_2\,|_{\Gamma_2} &= d(\sigma\cos\varphi - i\mu(w^\perp)\sin\varphi)\wedge d(\sigma\sin\varphi + i\mu(w^\perp)\cos\varphi)\\
&= (\sigma + i\,d\mu/d\varphi).
\end{aligned}
\tag{5}
$$

Formulas (4) and (5) imply

$$
\begin{aligned}
&\int_{\mathbb{R}^2} F(\xi)\,d\xi_1\,d\xi_2\\
&\quad= \int_{S^1}\int_0^\infty F(\sigma w + \mu(w^\perp)w^\perp)\varkappa(\sigma - |\mu(w^\perp)|)\left(\sigma + i\frac{d\mu}{d\varphi}\right)d\sigma\,d\varphi\\
&\quad= \int_{S^1}\int M_\theta^+ F(\xi + i\mu(\theta)\theta)\varkappa(|\xi| - |\mu(\theta)|)(|\xi| + i(\mathscr{D}\mu)(\xi,\theta))\,d\xi_\theta\,d\theta.
\end{aligned}
\tag{6}
$$

In the last formula we have $\theta = w^\perp$, $M_\theta^+ = \{\xi \in \mathbb{R}^2 : (\xi/|\xi|)^\perp = \theta\}$, $d\xi_\theta$ is a measure on the line $M_\theta = \{\xi \in \mathbb{R}^2 : \xi\cdot\theta = 0\}$, and

$$
(\mathscr{D}\mu)(\xi,\theta) = \frac{d}{dt}\left[\mu(\cos t\theta - \sin t(\xi/|\xi|))\right]\Big|_{t=0}.
$$

Taking $\nu(w) = -\mu(w^\perp)w^\perp$ and $M_\theta^- = \{\xi \in \mathbb{R}^2 : (\xi/|\xi|)^\perp = -\theta\}$, we get a formula of the form (6) with the inner integral taken over M_θ^-. Combining these two cases, we get

$$
\begin{aligned}
\int_{S^1}\int M_\theta F(\xi)|\xi|\,d\xi_\theta\,d\theta &= 2\int_{\mathbb{R}^2} F(\xi)\,d\xi_1\,d\xi_2\\
&= \int_{S^1}\int M_\theta F(\xi + i\mu(\theta)\theta)\varkappa(|\xi| - |\mu(\theta)|)(|\xi| + i(\mathscr{D}\mu)(\xi,\theta))\,d\xi_\theta\,d\theta.
\end{aligned}
\tag{7}
$$

Let $F\colon \mathbb{R}^n \to \mathbb{R}^1$. We have the following equality (see **[10]**):

$$
\int_{\mathbb{R}^n} F(\xi)d\xi_1\cdots d\xi_n = \frac{1}{m(S^{n-2})}\int_{S^{n-1}}\int L_\theta|\xi|F(\xi)\,d\xi_L\,d\theta,
\tag{8}
$$

where $d\xi_L$ is the Lebesgue measure on the hyperplane $L_\theta = \{\xi \in \mathbb{R}^n : \xi\cdot\theta = 0\}$.

Later we will need the following lemma.

LEMMA 2. *Let $f\colon T \to \mathbb{R}^1$ and $1 < r \le n$. Then*

$$
\int_{S^{n-1}}\int L_\theta f(\theta,\xi)\,d\xi_L\,d\theta = a_{n,r}\int_{G_{n,r}}\int_{S^{r-1}(M)}\int_{M_\theta}|\xi|^{n-r}f(\theta,\xi)\,d\xi_\theta\,d\theta_M\,dM,
\tag{9}
$$

where $G_{n,r}$ is the set of all r-dimensional subspaces in $\mathbb{R}^n$, dM is the normalized rotation-invariant measure on $G_{n,r}$, $S^{r-1}(M)$ is the radius 1 sphere in the r-dimensional subspace $M \in G_{n,r}$, $M_\theta = L_\theta \cap M$, $d\xi_\theta$ is the Lebesgue measure on the $(r-1)$-dimensional subspace M_θ, $d\theta_M$ is the measure on $S^{r-1}(M)$,

$$
a_{n,r} = \frac{(n-1)m(S^{n-1})m(B^{n-1})}{m(S^{r-1})m(S^{r-2})},
$$

$m(S^{n-1})$ is the volume of the sphere S^{n-1}, and $m(B^{n-1})$ is the volume of the $(n-1)$-dimensional ball B^{n-1}.

PROOF. Both the left- and the right-hand side in (9) are continuous linear functionals on the space $C_0(T)$ of continuous compactly supported functions on T. Denote these functionals by Φ_1 and Φ_2 respectively. Let U be an orthogonal linear transformation of $\mathbb{R}^n$ and $\lambda \neq 0$. Define $U_\lambda : T \to T$ by $U_\lambda(w, \xi) = (Uw, \lambda U\xi)$. Denote by U_λ^* the operator in $C_0(T)$ defined by $(U_\lambda^* f)(w, \xi) = f(Uw, \lambda U\xi)$. We have

$$\Phi_1(U_\lambda^* f) = |\lambda|^{1-n}\Phi_1(f), \qquad \Phi_2(U_\lambda^* f) = |\lambda|^{1-n}\Phi_2(f). \tag{10}$$

Since the transformations U_λ acts transitively on $T \setminus (S^{n-1} \times \{0\})$, formula (10) implies that there exists a constant $a_{n,r}$ such that $\Phi_1(f) = a_{n,r}\Phi_2(f)$ for all $f \in C_0(T)$. Taking $f(w, \xi) = \chi_{[0,1]}(|\xi|)$, we get the value of $a_{n,r}$ indicated in the lemma. □

LEMMA 3. *We have*

$$\int_{\mathbb{R}^n} F(\xi)d\xi_1 \cdots d\xi_n = \frac{1}{m(S^{n-2})} \int_{S^{n-1}} \int L_\theta \left[|\xi|^2 - \mu^2(\theta)\right]^{(n-2)/2}$$
$$\times |\xi|^{2-n} F(\xi + i\mu(\theta)\theta)(|\xi| + i(\mathscr{D}\mu)(\xi, \theta))\varkappa(|\xi| - |\mu(\theta)|)\, d\xi_L\, d\theta.$$

PROOF. Formula (8) and Lemma 2 imply that

$$\int_{\mathbb{R}^n} F(\xi)d\xi_1 \cdots d\xi_n = \frac{1}{m(S^{n-2})} \int_{S^{n-1}} \int L_\theta |\xi| F(\xi)\, d\xi_L\, d\theta$$
$$= \frac{a_{n,r}}{m(S^{n-2})} \int_{G_{n,2}} J(M)\, dM,$$

where

$$J(M) = \int_{S^1(M)} \int_{M_\theta} |\xi|^{n-2} F(\xi)|\xi|\, d\xi_\theta\, d\theta_M.$$

By formula (7),

$$J(M) = \int_{S^1(M)} \int_{M_\theta} |\xi + \mu(\theta)\theta|^{n-2} F(\xi + i\mu(\theta)\theta)$$
$$\times \varkappa(|\xi| - |\mu(\theta)|)(|\xi| + i(\mathscr{D}\mu)(\xi, \theta))\, d\xi_L\, d\theta.$$

Since $|\xi + \mu(\theta)\theta| = \sqrt{|\xi|^2 - \mu^2(\theta)}$, applying Lemma 2 once again, this time to the integral $\int_{G_{n,2}} J(M)\, dM$, we come to the conclusion of Lemma 3. □

§3. Inversion formulas for the operators R_ν and $\mathscr{P}_\mu$

For functions g and g_0 defined on $S^{n-1} \times \mathbb{R}^1$, by $g * g_0$ we will denote the convolution of these functions with respect to the linear variable,

$$g * g_0(w, p) = \int_{-\infty}^{\infty} g(w, t) g_0(w, p - t)\, dt,$$

and by $\widetilde{g}(w, \sigma)$ the Fourier transform of the function $g(w, p)$ with respect to the second variable. For a function $K : S^{n-1} \times \mathbb{R}^1 \to \mathbb{R}^1$ define

$$(R_{-\nu}^\# K)(x) = \int_{S^{n-1}} K(w, x \cdot w) e^{-\nu(w) \cdot x}\, dw.$$

We will need the following formulas (see **[10]**):

$$R^{\#}_{-\nu}(K * R_\nu f) = (R^{\#}_{-\nu} K) * f, \tag{11}$$

$$\widetilde{g}(w,\sigma) = (\widetilde{R_\nu f})(w,\sigma) = (2\pi)^{(n-1)/2}\widetilde{f}(\theta w + i\nu(w)); \tag{12}$$

here $\widetilde{f}$ is the Fourier transform of a function $f\colon \mathbb{R}^n \to \mathbb{R}^1$. Let us note that if $\nu_0(w) = \nu(w) - (\nu(w)\cdot w)w$, then

$$\begin{aligned}(R_\nu f)(w,p) &= \int_{x\cdot w = p} f(x)\exp\left[(\nu(w)\cdot w)(w\cdot x) + \nu_0(w)\cdot x\right] ds\\ &= e^{(\nu(w)\cdot w)p}(R_{\nu_0} f)(w,p).\end{aligned} \tag{13}$$

Formula (13) shows that it suffices to obtain an inversion formula for the operator R_{ν_0}. Since $\nu_0(w)\cdot w = 0$, below we will consider operators R_ν under the additional assumption

$$\nu(w)\cdot w = 0. \tag{14}$$

Let $f \in C_0^\infty(\mathbb{R}^n)$. For $K\colon S^{n-1}\times\mathbb{R}^1 \to \mathbb{R}^1$ we define the operator Λ_k by the formula

$$\widetilde{\Lambda_k(g)}(w,\sigma) = K(w,\sigma)\widetilde{g}(w,\sigma).$$

Formulas (4) and (12) show that

$$\begin{aligned}f(x) &= (2\pi)^{-n/2}\int_{\mathbb{R}^n}\widetilde{f}(\xi)e^{ix\xi}d\xi_1\cdots d\xi_n\\ &= (2\pi)^{(1/2)-n}\int_{S^{n-1}}\int_{\mathbb{R}^1}\widetilde{g}(w,\sigma)\varkappa(\sigma - |\nu(w)|)\sigma V(\sigma w)e^{i\sigma x\cdot w}\,d\sigma e^{-x\cdot\nu(w)}\,dw.\end{aligned} \tag{15}$$

Set $K(w,\sigma) = \sigma V(\sigma w)\varkappa(\sigma - |\nu(w)|)$. Equality (15) implies the following inversion formula:

$$f = (2\pi)^{1-n}R^{\#}_{-\nu}\Lambda_K R_\nu f. \tag{16}$$

When $n = 2$ and $\nu(w) = \mu(w^\perp)w^\perp$, where $\mu\colon S^1 \to \mathbb{R}^1$, the function K is given by

$$K(w,\sigma) = \left(\sigma_i\frac{d\mu}{\varphi}\right)\varkappa(\sigma - |\mu(w)|).$$

If $\mu(w)$ is the constant function taking the value μ, then the inversion formula is

$$f = (2\pi)^{-1}R^{\#}_{-\mu}\Lambda^+_\mu R_\mu f, \tag{17}$$

where $(\widetilde{\Lambda^+_\mu g})(w,\sigma) = \varkappa(\sigma - |\mu|)\sigma$.

Let $c\colon \mathbb{R}^1 \to \mathbb{R}^1$ be an odd function and $F(w,p) = c(p)$. One can easily verify that for a constant μ we have $R^{\#}_{-\mu}F = 0$. Together with (11) and (17), this implies that

$$f = (4\pi)^{-1}R^{\#}_{-\mu}\Lambda_\mu R_\mu f, \tag{18}$$

with $(\widetilde{\Lambda_\mu g})(w,\sigma) = \sigma\varkappa(|\sigma| - |\mu|)\sigma$. Formula (18) is well known and was first obtained in **[5]**.

Now we consider the inversion formula for the ray transform $\mathscr{P}_\mu$ in $\mathbb{R}^n$. For a function $g\colon T \to \mathbb{R}^1$ and $\xi \cdot \theta = 0$ denote

$$\widetilde{g}(w, \xi) = (2\pi)^{(1-n)/2} \int_{L_\theta} g(\theta, x) e^{-i\xi x}\, dx_L.$$

We have (see **[8]**)

$$\widetilde{g(\theta, \xi)} = (\widetilde{\mathscr{P}_\mu f})(\theta, \xi) = \sqrt{2\pi}\widetilde{f}(\xi + i\mu(\theta)\theta).$$

Lemma 3 and formula (19) imply

$$\begin{aligned} f(x) &= (2\pi)^{-n/2} \int_{\mathbb{R}^n} \widetilde{f}(\xi)\, d\xi_1 \cdots d\xi_n \\ &= \frac{m(S^{n-2})}{(2\pi)^{(n+1)/2}} \int_{S^{n-1}} \int_{L_\theta} [|\xi|^2 - \mu^2(\theta)]^{(n-2)/2} \widetilde{g}(\theta, \xi)(|\xi| + i(\mathscr{D}\mu)(\theta, \xi)) \\ &\qquad \times \varkappa(|\xi| - |\mu(\theta)|)|\xi|^{2-n} e^{ix\xi}\, dx_L e^{-x\mu(\theta)\theta}\, d\theta. \end{aligned}$$

This formula gives the following result.

THEOREM 1. *We have the equality*

$$f(x) = \frac{1}{2\pi m(S^{n-2})} (\mathscr{P}^{\#}_{-\mu} \Lambda_U \mathscr{P}_\mu f)(x), \tag{20}$$

where

$$U(\theta, \xi) = [|\xi|^2 - \mu^2(\theta)]^{(n-2)/2} |\xi|^{2-n} (|\xi| + i(\mathscr{D}\mu)(\theta, \xi)) \varkappa(|\xi| - |\mu(\theta)|),$$

$$(\mathscr{P}^{\#}_{-\mu} g)(x) = \int_{S^{n-1}} g(\theta, P_\theta x) e^{-\mu(\theta) x \cdot \theta}\, d\theta,$$

and P_θ is the orthogonal projection onto $\theta^\perp$.

For a constant function μ, the inversion formula (20) was established in **[8]**.

§4. The operator R_μ for $n = 2$ and a constant function μ

This case is particularly important in medical emission tomography. Numerical algorithms for the solution of the equation $R_\mu f = g$ are considered in **[6, 12, 13]**. In these papers it was noted that for a small number of projections ($N \sim 60$) and large diameter of the support of the function f ($\mu d \sim 6$) strong distortions appear on tomograms, which are mainly caused by the exponential (as $|x| \to \infty$) growth of error in the quadrature formula for the operator $R^{\#}_{-\mu}$:

$$(R^{\#}_{-\mu} F)(x) \sim \frac{2\pi}{N} \sum_{j=1}^{N} F(w_j, x \cdot w_j) e^{-\mu x \cdot w_j^\perp},$$

where $w_j = (\cos\varphi_j, \sin\varphi_j)$, $\varphi_j = (2\pi/N)(j - 1)$.

Here we show how to eliminate this growth of the error. Denote by $L_2(S^1 \times E)$ the Hilbert space of funtions $F(w, p)$ defined on the set $S^1 \times E$, where E is an interval in $\mathbb{R}^1$. Define the inner product by the formula

$$(F_1, F_2) = \int_{S^1} \int_E F_1(w, p)\overline{F_2(w, p)}\, dw\, dp.$$

Similarly to the ordinary Radon transform (see **[10]**), the operator R_μ acts continuously from the space $L_2(\Omega_a)$ to the space $L_2(S^1 \times [-a, a])$, $0 < a < \infty$, $\Omega_a = \{x \in \mathbb{R}^2 : |x| \leq a\}$. The operator $R^\#_{-\mu}$ is adjoint to R_μ and acts from $L_2(S^1 \times [-a, a])$ to $L_2(\Omega_a)$. The norms of the operators $R^\#_{-\mu}$ and R_μ tend to infinity as $a \to \infty$. Let $F \in L_2(S^1 \times [-a, a])$. Expanding F in a Fourier series with respect to the angle variable, we get

$$F(w, p) = \sum_{m=-\infty}^{\infty} F_m(p)e^{im\varphi} = \frac{1}{\sqrt{2\pi}} \sum_{m=-\infty}^{\infty} \left[\int_{\mathbb{R}^1} \widetilde{F}_m(\xi)e^{i\xi p}\, d\xi\right] e^{im\varphi}.$$

For $\alpha = \pm 1$ define operators $\mathscr{D}_\pm$ that project $F \in L_2(S^1 \times [-a, a])$ to the spaces of harmonics with positive ($\alpha = +1$) and negative ($\alpha = -1$) indices:

$$(\mathscr{D}_\alpha F)(w, p) = \sum_{m=0}^{\infty} \varkappa(\alpha m)F_m(p)e^{im\varphi}.$$

Next, define operators Q^μ_α by the formula

$$\widetilde{(Q^\mu_\alpha F)}(w, \xi) = \varkappa(\alpha\xi - \mu)\widetilde{F}(w, \xi).$$

THEOREM 2. *If $\mu \neq 0$, then the operator $Q^\mu_\alpha \mathscr{D}_\beta R_\mu$ (respectively, the operator $R^\#_\mu Q^\mu_\alpha \mathscr{D}_\beta)$) acts continuously from the space $L_2(R^2)$ to the space $L^2(S^1 \times \mathbb{R}^1)$ (respectively from $L^2(S^1 \times \mathbb{R}^1)$ to $L_2(R^2)$) if and only if $\alpha\beta = \operatorname{sgn}\mu$. If this is the case, then*

$$\|Q^\mu_\alpha \mathscr{D}_\beta R_\mu\| = \|R^\#_\mu Q^\mu_\alpha \mathscr{D}_\beta\| \leq \sqrt{2\pi/|\mu|}. \tag{21}$$

PROOF. We consider the operator $Q^\mu_+ \mathscr{D}_+ R_\mu$, $\mu > 0$. Define $g(w, p, \mu) = (R_\mu f)(w, p)$ and

$$g(w, p, \mu) = \sum_{m=-\infty}^{\infty} g_m(p, \mu)e^{im\varphi}.$$

In **[5, 6]** it is proved that

$$\widetilde{g}(\xi, \mu) = \left(\frac{\xi - \mu}{\sqrt{\xi^2 - \mu^2}}\right)^m \widetilde{g}(\sqrt{\xi^2 - \mu^2}, 0) \tag{22}$$

(the same branch of the square root is taken in both occurrences). We have

$$\begin{aligned} \|Q^\mu_+ \mathscr{D}_+ R_\mu f\|^2_{L_2(S^1 \times \mathbb{R}^1)} &= 2\pi \sum_{m=1}^{\infty} \left\| \left(\frac{\xi - \mu}{\sqrt{\xi^2 - \mu^2}}\right) \widetilde{g}(\sqrt{\xi^2 - \mu^2}, 0)\right\|^2_{L_2(\mu,\infty)} \\ &\leq \sum_{m=1}^{\infty} \left\|\widetilde{g}(\sqrt{\xi^2 - \mu^2}, 0)\right\|^2_{L_2(\mu,\infty)}. \end{aligned} \tag{23}$$

Since $\widetilde{g}(w,\xi,0)=\sqrt{2\pi}\widetilde{f}(\xi w)$ (see formula (12)), we have

$$\|f\|^2_{L_2(\mathbb{R}^2)}=\|\widetilde{f}\|^2_{L_2(\mathbb{R}^2)}=\sum_{m=-\infty}^{\infty}\int_0^{\infty}|\widetilde{g}_m(t,0)|^2\,dt. \tag{24}$$

Formulas (23) and (24) imply (21). On the other hand, if $\xi m<0$, then the factor $\left(\frac{\xi-m}{\xi+m}\right)^m$ tends to ∞ as $m\to\infty$, which implies that the operator $Q^{\mu}_{\alpha}\mathscr{D}_{\beta}R_{\mu}$ is unbounded if $\alpha\beta<0$. Theorem 2 is proved □

Below we will assume that $\mu>0$. Consider the action of the operator $R^{\#}_{-\mu}$ on an exponential function. Set $\chi_{\xi,m}(w,p)=e^{i(m\varphi+\xi p)}$. We have

$$(R^{\#}_{-\mu}\chi_{\xi,m})(x)=\int_0^{2\pi}\exp\{i[m\varphi+\xi(x_1\cos\varphi+x_2\sin\varphi)]\}$$
$$\times\exp[-\mu(-x_1\sin\varphi+x_2\cos\varphi)]\,d\varphi.$$

Denoting $x_1=r\cos\varphi$, $x_2=r\sin\varphi$, we get (see **[5]**) that for $|\xi|\neq\mu$

$$(R^{\#}_{-\mu}\chi_{\xi,m})(x)=2\pi i^m e^{im\theta}\left(\frac{\xi+\mu}{\sqrt{\xi^2-\mu^2}}\right)^m J_m(\sqrt{\xi^2-\mu^2},0), \tag{25}$$

where

$$J_m(z)=\frac{1}{2\pi}\int_0^{2\pi}e^{-i(m\varphi-z\sin\varphi)}\,d\varphi$$

is the Bessel function of order m. Passing in (25) to the limit as $\xi\to\mu$ and assuming that $m\geq 0$, we obtain

$$(R^{\#}_{-\mu}\chi_{\xi,m})(x)=\frac{2\pi i^m}{m!}(2\mu)^m|x|^m e^{im\theta}. \tag{26}$$

Formula (25) implies that

$$\lim_{|x|\to\infty}(R^{\#}_{-\mu}\chi_{\xi,m})(x)=\begin{cases}\infty, & |\xi|<\mu,\\ 0, & |\xi|>\mu.\end{cases} \tag{27}$$

Let us expand the function $g(w,p,\mu)=(R_{\mu}f)(w,p)$ in a Fourier series in φ and a Fourier integral in p:

$$g(w,p,\mu)=\sum_{m=-\infty}^{\infty}g_m(w,p)e^{im\varphi}=\frac{1}{\sqrt{2\pi}}\sum_{m=-\infty}^{\infty}\int_{\mathbb{R}^1}\widetilde{g}_m(\xi,\mu)e^{i\xi p}\,d\xi e^{im\varphi}.$$

Applying to $g(w,p,\mu)$ the inversion formula (18) and using (25), we obtain the following equality:

$$f(x)=\frac{1}{4\pi}(R^{\#}_{-\mu}\Lambda_{\mu}g)(x)=\sum_{m=-\infty}^{\infty}f_m(|x|)e^{im\varphi}, \tag{28}$$

where

$$f_m(r)=\frac{1}{\sqrt{2\pi}}\int_{|\xi|>\mu}\xi\widetilde{g}_m(\xi,\mu)c(\xi,mr)\,d\xi \tag{29}$$

and

$$c(\xi,m,r)=i^m\left(\frac{\xi+\mu}{\sqrt{\xi^2-\mu^2}}\right)^m J_m(\sqrt{\xi^2-\mu^2}r). \tag{30}$$

This formula, together with (22), implies

$$\widetilde{g}_m(\xi,\mu)c(\xi,m,r)=\widetilde{g}_m(-\xi,\mu)c(-\xi,m,r). \tag{31}$$

Formulas (30) and (31) show that if $\xi>0$, $m>0$, then replacing ξ by $-\xi$ in the product $\widetilde{g}_m(\xi,\mu)c(\xi,m,r)$ increases the modulus of the first factor and decreases the modulus of the second factor. Since $\widetilde{g}_m(\xi,\mu)$ is known only approximately, whereas $c(\xi,m,r)$ can be computed with any required precision, we can decrease the computation error using the formulas

$$\begin{gathered} f_m(r)=\sqrt{\frac{2}{\pi}}\int_{\Delta_m}\xi\widetilde{g}_m(\xi,\mu)c(\xi,m,r)\,d\xi,\\ \Delta_m=\begin{cases}[\mu,\infty), & m<0,\\ (-\infty,-\mu], & m>0.\end{cases}\end{gathered} \tag{32}$$

Formulas (28) and (32) can be rewritten in the operator form

$$f=(1/2\pi)(R^{\#}_{-\mu}\Lambda_\mu(Q_+\mathscr{D}_-+\tfrac{1}{2}\mathscr{D}_0+Q_-\mathscr{D}_+)g, \tag{33}$$

where

$$(\widetilde{Q_\alpha F})(w,\xi)=\varkappa(\alpha\xi)\widetilde{F}(w,\xi),\qquad (\mathscr{D}_0 g)(p)=\frac{1}{2\pi}\int_0^{2\pi}g(w,p)\,d\varphi.$$

The computation scheme based on (28) and (32) was realized on a computer by the author together with V. A. Dmitrichenko, S. D. Kalashnikov, and I. V. Ponomarev. A detailed discussion of this algorithm is given in their paper in the present collection.

§5. Cormack inversion formula

Let $T=S^1\times\mathbb{R}^1$. We will consider the spaces $H^s(T)$ and $H^s_+(T)$. The space $H^s(T)$ consists of functions $g\colon T\to\mathbb{R}^1$ with finite norm

$$\|g\|_{H^s(T)}=\int_0^{2\pi}\int_{-\infty}^{\infty}|\widetilde{g}(w,\sigma)|^2(1+\sigma^2)^s\,d\sigma\,d\varphi,$$

and

$$H^s_+(T)=\{g\in H^s(T):g(-w,-p)=g(w,p)\}.$$

If $f(x)=\sum_{-\infty}^{\infty}f_m(r)e^{im\theta}$, where $r=|x|$, $x_1=\cos\theta$, $x_2=\sin\theta$, then one can easily see that

$$g(w,p)=(R_\mu f)(w,p)=\sum_{-\infty}^{\infty}g_m(p)e^{im\varphi},$$

where

$$\begin{aligned} g_m(p)=\int_{|p|}^{\infty}f_m(r)\Big[&\exp(im\arccos(p/r)+\mu\sqrt{r^2-p^2})\\ &+\exp(-im\arccos(p/r)-\mu\sqrt{r^2-p^2})\Big]\frac{dr}{\sqrt{1-p^2/r^2}}.\end{aligned} \tag{34}$$

For $\mu = 0$, formula (34) turns into the well-known (see **[1, 14]**) formula

$$g_m(p) = (R_m f_m)(p) = 2\int_{|p|}^{\infty} f_m(r)T_m(p/r)\frac{dr}{\sqrt{1-p^2/r^2}}, \tag{35}$$

where $T_m(x) = \cos m \arccos x$ is the Chebyshev polynomial of the first kind. Formula (29) is the inversion formula for the integral operator (34). For $\mu = 0$, we obtain the inversion formula for the operator (35)

$$f_m(r) = (Q_m g_m)(r) = \frac{i^m}{\sqrt{2\pi}}\int_0^{\infty} \xi \widetilde{g}_m(\xi)J_m(\xi r)\,d\xi. \tag{36}$$

The operator $R = R_0$ can be extended from the space $C_0^\infty(\mathbb{R}^2)$ to the space

$$D = \left\{ f \in L_2(\mathbb{R}^2) : \int_0^{2\pi}\int_0^{\infty} |\widetilde{f}(\sigma w)|^2(1+\sigma)\,d\sigma\,d\varphi < \infty \right\}$$

If $f \in D$, then $g = Rf$ is given by the formula

$$\widetilde{g}(w,\sigma) = \widetilde{f}(\sigma w), \tag{37}$$

and the operator R establishes a one-to-one correspondence between D and the Banach space $H_+^{1/2}(T)$; the inverse operator Q, defined by (37), is continuous as an operator from $H_+^{1/2}(T)$ to $L_2(\mathbb{R}^2)$.

In **[1]** a series of inversion formulas (Cormack formulas) was considered for operators R_m applied to $f \in C_0^\infty$:

$$f_m(r) = (V_m g_m)(r) \int_r^{\infty} G_m(r,s)g_m'(s)\,ds + \int_0^r G_m^{(1)}(r,s)g_m'(s)\,ds, \tag{38}$$

where

$$G_m(r,s) = -\frac{1}{\pi r}\left[\left(s^2/r^2-1\right)^{-1/2} T_{|m|}(s/r) - P_{|m|}(s/r)\right],$$

$$G_m^{(1)}(r,s) = \frac{1}{\pi r}T_{|m|}(s/r), \qquad r > 0,$$

and $P_{|m|}$ is a polynomial of degree less than $|m|$, which is even for odd m and odd for even m. If $P_m(t) = \mathscr{U}_{|m|-1}(t)$, where $\mathscr{U}_m(t) = (\sin m \arccos t)/\sqrt{1-t^2}$ is the Chebyshev polynomial of the second kind, $\mathscr{U}_{-1} \equiv 0$, then

$$\begin{aligned} G_m(r,s) &= -\frac{1}{\pi r}\left(s^2/r^2-1\right)^{-1/2}\left[s/r + \sqrt{s^2/r^2-1}\right], \\ G_m^{(1)}(r,s) &= \frac{1}{\pi r}\mathscr{U}_{|m|-1}(s/r). \end{aligned} \tag{39}$$

One can easily show that

$$\int_r^{\infty} G_m^2(r,s)\,ds \le \gamma/r, \qquad \int_0^r \left[G_m^{(1)}(r,s)\right]^2 ds \le \gamma/r$$

for a constant γ and all $r > 0$. This implies that the operator V_m defined by formulas (38), (39) satisfies the estimate

$$|(V_m g_m)(r)| \le (\gamma/r)\|g_m'\|_{L_2(\mathbb{R}^1)}. \tag{40}$$

The Parseval formula for the Fourier-Bessel transform gives

$$(41)\quad \|Q_m g_m\|^2_{L_2(\mathbb{R}^1,r)} = \int_0^\infty \xi|\widetilde{g}_m(\xi)|^2\,d\xi \le \int_0^\infty (1+\xi)^2|\widetilde{g}_m(\xi)|^2\,d\xi = \|g_m\|_{H^1(\mathbb{R}^1)}.$$

The operators V_m and Q_m, being left inverse to the operator R_m in the space $C_0^\infty(\mathbb{R}^1)$, coincide on functions g in the image of R_m. The image of R_m in $C_0^\infty(\mathbb{R}^1)$ is determined by the relations (see **[16]**)

$$(42)\quad \begin{gathered} \int_{-\infty}^{\infty} p^k g_m(p)\,dp, \qquad 0 \le k < m, \\ g_m(-p) = (-1)^m g_m(p). \end{gathered}$$

Since the functionals (42) are not continuous on the space $H^1(\mathbb{R}^1)$, the set $R_m(C_0^\infty)$ is dense in $H^1_{+,m}(\mathbb{R}^1)$. Together with (40) and (41), this remark implies that the operators V_m and Q_m coincide on $H^1_{+,m}(\mathbb{R}^1)$. Therefore, formulas (28) and (29) are generalizations of Cormack formulas to the case $\mu \neq 0$.

References

1. F. Natterer, *The mathematics of computerized tomography*, Wiley, New York, 1985.
2. M. M. Lavrent′ev and Yu. E. Anikonov, *On a class of problems of integral geometry*, Dokl. Akad. Nauk SSSR **176** (1967), no. 6, 1240–1241; English transl. in Soviet Math. Dokl. **8** (1967).
3. F. Natterer, *Computerized tomography with unknown sources*, SIAM J. Appl. Math. **43** (1983), 1201–1212.
4. U. Heike, *Single-photon emission computed tomography by inverting the attenuated Radon transform with least-square collocation*, Inverse Problems **2** (1986), 307–330.
5. O. Tretyak and C. Metz, *The exponential Radon trasnform*, SIAM J. Appl. Math. **39** (1980), 341–357.
6. S. Bellini et al., *Compensation of tissue absorption in emission tomography*, IEEE Trans. Acoust. Speech Signal Process. **ASSP-27** (1979), no. 3, 213–218.
7. P. A. Kuchment and S. Ya. L′vin, *Paley-Wiener theorem for exponential Radon transform*, Dokl. Akad. Nauk SSSR **313** (1990), no. 6, 1329–1330; English transl. in Soviet Math. Dokl. **42** (1991).
8. I. A. Hazou and D. S. Solomon, *Inversion of the exponential X-ray transform*. I: *Analysis*, Math. Methods Appl. Sci. **10** (1988), 561–574.
9. ———, *Filtered backprojection and the exponential Radon transform*, J. Math. Pures Appl. (9) **141** (1989), 109–119.
10. F. Natterer, *On the inversion of the attenuated Radon transform*, Numer. Math. **32** (1979), 431–438.
11. P. Kuchment and I. Shneiberg, *Some inversion formulas in emission tomography*, Applicable Anal. (to appear).
12. I. A. Hazou and D. C. Solmon, *Inversion of the exponential X-ray transform*. II: *Numerics*, Math. Methods Appl. Sci. **13** (1990), 208–215.
13. G. Gillberg and T. Budinger, *Use of filtering methods to compensate for constant attenuation in single-photon emission computed tomography*, IEEE Trans. Biomedical Engrg. **BME-28** (1981), no. 2, 142–147.
14. A. N. Tikhonov, V. Ya. Arsenin, and A. A. Timonov, *Mathematical problems of computerized tomography*, "Nauka", Moscow, 1987. (Russian)
15. P. Kuchment and S. L′vin, *Paley-Wiener theorem for exponential Radon transform*, Acta Appl. Math. **18** (1990), 251–260.
16. I. M. Gel′fand, M. I. Graev, and N. Ya. Vilenkin, *Generalized functions*. Vol. 5: *Integral geometry and representation theory*, Fizmatgiz, Moscow, 1962; English transl., Academic Press, New York, 1966.

Amer. Math. Soc. Transl.
(2) Vol. **162**, 1994

On a New Reconstruction Algorithm in Emission Tomography

I. Ya. Shneĭberg, I. V. Ponomarev,
V. A Dmitrichenko, and S. D. Kalashnikov

§1.

The mathematical model of data gathering in single-photon emission tomography can be reduced to the weakened Radon transform (see **[1]**):

$$g_0(w, p) = \int_{x\cdot w=p} f(x)\exp\left\{-\int_{L(x)} \mu(y)\,dy\right\} dx, \tag{1}$$

where $f(x)$ is the density of the emission source at the point $x = (x_1, x_2)$, $\mu(y)$ is the attenuation coefficient at the point y, $w = (\cos\varphi, \sin\varphi)$ is a unit vector, and $L(x)$ is the segment of the straight line $x \cdot w = p$ between the point x and the boundary of the radiation absorbing object V. The function f vanishes outside the region V. In this paper we assume the attenuation coefficient μ to be constant. This assumption is justified, for example, for various types of biological tissue. The filtered backprojection algorithm is widely used in transmission tomography (see **[4]**). An analog of this algorithm for emission tomography is obtained in **[5]**. In this case, the equation (1) with a constant μ and a convex V can be reduced to the form

$$g(w, p) = (R_\mu)(w, p) = \int_{x\cdot w=p} f(x)e^{\mu x\cdot w^\perp}\,dx, \tag{2}$$

where

$$\begin{gathered} g(w, p) = g_0((w, p)e^{\mu c(w,p)}, \\ c(w, p) = \max\{t : pw + tw^\perp \in V\}, \qquad w^\perp = (-\sin\varphi, \cos\varphi). \end{gathered} \tag{3}$$

The operator R_μ is called the *exponential Radon transform*.

The inversion formula for R_μ has the form **[5]**

$$f = \frac{1}{4\pi} R^{\#}_{-\mu}\Lambda_\mu g, \tag{4}$$

where the operator Λ_μ acts on a function $g(w, p)$ by the formula

$$(\widetilde{\Lambda_\mu g})(w, \sigma) = \begin{cases} \sigma\widetilde{g}(w, \sigma), & |\sigma| > \mu, \\ 0, & |\sigma| < \mu, \end{cases}$$

and $\widetilde{g}(w, p)$ is the Fourier transform of the function $g(w, p)$ with respect to the

0065-9290/94/$1.00 + $.25 per page

linear variable p. The operator $R^{\#}_{-\mu}$ is adjoint to $R_{-\mu}$; it is called the *backprojection operator*:

$$(R^{\#}_{-\mu})(x) = \int_0^{2\pi} g(w, x \cdot w) e^{-\mu x \cdot w^{\perp}} \, d\varphi. \tag{5}$$

In the numerical realization of formula (4) the integral (5) is usually computed using the rectangle integration formula, and the operator Λ_μ is replaced by the convolution with a function $c_\mu(p)$ whose Fourier transform $\widetilde{c}_\mu(\sigma)$ is an approximation to the function $|\sigma|$ for $|\sigma| > \mu$ and vanishes, $\widetilde{c}_\mu(\sigma) = 0$, for $|\sigma| < \mu$.

Computer simulation (see **[6]**, **[8]**) shows that this algorithm produces good tomograms for $n > 120$ and $\mu d < 3$, where d the diameter of the support of the function f. The violation of these conditions lead to strong distortions of the tomograms, which are mainly caused by the exponential (as $|x| \to \infty$) increase of the error in the quadrature formula for the operator $R^{\#}_{-\mu}$. In **[7]**, a nice algorithm was presented in which the projection data $g = R_\mu f$ are used to compute the image $g_1 = Rf$ of the ordinary Radon transform ($\mu = 0$), and then the operator R^{-1} is applied to g_1. This algorithm is not so sensitive to the increase of the diameter of the support of f. In **[9]**, another formula for the inversion of the operator R_μ was suggested. Here we show that this formula yields an economical algorithm that produces good tomograms for an object of large diameter $\mu d \approx 6$ with $N = M = 64$.

Let us expand the function $g(w, p) = (R_\mu f)(w, p)$ in a Fourier series with respect to φ and a Fourier integral with respect to p:

$$g(w, p) = \sum_{m=-\infty}^{\infty} g_m(p) e^{im\varphi} = \frac{1}{\sqrt{2\pi}} \sum_{m=-\infty}^{\infty} \int_{\mathbb{R}^1} \widetilde{g}_m(\xi) e^{i\xi p} \, d\xi \, e^{im\varphi}.$$

For a real-valued function f we have (see **[9]**)

$$f(x) = f_0(|x|) + 2\,\mathrm{Re} \sum_{m=-\infty}^{-1} f_m(|x|) e^{im\theta}, \tag{6}$$

where

$$\begin{aligned} f_m(r) &= \frac{1}{\sqrt{2\pi}} \int_\mu^\infty \xi \widetilde{g}_m(\xi) c(\xi, m, r) \, d\xi, \\ c(\xi, m, r) &= \frac{1}{2\pi} (R^{\#}_{-\mu} e^{i(m\varphi + \xi p)})(a_r) \\ &= \frac{1}{2\pi} \int_0^{2\pi} \exp[i(m\varphi + \xi r \cos\varphi) + \mu r \sin\varphi] \, d\varphi \\ &= \left(\frac{\xi + \mu}{\xi - \mu} \right)^{m/2} i^m I_m(\sqrt{\xi^2 - \mu^2} r), \end{aligned} \tag{7}$$

$x = r(\cos\varphi, \sin\varphi)$, $a_r = (r, 0)$, and I_m is the Bessel function of order m.

Let us note that the action of the operator $R^{\#}_{-\mu}$ on an exponential function $e^{i(m\varphi + \xi p)}$ was earlier considered in **[7]**.

The choice of negative values of m in (6) is related to the desire to avoid the multiplication of the imprecisely defined function $\widetilde{g}_m(\xi)$ by large factors.

In the case when the function $g(w, p)$ is defined only at the nodes of the lattice, i.e., at the points $p_j - jh$, $j = -M/2 + 1, \ldots, M/2$, $w_k = (\cos\varphi_k, \sin\varphi_k)$, $\varphi_k = (k-1)2\pi/M$, $k = 1, \ldots, N$, $M = 2^{n_1}$, $N = 2^{n_2}$, we have

$$g_m(p) = \frac{1}{2\pi}\int_0^{2\pi} g(w, p)e^{-im\varphi}\,d\varphi \sim \frac{1}{N}\sum_{j=1}^{N} g(w_j, p)e^{-im\varphi_j} \tag{8}$$

and

$$\widetilde{g}_m(\xi) \sim \frac{h}{\sqrt{2\pi}} \sum_{j=-(M/2)+1}^{M/2} g_m(jh)e^{-i\xi jh}. \tag{9}$$

In computing integrals of the form (7) one usually applies a filter $0 \le W(\xi) \le 1$, $0 \le \xi \le B$, that suppresses the influence of high frequency components. Here B is the cutoff frequency that is determined by the Nyquist condition $Bh \le \pi$. We have

$$f_m(r) \sim \frac{1}{\sqrt{2\pi}}\int_\mu^B W(\xi)\xi\widetilde{g}(\xi)c(\xi, m, r)\,d\xi. \tag{10}$$

Substituting (9) into (10), we get

$$f_m(r) \sim \frac{h}{4\pi^2} \sum_{j=-(M/2)+1}^{M/2} g_m(jh)\alpha(m, j, r),$$

where

$$\begin{aligned}\alpha(m, j, r) &= 2\pi\int_\mu^B W(\xi)\xi e^{-i\xi jh}c(\xi, m, r)\,d\xi \\ &= \int_0^{2\pi} e^{im\varphi}\left(\int_\mu^B W(\xi)\xi e^{-i\xi jh}\exp(i\xi r\cos\varphi + \mu r\sin\varphi)\,d\xi\right)d\varphi.\end{aligned}$$

The reconstruction of $f(x)$ is first computed at the nodes of the radial lattice $r_h = sh$, $s = 0, \ldots, M/2$, $\theta_k = (k-1)2\pi/N$, $k = 1, \ldots, N$. After that, values at the nodes of the square lattice are reconstructed using the bilinear interpolation, and the visualization of the image is performed.

In computations of $g_m(p_j)$ using (8) and of $f(x)$ using (6), the fast Fourier transform was applied. Good results were obtained for the rectangular filter $W(\xi) \equiv 1$ with the cutoff frequency $B \sim 2/h$. Coefficients $\alpha(m, j, r)$ were computed in advance and stored in a hard disk.

To test the new algorithm we selected the following objects:

1. The function f is the characteristic function of the disk of diameter 20 cm. The projection data $g = R_\mu f$ have been computed analytically.

2. Projection data corresponding to one plane section were obtained in a tomographic gamma-ray camera. Emission sources in 17 cylindric capsules were placed into the cylinder of diameter 20 cm. The media absorption coefficient is $\mu \sim 0.15\ \text{cm}^{-1}$.

3. The function f is the characteristic function of the system of 17 rectangles located inside a circle of diameter 40 cm. The location of rectangles correspond to the location of capsules for the object 2. Projection data were computed analytically.

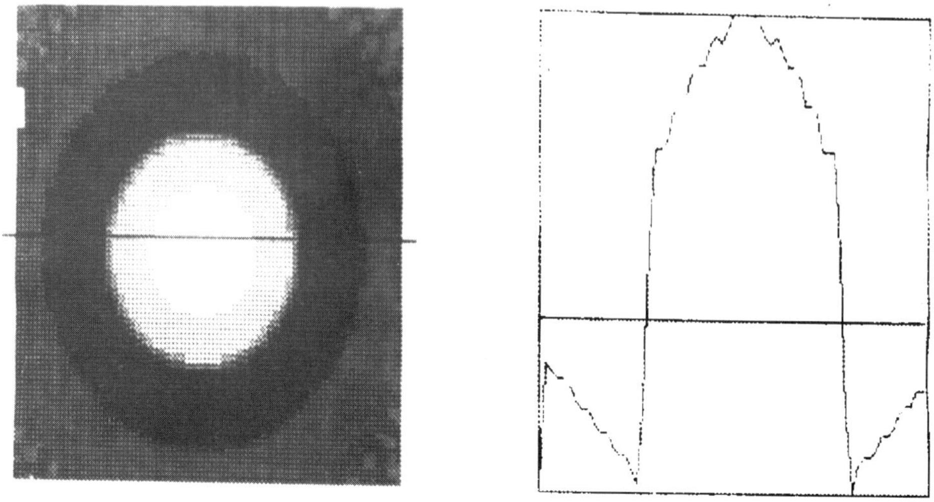

FIGURE 1a. In the backprojection, $\mu = 0$. min $= -0.58$, max $= 1.3$.

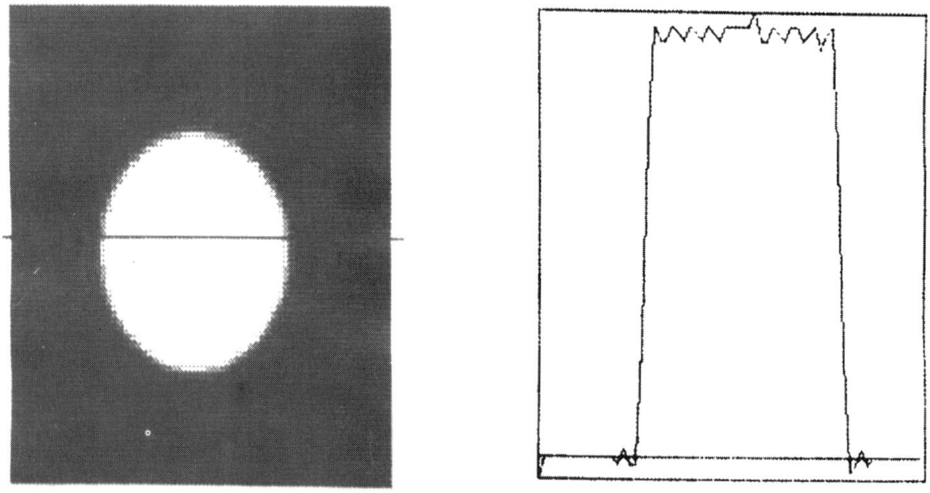

FIGURE 1b. In the backprojection, $\mu = 0$. min $= -0.06$, max $= 1.4$.

The projection data $g(w, p)$ for all these objects were determined at the above lattice with the parameters $N = M = 64$, $h = 40/M$. The absorption coefficient was taken to be $\mu \sim 0.15\ \text{cm}^{-1}$. The diameter of the vision field, the number of projections, and the attenuation coefficient correspond to the capacity of the tomographic gamma-ray camera. To apply the fast Fourier transform it is necessary to have $N = 2^n$. The values of the source density function $f(x)$ were determined on a rectangular lattice of size 64×64 that covers the support of the function f.

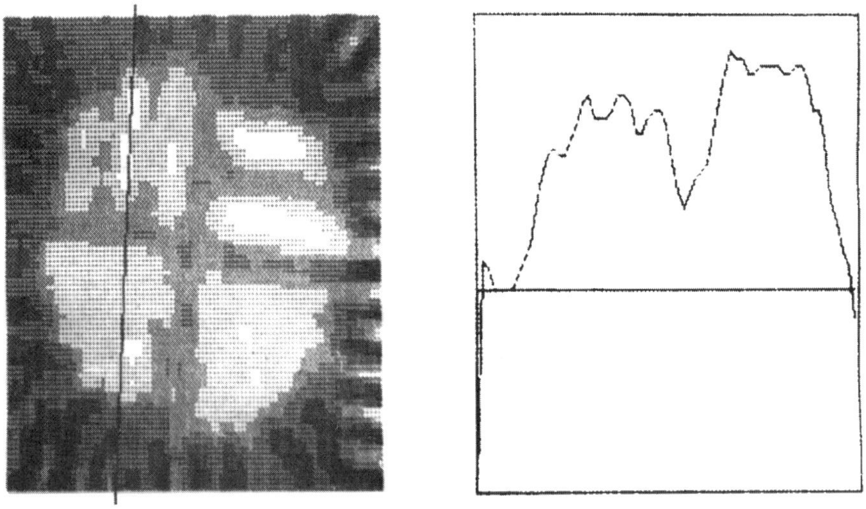

FIGURE 2a. In the backprojection, $\mu = 0.15$. min $= -115.1$, max $= 150.4$.

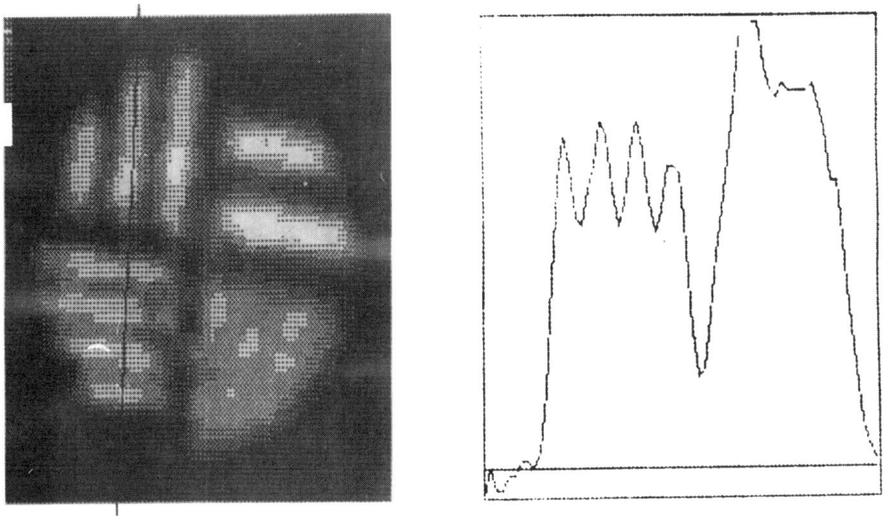

FIGURE 2b. In the backprojection, $\mu = 0.15$. min $= -12.8$, max $= 153.7$.

In Figures 1–3 the tomograms of the objects described in 1–3 above are presented. These tomograms are obtained using: a) the previously known backprojection algorithm BKFIL and b) the new algorithm described in this paper. Each tomogram is accompanied by the graph of the function f along a line shown in the corresponding figure. Also, the minimal (min) and the maximal (max) values of the reconstructed array are given; these values correspond to the bottom and top of the rectangle containing the graph.

For the object 2 the transition from the weakened to the exponential Radon transform was performed (using formula (3)). This transition can be considered as

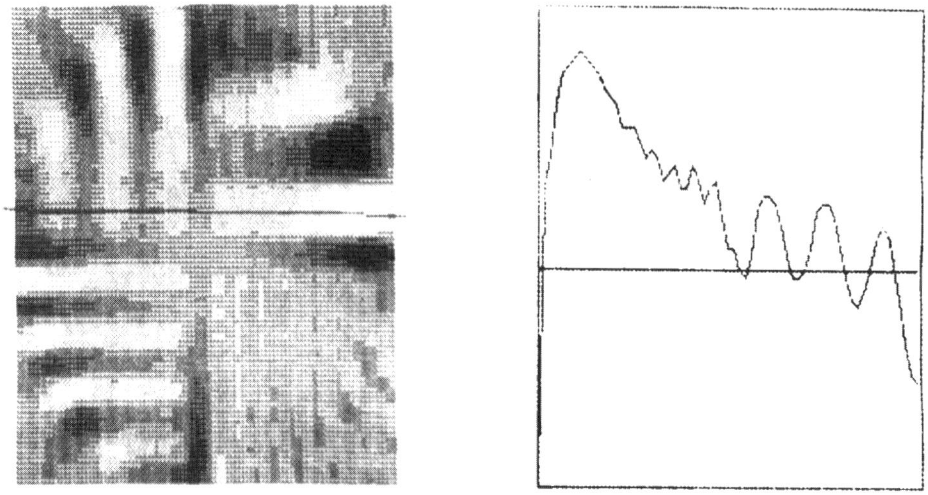

FIGURE 3a. In the backprojection, $\mu = 0$. min $= -3.17$, max $= 3.63$.

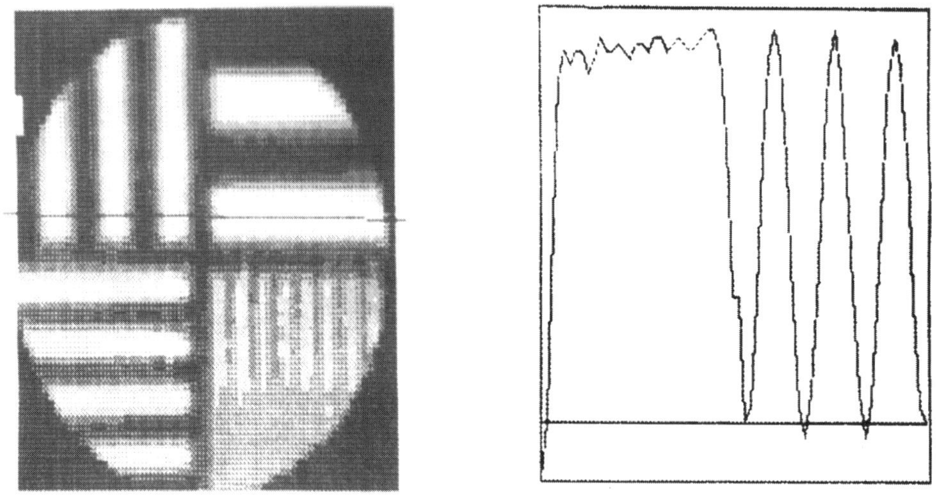

FIGURE 3b. In the backprojection, $\mu = 0$. min $= -0.16$, max $= 1.3$.

the account of the absorption when the value $g_0(w, p)$ of the projection data is divided by the attenuation coefficient $e^{-\mu c(w,p)}$ for the beam of gamma-quanta from the point (p, w) in the direction $w^{\perp}$. For small objects (with $\mu d < 3$, where d is the diameter of the support of the function) the application of the operator $R_0^{\#}\Lambda_\mu$ to the exponential transform $g = R_\mu f$ yields a good tomogram with the proper intensity distribution. For larger objects such rough account proves to be insufficient (see Figures 1a and 3a).

Let us note that the application of the backprojection algorithm BKFIL with $\mu = 0.15$ to the object 3 leads to large distortion, so we omit the corresponding tomogram. If we use a smoother filter in the algorithm BKFIL and discard negative entries in the reconstruction array, we can improve the quality of the tomogram shown in Figure 2a.

§2.

The mathematical model of projection data that lead to the exponential Radon transform is based on several simplifying assumptions. In particular, it does not take into account the Poisson noise and the scattering of gamma-rays.

To verify that this model is adequate in each particular case, we can use the conditions to the image of the exponential Radon transform $g = R_\mu f$ from **[5]** and [7]. It is proved in **[10]** that for $\mu \neq 0$ the equalities

$$(\xi + \mu)^m \widetilde{g}_m(\xi) = (-\xi + \mu)^m \widetilde{g}(-\xi) \tag{11}$$

give a set of necessary and sufficient conditions for g to belong to the image of the operator R_μ in the space $C_0^\infty(\mathbb{R}^2)$. For $\mu = 0$, equalities (11) become the symmetry condition $g(w, p) = g(-w, -p)$ that is satisfied for all functions from the image of the Radon transform R. For $m = 0$, (11) means that the function

$$g_0(p) = \int_0^{2\pi} g(w, p)\, dp$$

is even. Let us remark that for $\mu \neq 0$ the function $g(w, p)$ itself is not even. To compute $\widetilde{g}_m(\xi)$ we can use the quadrature formula

$$\widetilde{g}(\xi) \sim \frac{1}{MN} \sum_{j=0}^{N-1} \sum_{k=0}^{M-1} g(w_j, p_k) e^{i(jm/N + k\xi/N)}.$$

According to the Nyquist rule, the frequencies $\xi = \xi_L$ are computed by the formula $\xi_L = 2\pi L/h$, $L = -M/2 + 1, \ldots, M/2$. Let us note that $g_0(w_j, p_k)$ from (3) corresponds to the number of quanta registered by the detector in the direction of the line $p_j w_k + t w_k^\perp$.

Denote by d_1 and d_2 the variances of the real and of the imaginary part of $\widetilde{g}_m(\xi)$. Assuming that $g_0(w_j, p_k)$ are independent real-valued random variables with variances $\leq d$, we obtain

$$d_1 \leq \frac{d}{M^2 N^2} \sum_{j=0}^{N-1} \sum_{k=0}^{M-1} e^{2\mu c(w_j, p_k)} \cos^2(jm/N + k\xi_L/N).$$

For d_2, there exists a similar estimate. If the absorption region is a disk of radius r we get

$$c(w_j, p_k) = \begin{cases} \sqrt{r^2 - p_k^2}, & |p_k| \leq r, \\ 0 & |p_k| > r. \end{cases}$$

We have

$$d_1 \leq d\gamma(\mu r, m, L),$$

where

$$\gamma(\mu r, m, L) = \frac{1}{M^2N^2}\sum_{k=0}^{M-1} \exp\left(2\mu r\sqrt{(1-(p_k/r)^2}\right)\sum_{j=0}^{N-1}\cos^2(jm/N + k\xi_L/N).$$

Let us analyze in more detail the relation (11) for the object 2. In this case the parameter d must be estimated from experimental data. In accordance with the Poisson distribution, which describes the behavior of gamma-radiation quanta, d coincides with the average value of the parameter measured by the detector, and in our case it does not exceed 800. The coefficient γ achieves its maximal value at $L = m = 0$, and this maximal value equals $3.6 \cdot 10^{-3}$ (calculated on a computer). When L and m grow, γ decreases, although slower than the Fourier coefficients of the projection data. Let us present the table for values of $X = X_{L,m} = \widetilde{g}_m(\xi_L)/\widetilde{g}_m(-\xi_L)$ obtained by the above formulas for object 2, as well as the corresponding coefficients $S = S_{L,m} = ((-\xi_L + \mu)/(\xi_L + \mu))^m$.

The above values of X and S show that in spite of the Poisson noise, the relation (11) is rather accurate even for actual data.

TABLE. $m = 1$

L	1	2	3	4	5
S	0.01	-0.33	-0.49	-0.71	-0.66
X	$-0.05 - 0.04i$	-0.30	$-0.51 + 0.02i$	$-0.7 - 0.08i$	$-0.81 + 0.12i$

Large differences between X and S and the distribution of X and S over various harmonics can provide information about the character of perturbations in the data gathering that lead to deviations from the exponential Radon transform model.

REMARK. When this paper was submitted for publication, we learned about the interesting paper **[11]**, in which a similar reconstruction algorithm is considered. Let us note that our algorithm has the following differences from the algorithm in **[11]**.

(1) For the reconstruction, it suffices to use $\widetilde{g}_m(\xi)$ only for $m \geq 0$ and $\xi < 0$. This allows us to substantially descrease the errors caused by the discretization and the presence of noise.

(2) In the numerical realization of the algorithm, the result of filtration of basic functions is determined in advance. This allows us to compute the Fourier transforms of projected data with respect to the angle variable only.

References

1. V. A. Kostylev, S. D. Kalashnikov, and L. Ya. Fishman, *Emission gamma tomography*, Energoatomizdat, Moscow, 1988. (Russian)
2. V. V. Pikalov and N. G. Preobrazhenskiĭ, *Reconstruction tomography in gas dynamics and plasma physics*, "Nauka", Moscow, 1987. (Russian)
3. G. A. Fedorov and S. A. Tereshchenko, *Computation emission tomography*, Energoatomizdat, Moscow, 1990. (Russian)
4. F. Natterer, *The mathematics of computerized tomography*, Wiley, New York, 1985.
5. O. Tretyak and C. Metz, *The exponential Radon transform*, SIAM J. Appl. Math. **39** (1980), 341–357.
6. G. T. Gullberg and T. F. Budinger, *The use of filtering methods to compensate for constant attenuation in single-photon emission computed tomography*, IEEE Trans. Biomedical Engrg. **BME-28** (1981), no. 2, 142–157.

7. S. Bellini, M. Piacentini, C. Cafforio, and F. Rocca, *Compensation of tissue absorption in emission tomography*, IEEE Trans. Acoust. Speech Signal Process. **ASSP-27** (1979), no. 3, 213–218.
8. I. Hazon and D. Solmon, *Inversion of the exponential X-ray transform*. II: *Numerics*, Math. Methods Appl. Sci. **13** (1990), 208–215.
9. I. Ya. Shneĭberg, *Exponential Radon transform*, in this volume.
10. P. Kuchment and B. L′vin, *Paley-Wiener theorem for exponential Radon transform*, Acta Appl. Math. **18** (1990), 251–260.
11. W. Hawkins, P. Leichner, and Nai-Chuen Yang, *The circular harmonic transform for SPECT reconstruction and boundary conditions on the Fourier trasnform of the sinogram*, IEEE Trans. Medical Imaging **MI-7** (1988), no. 2, 135–148.

Institute of Forest Technology, Voronezh 394000, Russia

Institute of Medical Technology, Moscow 125422, Russia

Amer. Math. Soc. Transl.
(2) Vol. **162**, 1994

Examples of Nonuniqueness in Problems Related to the Generalized Radon Transform and Emission Tomography with Absorption

L. Vertgeĭm

Let $\varphi\colon \mathbb{R}^2 \to \mathbb{R}$. The *generalized Radon transform* of a function φ with weight ρ is defined by the formula

$$R_\rho\varphi(p,\omega) = \int_{r\cdot\omega=p} \rho(r,\omega^\perp)\varphi(r)\,ds, \tag{1}$$

where $r=(x,y)$, $p\in\mathbb{R}$, $\omega=(\cos\theta,\sin\theta)$, $\omega^\perp=(-\sin\theta,\cos\theta)$, and ds is the length form on the line.

§1.

A weight ρ is said to be *invariant under rotations* if

$$\rho(\Pi r,\Pi\omega)\equiv\rho(r,\omega) \tag{2}$$

for any rotation Π around the origin. It is shown in **[2]** that the generalized Radon transform is invertible in the class of functions with compact support for any weight ρ that is sufficiently smooth and invariant under rotations. Let us prove that this is not so for functions from the Schwartz space and, more generally, for functions that decrease arbitrarily strongly at infinity.

STATEMENT 1. *Let*

$$\varphi(r) = f(|r|^2)\cos(ph(|r|)), \tag{3}$$

where f is a positive smooth function with a given decrease rate at infinity. Let a smooth positive convex function h be such that for any $t>0$

$$h'(t) \geq \left(f(t)\Big/\int_{-\infty}^{+\infty} f(t+\xi^2)\,d\xi\right)^2 \tag{4}$$

and for any $\tau\geq 0$ the function

$$t\mapsto h'(t)\sqrt{(t-\tau)/(h(t)-h(\tau))} \tag{5}$$

monotonically increases for $t>\tau$.

Then for any $\varepsilon > 0$ there exists a weight ρ that is smooth, invariant under rotations, and satisfies the conditions

$$1-\varepsilon < \rho < 1+\varepsilon, \tag{6}$$

$$R_\rho \varphi \equiv 0. \tag{7}$$

Proof. Since a function $\varphi(r)$ of the form (3) depends on $|r|$ only, it suffices to find a smooth function $g(x,y)$ such that $1-\varepsilon < g < 1+\varepsilon$ and

$$\int_{-\infty}^{+\infty} g(x,y)\varphi(x,y)\,dx = 0 \tag{8}$$

for any y. Let Π_ω be the rotation moving ω to $(1,0)$. Then any weight ρ of the form

$$\rho(r,\omega) = g(\Pi_\omega r) \tag{9}$$

will satisfy the desired conditions.

We look for a function g of the form

$$g(x,y) = 1 + k(y)\cos(ph(x^2+y^2)) \tag{10}$$

with the factor $k(y)$ that is determined by the condition (8):

$$k(y) = -\frac{\int_{-\infty}^{+\infty} f(x^2+y^2)\cos(ph(x^2+y^2))\,dx}{\int_{-\infty}^{+\infty} f(x^2+y^2)\cos^2(ph(x^2+y^2))\,dx}. \tag{11}$$

To estimate $k(y)$ we need the following result.

Lemma. *Let $F\colon \mathbb{R}_+ \to \mathbb{R}_+$ be a positive smooth decreasing function such that $F \to 0$ at infinity, and let $H\colon \mathbb{R}_+ \to \mathbb{R}_+$ be a smooth decreasing function satisfying the following conditions: $H(0) = 0$, $H'(0) > 0$, and the function $H'(x)\sqrt{x/H(x)}$ increases. Then there exists a constant C, independent of F, H, and p, such that*

$$\left|\int_{-\infty}^{+\infty} F(x^2)e^{ipH(x^2)}\,dx\right| \le CF(0)/\sqrt{pH'(0)}.$$

Proof. Making the change of variable $t^2 = H(x^2)$, we transform the integral to the form

$$2\int_0^{+\infty} \widetilde{F}(t)e^{ipt^2}\,dt,$$

where

$$\widetilde{F}(t) = F(H^{-1}(t^2))t\Big/\left(\sqrt{H^{-1}(t^2)}H'(H^{-1}(t^2))\right).$$

The function $\widetilde{F}(t)$ decreases by the condition of the lemma, and we have $\widetilde{F}(0) = F(0)/\sqrt{H'(0)}$.

Setting $\Phi(\tau) = \int_0^\tau e^{it^2}\,dt$ and integrating by parts, we get

$$\int_0^{+\infty} \widetilde{F}(t)e^{ipt^2}\,dt = -\frac{1}{\sqrt{p}}\int_0^{+\infty} \widetilde{F}'(t)\Phi(\sqrt{p}t)\,dt = \frac{1}{\sqrt{p}}\Phi(\xi)\widetilde{F}(0),$$

Since Φ is bounded, we obtain the required estimate. □

Using the lemma and taking into account the conditions imposed on f and h, we have

$$\left| -\int_{-\infty}^{+\infty} f(x^2+y^2)\cos(ph(x^2+y^2))\,dx \right| \le Cf(y^2)/\sqrt{ph'(y^2)},$$

and a similar estimate with p replaced by $2p$. Using the condition (4) with a sufficiently large p, we obtain a uniform estimate $|k(y)| < \varepsilon$. The desired weight ρ is constructed. □

Let us note that for a given function f one can always find a function h such that both h and its derivative increase so fast that conditions (4) and (5) are satisfied. To give an example, consider the function $\varphi(r) = e^{-|r^2|}\cos(p|r|^2)$. In this case we can perform all computations explicitly, obtaining

$$g(x,y) = 1 + k(y)\cos(p(x^2+y^2)),$$

$$k(y) = \frac{-2(1+p^2)^{-1/4}\cos(py^2 + (1/2)\arctan p)}{1 + (1+4p^2)^{-1/4}\cos(2py^2 + (1/2)\arctan p)}.$$

§2.

The emission tomography problem with absorption reduces (see **[1]**) to the generalized Radon transform with the weight

$$\rho(r,\omega) = \exp\left[-\int_0^{+\infty}\mu(r+t\omega,\omega)\,dt\right], \tag{12}$$

where $\mu(r,\omega) \ge 0$ is the absorption coefficient at the point r in the direction ω.

Let us present an example that shows that in a general case a source function $\varphi(r)$ belonging to the class of functions satisfying an arbitrarily strong decrease condition at infinity cannot be uniquely reconstructed from the emission tomography data with absorption, i.e., from its generalized Radon transform with the weight (12).

STATEMENT 2. *Let*

$$\varphi(r) = f(|r|)\cos|r|, \tag{13}$$

where f is a positive smooth function that is monotonically increasing with an arbitrary given rate of increase at infinity. Then there exists a smooth absorption coefficient $\mu(r,\omega) \ge 0$ such that $R_\rho(\varphi) \equiv 0$ for the corresponding weight ρ.

PROOF. First, let us try to find an appropriate weight ρ. Let us analyze necessary and sufficient conditions for the representability of ρ in the form (12) with a smooth μ:

$$\rho \text{ is smooth and } 0 < \rho \le 1; \tag{14}$$

$$\begin{gathered}\text{the function } t \mapsto \rho(r+t\omega,\omega) \text{ increases}\\ \text{(nonstrictly) and tends to 1 as } t \to +\infty.\end{gathered} \tag{15}$$

The function μ can be reconstructed from ρ by the formula

$$\mu(r,\omega) = \frac{1}{\rho(r,\omega)}\frac{d}{d\tau}\rho(r+\tau\omega,\omega)\Big|_{\tau=0}. \tag{16}$$

Taking into account the form (13) of the function μ, let us look for ρ in the class of rotation invariant weights. As before, it suffices to find a smooth function $g(x,y)$ satisfying (8) and define ρ by (9). The function g must satisfy the following additional conditions:

$$g>0 \text{ and } g(\cdot,y) \text{ is nonstrictly increasing for any given } y; \tag{17}$$

$$g\le 1 \text{ and } g(x,y)\to 1 \text{ as } x\to+\infty. \tag{18}$$

Denote

$$\Phi(x,y)=\int_x^{+\infty}\varphi(t,y)\,dt, \qquad G(x,y)=\frac{\partial g}{\partial x}(x,y).$$

Then conditions (8), (17), (18) are satisfied provided that

$$g(-\infty,y)\Phi(-\infty,y)+\int_{-\infty}^{+\infty}G(x,y)\Phi(x,y)\,dx=0, \tag{19}$$

$$g(-\infty,y)>0, \qquad G\ge 0, \tag{20}$$

$$\int_{-\infty}^{+\infty}G(x,y)\,dx=1-g(-\infty,y). \tag{21}$$

First, let us construct a function $\widetilde{g}$ satisfying (8) and (17). We set $\widetilde{g}(-\infty,y)\equiv 1$ and

$$\widetilde{g}(x,y)=\int_{-\infty}^{x}\widetilde{G}(t,y)\,dt, \tag{22}$$

and look for a smooth function $\widetilde{G}\ge 0$ satisfying (19). Let us note that Φ possesses the following property: for any y the function $\Phi/(\cdot,y)$ changes sign. This follows from the property that integrals of the function $x\mapsto\varphi(x,y)$ between two consecutive zeros on the positive halfline decrease in modulus and have interleaving signs.

Now we perform the following local construction. Let $\Phi(x_+,y_0)>0$, $\Phi(x_-,y_0)<0$ for some y_0. By continuity,

$$\begin{aligned}\Phi>0 &\quad\text{on } (x_+-\delta,x_++\delta)\times(y_0-\delta,y_0+\delta),\\ \Phi<0 &\quad\text{on } (x_--\delta,x_-+\delta)\times(y_0-\delta,y_0+\delta).\end{aligned}$$

for some $\delta>0$. We are looking for a function $\widetilde{G}_{y_0}(x,y)=\alpha_+(y)\Delta(x-x_+)+\alpha_-(y)\Delta(x-x_-)$ such that (19) holds for $y_0-\delta<y<y_0+\delta$. The coefficients $\alpha_\pm$ are unknown, and the function Δ satisfies the conditions

$$\Delta\ge 0,\quad \Delta\in C^\infty(\mathbb{R}),\quad \operatorname{supp}\Delta\subset(-\delta,\delta),\quad \int_{-\infty}^{+\infty}\Delta(t)\,dt=1.$$

The condition (19) takes the form

$$\begin{aligned}&\alpha_+(y)I_+(y)+\alpha_-(y)I_-(y)=-\Phi(-\infty,y),\\ &I_\pm(y)=\int_{-\infty}^{+\infty}\Delta(x-x_\pm)\Phi(x,y)\,dx.\end{aligned} \tag{23}$$

It is clear that for $y_0-\delta<y<y_0+\delta$ the functions $I_\pm(y)$ are smooth and $I_+(y)>0$, $I_-(y)<0$. Evidently, the equation (23) has solutions $\alpha_+,\alpha_-\ge 0$ that are smooth inside the interval $(y_0-\delta,y_0+\delta)$, namely

$$\alpha_+(y)=-\lambda I_-(y)-\Phi(-\infty,y)/I_+(y), \qquad \alpha_-(y)=\lambda I_+(y)$$

for a sufficiently large $\lambda>0$.

Now it remains to glue all these local solutions $\widetilde{G}_{y_0}$ together using a smooth decomposition of unity on $\mathbb{R}$ that is subordinate to the covering

$$\mathbb{R} = \bigcap_{y_0} (y_0 - \delta(y_0), y_0 + \delta(y_0)).$$

The resulting function $\widetilde{G}$ is smooth and satisfies (29) and (20), and the smooth function $\widetilde{g}$ obtained by (22) satisfies (8) and (17). Defining $g(x, y) = \widetilde{g}(x, y)/\widetilde{g}(+\infty, y)$, we see that g satisfies (8), (17), and (18). Defining ρ from (9) and μ from (16), we obtain the desired smooth absorption coefficient.

In conclusion we remark that this absorption coefficient is nonisotropic, i.e., $\mu(r, \omega)$ indeed depends on ω. Therefore, the problem of invertibility in the case when μ depends only on r remains open. $\square$

References

1. F. Natterer, *The mathematics of computerized tomography*, Wiley, New York, 1986.
2. E. T. Quinto, *The invertibility of rotation invariant Radon transforms*, J. Math. Anal. Appl. **91** (1983), 510–522; **94** (1983), 602–603.

Recent Titles in This Series

(Continued from the front of this publication)

(See the AMS catalog for earlier titles)